Planning, Implementing, and Evaluating Health Promotion Programs

A Primer

FOURTH EDITION

James F. McKenzie

Ball State University

Brad L. Neiger

Brigham Young University

Jan L. Smeltzer

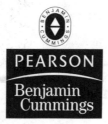

PEARSON

Benjamin Cummings

San Fransicso   Boston   New York
Cape Town   Hong Kong   London   Madrid   Mexico City
Montreal   Munich   Paris   Singapore   Sydney   Tokyo   Toronto

Publisher: *Daryl Fox*
Acquisitions Editor: *Deirdre McGill Espinoza*
Developmental Manager: *Claire Alexander*
Editorial Assistant: *Alison Rodal*
Production Supervisor: *Steven Anderson*
Managing Editor: *Deborah Cogan*
Manufacturing Buyer: *Stacey Weinberger*
Marketing Manager: *Sandra Lindelof*
Cover Designer: *Yvo Riezebos Design*
Production and Composition: *WestWords, Inc.*
Copy Editor: *LeAnn Paskett*
Proofreader: *Suzi Wilson*
Cover Printer: *Phoenix Book Tech*
Text Printer: *Phoenix Book Tech*
Cover Photo: *Getty Images*

ISBN 0-8053-6010-7

Library of Congress Cataloging-in-Publication Data

McKenzie, James F., 1948–
    Planning, implementing, and evaluating health promotion programs : a primer / James F.
McKenzie, Brad L. Neiger, Jan L. Smeltzer.—4th ed.
        p. ; cm.
    Includes bibliographical references and index.
    ISBN 0-8053-6010-7 (pbk.)
1. Health promotion—Planning. 2. Health promotion—Evaluation. 3. Health planning—
    Methodology. I. Neiger, Brad L. II. Smeltzer, Jan L. III. Title.
    [DNLM: 1. Health Promotion. 2. Health Education. 3. Health Planning.
4. Program Evaluation. WA 525 M4785p 2005]
    RA427.8.M39 2005
    613'.068—dc22

2004004984

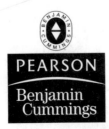

PEARSON

Benjamin
Cummings

2 3 4 5—PBT—07 06 05 04
www.aw-bc.com

This book is dedicated to nine special people—
Bonnie, Anne, Greg, Sherry, Lindsay, Jack,
Chelsea, Hilary, and Mike—

and to our teachers and mentors—
Marshall H. Becker (deceased), Mary K. Beyrer, Noreen Clark,
Nancy Kinney, Enrico A. Leopardi, Terry W. Parsons,
Glenn E. Richardson, Irwin M. Rosenstock (deceased),
Yuzuru J. Takeshita, and Doug Vilnius

CONTENTS

CHAPTER 5

Measurement, Measures, Data Collection, and Sampling 98

CHAPTER 14
Evaluation Approaches, Framework, and Designs 304

CHAPTER 15
Data Analysis and Reporting 328

This book is written for students who are enrolled in their first professional course in health promotion program planning. It is designed to help them understand and develop the skills necessary to carry out program planning regardless of the setting. The book is unique among the health promotion planning textbooks on the market in that it provides readers with both theoretical and practical information. A straightforward, step-by-step format is used to make concepts clear and the full process of health promotion planning understandable. This book provides, under a single cover, material on all three areas of program development: planning, implementing, and evaluating.

Learning Aids

Each chapter of the book includes chapter objectives, a list of key terms, presentation of content, chapter summary, review questions, activities, and weblinks. In addition, many of the key concepts are further explained with information presented in boxes, figures, tables, and the appendixes.

Chapter Objectives

The chapter objectives identify the content and skills that should be mastered after reading the chapter, answering the review questions, completing the activities and using the weblinks. Most of the objectives are written using the cognitive and psychomotor (behavior) educational domains. For most effective use of the objectives, we suggest that they be reviewed before reading the chapter. This will help readers focus on the major points in each chapter and will facilitate answering the questions and completing the activities at the end.

Key Terms

Key terms are introduced in each chapter of the textbook and are important to the understanding of the chapter. The terms are presented in a list at the beginning of each chapter and then are printed in boldface at the appropriate points within the chapter. Again, as with the chapter objectives, we suggest that readers skim the list before reading the chapter. Then as the chapter is read, particular attention should be paid to the definition of each term.

Presentation of Content

Although each chapter in this book could be expanded—in some cases, entire books have been written on topics we have covered in a chapter or less—we believe that each chapter contains the necessary information to help students understand and develop many of the skills required to be a successful health promotion planner, implementor, and evaluator.

Chapter Summary

At the end of each chapter, readers will find a one- or two-paragraph review of the major concepts contained in the chapter.

Review Questions

The purpose of the questions at the end of each chapter is to provide readers with some feedback regarding their mastery of the content. We have endeavored to ask questions that would reinforce the chapter objectives and key terms presented in each chapter.

Activities

Each chapter also includes several activities that will allow students to put their new knowledge and skills to use. The activities are presented in several different formats for the sake of variety and to appeal to the different learning styles of students. It should be noted that, depending on the ones selected for completion, the activities in one chapter can build on those in a previous chapter and lead to the final product of a completely developed health promotion program.

Weblinks

The final portion of each chapter consists of a list of links on the World Wide Web. These links allow students to explore a number of different websites that are available to support planning, implementing, and evaluating efforts.

New to This Edition

In revising this textbook, we incorporated as many suggestions from reviewers, colleagues, and former students as possible. In addition to updating material throughout the text, the following points reflect the major changes in this new edition:

- Chapter 1 has been updated and expanded to include new definitions from the *Report of the 2000 Joint Committee on Health Education and Promotion Terminology,* and additional information about the Certified Health Education Specialists (CHES) and Competencies Update Project (CUP).

- Chapter 2 on planning models still includes presentations of the Generalized Model for Program Planning, PRECEDE-PROCEED, MATCH, CDCynergy, and SMART models, but also now includes presentations of these newer planning models—A Systematic Approach to Health Promotion, Mobilizing for Action through Planning and Partnerships (MAPP), Assessment Protocol for Excellence in Public Health (APEX-PH), SWOT Analysis, Healthy Communities, The Health Communication Model, and Healthy Plan-IT.

- Chapter 3 on starting the planning process has been expanded to include greater insight into working with program stakeholders.

- Chapter 4 has been expanded to address benefits and barriers of comprehensive versus categorical and practitioner versus consumer-driven assessments.

- Chapter 5 includes expanded discussions of measures, measurement, and data collection, and sampling.

- Chapter 6 includes additional information on *Healthy People 2010.*

- A complete updating of Chapter 7, including the addition of several new and emerging theories.

- Chapter 8 on interventions has been completely reorganized and now uses terminology consistent with the terminology used by the Centers for Disease Control and Prevention to describe interventions.

- Chapter 9 includes more information on community building.

- Chapter 11 has been modified to better identify differences between true marketing campaigns compared with more basic promotional or advertising strategies.

- Chapter 12 has been completely reorganized and now presents a single generic model for implementing a program that includes more information on implementation timelines.

- Chapter 14 has been completely updated and now presents a new classification system for approaches to evaluation.

- A revised instructors' manual and testbank have been created.

- PowerPoint© presentations, by the author, are available online.

- The replacement of the term "target population/audience" throughout the book with priority population/audience.

- And finally, but by no means the least, the addition of a new coauthor, Brad L. Neiger, who brings a wealth of knowledge and practical experience to the book.

Students will find this book easy to understand and use. We are confident that if the chapters are carefully read and an honest effort is put into completing the activities, and visiting the weblinks, students will gain the essential knowledge and skills for program planning, implementation, and evaluation.

Acknowledgments

A project of this nature could not have been completed without the assistance and understanding of many individuals. First, we thank all our past and present students, who have had to put up with our "working drafts" of the manuscript.

Second, we are grateful to those professionals who took the time and effort to review and comment on various editions of this book. For the first edition, they included Vicki Keanz, Eastern Kentucky University; Susan Cross Lipnickey, Miami University; Fred Pearson, Ricks College; Kerry Redican, Virginia Tech; John Sciacca,

Northern Arizona University; and William K. Spath, Montana Tech. For the second edition, reviewers included Gordon James, Weber State; John Sciacca, Northern Arizona University; and Mark Wilson, University of Georgia. For the third edition, reviewers included Joanna Hayden, William Paterson University; Raffy Luquis, Southern Connecticut State University; Teresa Shattuck, University of Maryland; Thomas Syre, James Madison University; and Esther Weekes, Texas Women's University. For this edition, the reviewers include Robert G. LaChausse, California State University, San Bernardino; Julie Shepard, Director of Health Promotion, Adams County Health Department; Sherm Sowby, California State University, Fresno; and William Kane, University of New Mexico.

Third, we thank our friends for providing valuable feedback on various editions of this book: Robert J. Yonker, Ph.D., Professor Emeritus in the Department of Educational Foundations and Inquiry, Bowling Green State University; Lawrence W. Green, Dr.P.H., Distinguished Fellow/Office of Extramural Research, Public Health Practice Program Office, Centers for Disease Control and Prevention; Bruce Simons-Morton, Ed.D., M.P.H., Chief, Prevention Research Branch, National Institute of Child Health and Human Development, National Institutes of Health; and Jerome E. Kotecki, H.S.D., Professor, Department of Physiology and Health Science, Ball State University.

Fourth, we would like to thank the staff of the High Library at Elizabethtown College Elizabethtown, Pennsylvania, especially Sylvia T. Morra, Acting Director, and Naomi Hershey for their assistance in making this project possible.

Fifth, we appreciate the work of Benjamin Cummings employees Deirdre McGill Espinoza, senior acquisitions editor for health and kinesiology and her assistant, Alison Rodal. We also appreciate the careful work of Jami Darby at WestWords, Inc.

Finally, we express our deepest appreciation to our families for their support, encouragement, and understanding of the time that writing takes away from our family activities.

J. F. M.
B. L. N.
J. L. S.

Health Education, Health Promotion, Health Educators, and Program Planning

Chapter Objectives

After reading this chapter and answering the questions at the end, you should be able to:

- Explain the relationship among health behavior, health education, and health promotion.
- Explain the difference between health education and health promotion.
- Write your own definition of health education.
- Explain the role of the health educator as defined by the Role Delineation Project.
- Explain how a person becomes a Certified Health Education Specialist.
- Explain how the Framework for Competency-Based Health Education is used by colleges and universities, the National Commission for Health Education Credentialing, Inc. (NCHEC), the National Council for the Accreditation of Teacher Education (NCATE), and the SOPHE/AAHE Baccalaureate Program Approval Committee (SABPAC).
- Explain how the Framework has been expanded for advanced-level health practitioners.
- Identify the assumptions upon which health education is based.
- Name the generic components for developing a program.

Key Terms

advanced-level practitioners	health behavior	Healthy People
entry-level health educator	health education	health promotion
Framework	health educator	Role Delineation Project

Looking back over the twentieth century, we see that much progress was made in the health and life expectancy of Americans: "People are living longer than previously and with greater freedom from the threat of disease" (Breslow, 1999, p. 1031). Since 1900, we have seen a sharp drop in infant mortality (Hoyert, Kochanek, & Murphy, 1999); the eradication of smallpox; the elimination of poliomyelitis in the Americas; the control of measles, rubella, tetanus, diphtheria,

Haemophilus influenzae type b, and other infectious diseases; better family planning (CDC, 1999d), and an increase of 29.4 years in the average life span of a person in the United States (Pastor, Makuc, Reuben, & Xia, 2002). Over this same time, we have witnessed disease prevention change "from focusing on reducing environmental exposures over which the individual had little control, such as providing potable water, to emphasizing behaviors such as avoiding use of tobacco, fatty foods, and a sedentary lifestyle" (Breslow, 1999, p. 1030). In fact, in the latter part of the twentieth century, it was reported that better control of behavioral risk factors alone—such as lack of exercise, poor diet, use of tobacco and drugs, and alcohol abuse—could prevent between 40 and 70% of all premature deaths, one-third of all acute disabilities, and two-thirds of chronic disabilities (USDHHS, 1990b). As we begin the twenty-first century, behavior patterns continue to "represent the single most prominent domain of influence over health prospects in the United States" (McGinnis, Williams-Russo, & Knickman, 2002, p. 82) (see Table 1.1).

Though the focus on good health, wellness, and **health behavior** (those behaviors that impact a person's health) seem commonplace in our lives today, it was not until the last fourth of the twentieth century that health promotion was recognized for its potential to help control injury and disease and to promote health.

> Most scholars, policymakers, and practitioners in health promotion would pick 1974 as the turning point that marks the beginning of health promotion as a significant component of national health policy in the twentieth century. That year Canada published its landmark policy statement, *A New Perspective on the Health of Canadians* (Lalonde, 1974). In the United States, Congress passed PL 94-317, the Health Information and Health Promotion Act, which created the Office of Health Information and Health Promotion, later renamed the Office of Disease Prevention and Health Promotion. (Green 1999, p. 69).

This led the way for the U.S. government's publication *Healthy People: The Surgeon General's Report on Health Promotion and Disease Prevention* (*Healthy People*, 1979). This document brought together much of what was known about the relationship of

Table 1.1 Comparison of most common causes of death and actual causes of death

Most common causes of death, United States, 2002*	Actual causes of death, United States, 2000**
1. Diseases of the heart	1. Tobacco
2. Malignant neoplasms (cancers)	2. Poor diet and physical inactivity
3. Cerebrovascular diseases (stroke)	3. Alcohol consumption
4. Chronic lower respiratory diseases	4. Microbial agents
5. Unintentional injuries (accidents)	5. Toxic agents
6. Diabetes mellitus	6. Motor vehicles
7. Influenza and pneumonia	7. Firearms
8. Alzheimer's disease	8. Sexual behavior
9. Nephritis, nephrotic syndrome, and nephrosis	9. Illicit drug use
10. Septicemia	

Sources: * Kochanek, K.D., & Smith, B.L. (2004).
   ** Mokdad, Marks, Stroup and Gerberding (2004).

personal behavior and health status. The document also presented a "personal responsibility" model that provided Americans with a prescription for reducing their health risks and increasing their chances for good health.

It may not have been the content of *Healthy People* that made the publication so significant, because several publications written before it provided a similar message. Rather, *Healthy People* was important because it summarized the research available up to that point, presented it in a very readable format, and made the information available to the general public. *Healthy People* was then followed by the release of the first set of health goals and objectives for the nation, titled *Promoting Health/Preventing Disease: Objectives for the Nation* (USDHHS, 1980). These goals and objectives, now in their third generation (USDHHS, 2000) have defined the nation's health agenda and guided its health policy since their inception. And, in part, they have kept the importance of good health visible to all Americans.

This focus on good health has given many people in the United States a desire to do something about their health. This desire, in turn, has created a greater need for good health information that can be easily understood by the average person. One need only look at the current best-seller list, read the daily newspaper, observe the health advertisements delivered via the electronic mass media, or consider the increase in the number of health-promoting facilities (not illness or sickness facilities) to verify the interest that American consumers have in health. Because of the increased interest in health, health professionals are now faced with providing the public with the information and the skills needed to make quality health decisions.

Health Education and Health Promotion

In the simplest terms, **health education** is the process of educating people about health. However, two more formal definitions of health education have been frequently cited in the literature. The first comes from the *Report of the 2000 Joint Committee on Health Education and Promotion Terminology* (Joint Committee on Terminology, 2001). The committee defined health education as "Any combination of planned learning experiences based on sound theories that provide individuals, groups, and communities the opportunity to acquire information and the skills needed to make quality health decisions" (p. 99). The second definition was presented by Green and Kreuter (1999), who defined health education as

> any combination of learning experiences designed to facilitate voluntary actions conducive to health. *Combination* emphasizes the importance of matching the multiple determinants of behavior with multiple learning experiences or educational interventions. *Designed* distinguishes health education from incidental learning experiences as a systematically planned activity. *Facilitate* means predispose, enable, and reinforce. *Voluntary* means without coercion and with full understanding and acceptance of the purposes of the action. *Actions* means behavioral steps taken by an individual, group, or community to achieve an intended health effect or to build their capacity for health (p. 27).

Another term that is closely related to health education, and sometimes incorrectly used in its place, is **health promotion.** *Health promotion* is a broader term than *health education.* The Joint Committee on Terminology (2001) defined *health promotion* as "Any planned combination of educational, political, environmental, regulatory, or organizational mechanisms that support actions and conditions of living conducive to the health of individuals, groups, and communities" (p. 101). While Green and Kreuter (1999) define *health promotion* as "the combination of educational and ecological supports for actions and conditions of living conducive to health." In this definition "*combination* again refers to the necessity of matching multiple determinants of health with multiple interventions or sources of support" (p. 27). *Educational* refers to health education as defined by Green and Kreuter (1999). "*Ecological* refers to the social, political, economic, organizational, policy, regulatory, and other environmental circumstances interacting with behavior in affecting health" (Green & Kreuter, 1999, p. 27).

To help us to further understand and operationalize the term *health promotion,* Breslow (1999) has stated, "Each person has a certain degree of health that may be expressed as a place in a spectrum. From that perspective, promoting health must focus on enhancing people's capacities for living. That means moving them toward the health end of the spectrum, just as prevention is aimed at avoiding disease that can move people toward the opposite end of the spectrum" (p. 1031). According to these definitions of health promotion, health education is an important component of health promotion and firmly implanted in it (see Figure 1.1). "Without health education, health promotion would be a manipulative social engineering enterprise" (Green & Kreuter, 1999, p. 19).

The effectiveness of health promotion programs can vary greatly. However, the success of a program can usually be linked to the planning that takes place before implementation of the program. Programs that have undergone a thorough planning process are usually the most successful. As the old saying goes, "If you fail to plan, your plan will fail."

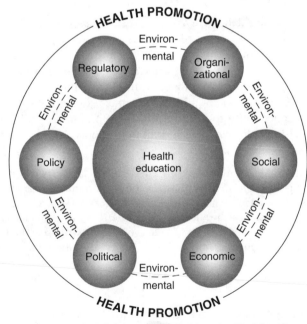

Figure 1.1 Relationships of health education and health promotion

Health Educators

The individuals best qualified to plan health promotion programs are health educators. A **health educator** is "A professionally prepared individual who serves in a variety of roles and is specifically trained to use appropriate educational strategies and methods to facilitate the development of policies, procedures, interventions, and systems conducive to the health of individuals, groups, and communities" (Joint Committee on Terminology, 2001, p. 100). Today, health educators can be found working in a variety of settings, including schools (K-12, colleges, and universities), community health agencies (governmental and nongovernmental), worksites (business, industry, and other work settings), and health care settings (e.g., clinics, hospitals, and managed care organizations).

The role of the health educator in the United States as we know it today is one that has evolved over time based on the need to provide people with educational interventions to enhance their health. The earliest signs of the role of the health educator appeared in the mid-1800s with school hygiene education, which was closely associated with physical activity. By the early 1900s, the need for health education spread to the public health arena, but it was the writers, journalists, social workers, and visiting nurses who were doing the educating—not health educators as we know them today (Deeds, 1992). As we gained more knowledge about the relationship between health, disease, and health behavior, it was obvious that the writers, journalists, social workers, visiting nurses, and primary caregivers—mainly physicians, dentists, other independent practitioners, and nurses—were unable to provide the needed health education. The combination of the heavy workload of the primary caregivers, the lack of formal training in the process of educating others, and the need for education at all levels of prevention (see Figure 1.2) created a need for health educators.

As the role of the health educator grew over the years, there was a movement by those in the discipline to clearly define their role so that people inside and outside the profession would have a better understanding of what the health educator did. In 1978, the **Role Delineation Project** began (National Task Force [on the Preparation and Practice of Health Educators, Inc.], 1985). Through a comprehensive process, this project yielded a generic role for the **entry-level health educator**— that is, responsibilities for health educators taking their first job regardless of their work setting. In more recent years, the list of responsibilities has become known as *"A Competency-Based Framework for Professional Development of Certified Health Education Specialists,"* or just simply the ***Framework*** (NCHEC, 1996). The *Framework* comprises seven major areas of responsibility and several different competencies and subcompetencies, which further delineate the responsibilities. The seven major areas of responsibility identified through the Role Delineation Project and still in use today include:

1. Assessing individual and community needs for health education.
2. Planning effective health education programs.
3. Implementing health education programs.
4. Evaluating the effectiveness of health education programs.
5. Coordinating provision of health education services.

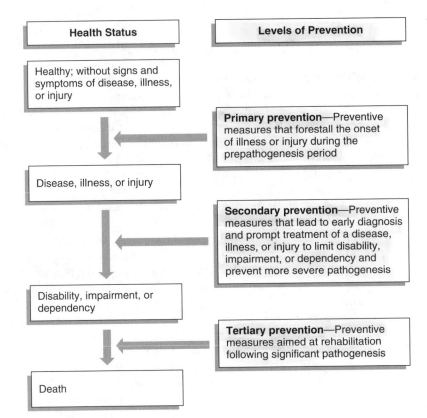

Figure 1.2 Levels of prevention
Source: Adapted from Pickett and Hanlon (1990).

6. Acting as a resource person in health education.

7. Communicating health and health education needs, concerns, and resources (National Task Force, 1985, pp. 15–16).

In reviewing the seven areas of responsibility, it is obvious that four of the seven are directly related to program planning, implementation, and evaluation and that the other three could be associated with these processes, depending on the type of program being planned. In effect, these responsibilities distinguish health educators from other professionals who try to provide health education experiences.

The importance of the defined role of the health educator is becoming greater as the profession of health promotion continues to mature. This is exhibited by its use in several major professional activities. First, the *Framework* has provided a guide for all colleges and universities to use when designing and revising their curricula in health education to prepare future health educators. Second, the *Framework* was used by the National Commission for Health Education Credentialing, Inc. (NCHEC) to develop the core criteria for certifying individuals as health educators (Certified Health Education Specialists, or CHES). The first group of individuals (N=1,558) to receive the CHES credential did so between October 1988 and December 1989, during the charter certification period. "Charter certification allowed qualified individuals to be certi-

---

Box 1.1 *Eligibility Guidelines to sit for the CHES Examination*

Eligibility to sit for the CHES examination is based exclusively on academic qualifications. An individual is eligible to sit for the examination if he/she has:
A bachelor's, master's or doctoral degree from an accredited institution of higher education; AND one of the following:

- An official transcript (including course titles) that clearly shows a major in health education, e.g., Health Education, Community Health Education, Public Health Education, School Health Education, etc.
  OR
- An official transcript that reflects at least 25 semester hours or 37 quarter hours of course work with specific preparation addressing the areas of responsibility of Health Education Specialists.

Source: National Commission for Health Education Credentialing, Inc. Reprinted by permission.

---

fied based on their academic training, work experience, and references without taking the certification exam" (Cottrell, Girvan, & McKenzie, 2002, p. 163). In 1990, using a criterion-referenced examination based on the *Framework,* the nationwide testing program to certify health educators was begun by NCHEC, Inc. During that first year, 648 passed the examination and received the CHES credential (AAHE, NCHEC, & SOPHE, 1999). As of January 2004, between 10,000 and 11,000 individuals have received the CHES credential. Currently, the CHES examination is given twice a year in April and October. Box 1.1 presents the current eligibility guidelines in order to be able to sit for the examination.

Third, the *Framework* is used by program accrediting and approval bodies to review college and university academic programs in health education. The National Council for the Accreditation of Teacher Education (NCATE) uses the *Framework* to review and accredit teacher preparation programs in health education at institutions of higher education. Also, a joint committee of the Society for Public Health Education, Inc. (SOPHE) and the American Association for Health Education, known as the SOPHE/AAHE Baccalaureate Program Approval Committee (SABPAC), uses the *Framework* to review and approve undergraduate health education programs via self-study and external reviewers.

The use of the *Framework* by the profession to guide academic curricula, provide the core criteria for the health education specialist examination, and form the basis of program approval processes (AAHE, NCHEC, & SOPHE, 1999) has done much to advance the health education profession. "In 1998 the U.S. Department of Commerce and Labor formally acknowledged 'health educator' as a distinct occupation. Such recognition was justified, based to a large extent, on the ability of the profession to specify its unique skills" (AAHE, NCHEC, & SOPHE, 1999, p. 9).

Prior to the recognition of "health educator" as a singular occupational classification code by the U.S. Department of Commerce and Labor, the initial responsibilities of the health educator that had served the profession so well were beginning to show their age and did not express the responsibilities and competencies of a health educator with an advanced degree in the field. As early as 1992, a Joint Committee for Graduate Standards was established by the Association for the Advancement of Health Education (now known as the American Association for Health Education (AAHE)) and the Society for Public Health Education (SOPHE) to help define the role of an **advanced-level practitioner.** Over the course of the next few years, the joint committee, with the help of many professionals, completed its work and submitted its final report and graduate competencies to the boards of AAHE and SOPHE. Both boards accepted the report in 1996. Then, in July 1997, the National Commission for Health Education Credentialing's (NCHEC) Board of Commissioners endorsed the competencies (AAHE, NCHEC, & SOPHE, 1999). The three responsibilities for advanced-level practitioners that were added to the existing seven for entry-level health educators included:

8. Applying appropriate research principles and techniques to health education.
9. Administering health education programs.
10. Advancing the profession of health education.

Even with the addition of the three responsibilities and their associated competencies/subcompetencies for advanced-level practitioners, there was a general feeling within the profession that there was a need to reverify the entry-level responsibilities and competencies/subcompetencies to ensure they reflected current practice and to further integrate, refine, and validate the advanced-level responsibilities and competencies/subcompetencies. Thus in March 1998, the NCHEC, Inc., along with ten other health education related organizations initiated the National Health Educator Competencies Update Project (CUP). The specific objectives of the CUP were to:

- Determine the degree to which the responsibilities, competencies, and subcompetencies for entry-level health educators are still valid as determined by their ability to accurately reflect the current scope of health education practice and their generic applicability across practice settings.

- Specify the role of the advanced-level health educator and further verify the responsibilities, competencies, and subcompetencies as determined by their ability to accurately reflect the current scope of health education practice and their generic applicability across practice settings.

- Realign the responsibilities, competencies, and subcompetencies for entry- and advanced-level health educators to accurately reflect the current scope of health education practice and their generic applicability across practice settings (NCHEC, 2003a, ¶ 4).

The CUP consisted of three major phases: 1) preliminary research to provide a solid, scientific foundation for the project, 2) pilot research to prepare for the main study, and 3) the final project in which a 19-page questionnaire was completed by more than 4,000 practicing health educators from every state in the United States (including the District of Columbia) and from a wide array of work settings (i.e., community, school, college/university, health care, business/industry). At the time of the writing of this book, the data from the 4,000 plus questionnaires were being analyzed and it was projected that the preliminary reporting of the results would be completed in 2004 (NCHEC, 2003a). For more information about the development of the project, contact the NCHEC. (*Note:* Its website address is noted at the end of the chapter in Weblinks.)

Assumptions of Health Promotion

So far, we have discussed the need for health, what health education and health promotion are, and the role health educators play in delivering successful health promotion programs. We have not yet discussed the assumptions that underlie health promotion—all the things that must be in place before the whole process of health promotion begins. In the mid-1980s, Bates and Winder (1984) outlined what they saw as four critical assumptions of health education. Their list has been modified by adding several items, rewording others, and referring to them as "assumptions of health promotion." This expanded list of assumptions is critical to understanding what we can expect from health promotion programs. Health promotion is by no means the sole answer to the nation's health care problem or, for that matter, the sole means of getting the smoker to stop smoking or the nonexerciser to exercise. Health promotion is an important part of the health care system, but it does have limitations. Here are the assumptions:

1. Health status can be changed.
2. "Health and disease are determined by dynamic interactions among biological, psychological, behavioral, and social factors" (Pellmar, Brandt, & Baird, 2002, p. 217).
3. Disease occurrence theories and principles can be understood (Bates & Winder, 1984).
4. Appropriate prevention strategies can be developed to deal with the identified health problems (Bates & Winder, 1984).
5. "Behavior can be changed and those changes can influence health" (Pellmar et al., 2002, p. 213).
6. "Individual behavior, family interactions, community and workplace relationships and resources, and public policy all contribute to health and influence behavior change" (Pellmar et al., 2002, p. 217).
7. "Initiating and maintaining a behavior change is difficult" (Pellmar et al., 2002, p. 217).
8. Individual responsibility should not be viewed as victim blaming.
9. For health behavior change to be permanent, an individual must be motivated and ready to change.

The importance of these assumptions is made clearer if we refer to the definitions of health education and health promotion presented earlier in the chapter. Implicit in those definitions was a goal of having program participants voluntarily adopt actions conducive to health. To achieve such a goal, the assumptions must indeed be in place. We cannot expect people to adopt lifelong healthenhancing behavior if we force them into such change. Nor can we expect people to change their behavior just because they have been exposed to a health promotion program. Health behavior change is very complex, and health educators should not expect to change every person with whom they come in contact. However, the greatest chance for success will come to those who have the knowledge and skills to plan, implement, and evaluate appropriate programs.

Program Planning

Since many of health educators' responsibilities are involved in some way with program planning, implementation, and evaluation, health educators need to become well versed in these processes. "Planning an effective program is more difficult than implementing it. Planning, implementing, and evaluating programs are all interrelated, but good planning skills are prerequisite to programs worthy of evaluation" (Breckon, Harvey, & Lancaster, 1998, p. 145). All three processes are very involved, and much time, effort, practice, and on-the-job training are required to do them well. Even the most experienced health educators find program planning challenging because of the constant changes in settings, resources, and priority populations.

The remaining chapters of this book present a process that health educators can use to plan, implement, and evaluate successful health promotion programs and will introduce you to the necessary knowledge and skills to carry out these tasks.

SUMMARY

The increased interest in personal health and the flood of new health information have created a need to provide quality health promotion programs. Individuals are seeking guidance to enable them to make sound decisions about behavior that is conducive to their health. Those best prepared to help these people are health educators who receive appropriate training. Properly trained health educators are aware of the limitations of the discipline and understand the assumptions on which health promotion is based.

REVIEW QUESTIONS

1. Explain the role *Healthy People* played in the relationship between the American people and health.
2. How is *health education* defined by the Joint Committee on Terminology (2001)?
3. What are the key phrases in the definition of health education presented by Green and Kreuter (1999)?
4. What is the relationship between health education and health promotion?
5. Why is there a need for health educators?
6. What is the Role Delineation Project?
7. How is the *Framework* for Competency-Based Health Education used by colleges and universities? By NCHEC? By NCATE? By SABPAC?
8. How does one become a Certified Health Education Specialist (CHES)?
9. What are the seven major responsibilities of entry-level health educators? What are the additional three responsibilities for the advanced-level health educators?
10. What is the National Health Educator Competencies Update Project (CUP)?
11. What assumptions are critical to health promotion?

ACTIVITIES

1. Based on what you have read in this chapter and your knowledge of the profession of health education, write your own definitions for *health, health education, health promotion,* and *health promotion program.*

2. Write a response indicating what you see as the importance of each of the nine assumptions presented in the chapter. Write no more than one paragraph per assumption.

3. With your knowledge of health promotion, what other assumptions would you add to the list presented in this chapter? Provide a one-paragraph rationale for each.

4. If you have not already done so, go to the government documents section of the library on your campus and read *Healthy People: The Surgeon General's Report on Health Promotion and Disease Prevention (Healthy People,* 1979).

WEBLINKS

1. **http://www.aahperd.org/aahe/template.cfm**
   American Association for Health Education (AAHE)

   This is the website for the AAHE which has been instrumental in the development of the profession over the years. This site includes much information about the profession as well as the NCATE accreditation process.

2. **http://www.nchec.org/**
   The National Commission for Health Education Credentialing, Inc. (NCHEC)

   This is the website for the NCHEC, Inc. It provides the most current information about the CHES credential and the CUP.

3. **http://www.sophe.org/sophemain.html**
   Society for Public Health Education (SOPHE)

   This is the website for SOPHE which has been instrumental in the development of the profession since it was founded in 1950. This site includes much information about the profession including SABPAC approval and continuing education credit to maintain the CHES credential.

4. **http://www.nap.edu/catalog/9838.html**
   The National Academies Press (NAP)

   At this website, the Institute of Medicine's (IOM) report titled Health and Behavior: The Interplay of Biological, Behavioral, and Societal Influences can be accessed. This report has much to say about the assumptions of health promotion.

Part I

Planning a Health Promotion Program

The chapters in this section of the book provide the basic information needed to plan a health promotion program. Each chapter presents readers with the tools they will need to develop a successful program in a variety of settings. The chapters and topics presented in this section are:

CHAPTER 2

Models for Program Planning in Health Promotion

Chapter Objectives

After reading this chapter and answering the questions at the end, you should be able to:

- Explain the value of using a model in planning a program.
  - Identify the models commonly used in planning health promotion programs and briefly explain each.
  - Identify the basic components of the planning models presented.
  - Apply a model to a program you are planning.

Map it   *4 areas charactos of ethics why we need it*

Key Terms

administrative and policy assessment

APEX-PH

behavioral and environmental assessment

CDCynergy or Cynergy

educational and ecological assessment

enabling factors

epidemiological assessment

evaluation

formative research

health communication

Health Communication Model

Healthy Communities

Healthy Plan-It

impact evaluation

implementation

MAPP

MATCH

message concepts

outcome evaluation

PACE-EH

PRECEDE-PROCEED

predisposing factors

process evaluation

reinforcing factors

SMART

social assessment

social marketing

SWOT

A Systematic Approach to Health Promotion

Three Fs of Program Planning

In regards to ethics + education

As noted in Chapter 1, a major portion of the role of the health educator is associated with planning, implementing, and evaluating programs. Good health promotion programs are not created by chance; they are the product of much effort and are usually based on a systematic planning model. Models are the means by which structure and organization are given to the planning process. They provide planners with direction and a framework on which to build. Many different planning models have been developed, some of which are used more frequently than others.

Although many of the models have common elements, those elements may have different labels. In fact, "the underlying principles that guide the development of the various models are similar; however, there are important differences in sequence, emphasis, and the conceptualization of the major components that make certain models more appealing than others to individual practitioners" (Simons-Morton, Greene, & Gottlieb, 1995, pp. 126–127). It is important to remember that there are no perfect planning models. Planners may have to adapt them to fit the needs of the planning situation and the cultural characteristics of the priority population, setting, and health problem (Kline & Huff, 1999).

Most planners find occasions when it is not feasible to use a model in its entirety or when it is necessary to combine parts of different models to meet specific needs and situations. What is most critical for any student, practicing health educator, or planner is a working knowledge of the basic steps that most planning models have in common. The Generalized Model for Program Planning (see Figure 2.1) outlines these common steps: understanding and engaging, assessing needs, setting goals and objectives, developing an intervention, implementing the intervention, and evaluating the results.

Pay particular attention to the models presented in this chapter and see how they integrate these basic steps in one form or another. With an understanding and appreciation for the steps presented in this book, all other planning models will become much easier to use in health promotion settings. Then, when you need to make adjustments in the middle of a planning process, you will be able to identify and preserve the critical planning components.

Selecting a specific planning model to apply will be based on many things: 1) the preferences of stakeholders (e.g., decision makers, program partners, consumers); 2) how much time is available for planning purposes; 3) how many resources are available for data collection and analysis; 4) the degree to which clients are actually involved as partners in the planning process or the degree to which your planning efforts will be consumer-oriented (i.e., planning is based on the wants and needs of consumers); and 5) preferences of a funding agency (in the case of a grant or contract award).

Three important criteria labeled the **Three Fs of Program Planning:** *fluidity, flexibility,* and *functionality,* should help guide the selection of your model and govern the application of its use. *Fluidity* suggests that steps in the planning process are sequential, or that they build upon one another. It may not be critical if a step is missed, but it is a problem if certain steps are performed out of sequence. The appropriate sequence of steps is diagrammed in the Generalized Model for Program Planning. For example, a planner cannot develop goals and objectives until a needs assessment has been performed, and a priority health problem has been identified.

Flexibility means that planning is adapted to the needs of stakeholders. Due to various circumstances, planning is usually modified as the process unfolds. Strict adherence to a model in light of unique circumstances will generally lead to frustration among partners and a less than desirable outcome. *Functionality* means that the out-

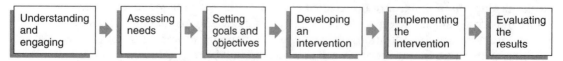

Figure 2.1 A generalized model for program planning

come of planning is improved health conditions, not the production of a program plan itself. A model is only a tool to help planners accomplish their real work.

The remainder of this chapter will present prominent models used by planners in health promotion settings. Four models, PRECEDE-PROCEED, MATCH, CDCynergy, and SMART, will be presented in detail. These models represent a wide range of planning approaches even though they share planning elements displayed in the Generalized Model. Others, which may be just as good from a theoretical framework, but used less widely, will be briefly presented and referenced.

PRECEDE-PROCEED

Currently, the most widely known model in program planning is the **PRECEDE-PROCEED** model. "PRECEDE is an acronym for *p*redisposing, *r*einforcing, and *e*nabling *c*onstructs in *e*ducational/*e*cological *d*iagnosis and *e*valuation" (Green & Kreuter, 1999, p. 34). "PROCEED stands for *p*olicy, *r*egulatory, and *o*rganizational *c*onstructs in *e*ducational and *e*nvironmental *d*evelopment" (Green & Kreuter, 1999, p. 34).

PRECEDE-PROCEED has been the basis for many professional projects at the national level. This model is well received professionally because it is theoretically grounded and comprehensive in nature; it combines a series of phases in the planning, implementation, and evaluation process.

PRECEDE-PROCEED was developed over the course of about 20 years. The Precede framework was created in the early 1970s (Green, 1974) and evolved as a planning model during the late 1970s (Green, 1975, 1976; Green, Levine, & Deeds, 1975; Green et al., 1978; Green et al., 1980). "The identification of priorities and the setting of objectives in the Precede phases provide the objectives and criteria for policy, implementation, and evaluation in the Proceed phases" (Green & Kreuter, 1999, p. 35).

The Proceed framework was developed in the 1980s (Green, 1979, 1980, 1981a, 1981b, 1982, 1983a, 1983b, 1984a, 1984b, 1984c, 1984d, 1986a, 1986b, 1986c, 1986d, 1986e, 1987a, 1987b; Green & Allen, 1980; Green & McAlister, 1984; Green, Mullen, & Friedman, 1986; Green, Wilson, & Lovato, 1986; Green, Wilson, & Bauer, 1983) and "is essentially an elaboration and extension of the administrative diagnosis step of PRECEDE, which was the final and least developed link in the PRECEDE framework" (Green & Kreuter, 1991, p. 25). It was influenced by the participation of Green and Kreuter in national policy initiatives and the development of community health promotion programs such as Planned Approach to Community Health (PATCH) (Green & Kreuter, 1992).

Though the basic components of the PRECEDE-PROCEED model have remained constant over the years, the model has been revised and updated as the practice of health promotion has advanced. For example, as Precede was used in the 1980s, it became apparent that the model needed to be expanded and thus the addition of Proceed. One subtle change to the most recent version of the model (Green & Kreuter, 1999) was removing the word *diagnosis* in the first five phases of the model and replacing it with *assessment*. Though Green and Kreuter still feel diagnosis to be the appropriate denotation, this change came as the result of many of the model's users feeling uncomfortable with the term *diagnosis*, associating the model with clinical procedures. It also suggests that all assessments must start with or find a problem, which is not the case. As Green and Kreuter (1999) point out, in assets-based approaches to community assessment, planning builds on the strengths within the community.

The Nine Phases of PRECEDE-PROCEED

As shown in Figure 2.2, PRECEDE-PROCEED is composed of nine phases or steps. At first glance, the model seems complicated, but on close examination, the continuous series of steps reveals a logical sequence for program planning. The underlying approach of this model is to begin by identifying the desired outcome, to determine what causes it, and finally to design an intervention aimed at reaching the desired outcome. In other words, PRECEDE-PROCEED begins with the final consequences and works backward to the causes. Once the causes are known, an intervention can be designed.

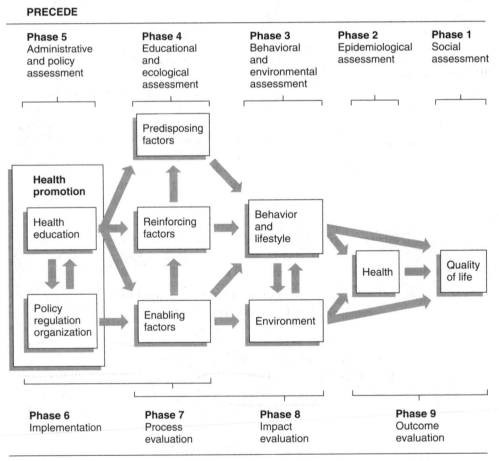

Figure 2.2 The PRECEDE-PROCEED model for health promotion planning and evaluation

Source: From *Health Promotion Planning: An Educational and Ecological Approach, Third Edition* by Lawrence W. Green and Marshall W. Kreuter. Copyright © 1999 by Mayfield Publishing Company. Reprinted by permission of the publisher.

Phase 1 in the model is called **social assessment** and seeks to subjectively define the quality of life (problems and priorities) of those in the priority population. The designers of this model suggest that this is best accomplished by involving individuals in the priority population in a self-study of their own needs and aspirations. Some of the social indicators of quality of life include absenteeism, alienation, crime, discrimination, happiness, illegitimacy, riots, self-esteem, unemployment, and welfare.

Phase 2, **epidemiological assessment,** is the step in which the planners use data to identify and rank the health goals or problems that may contribute to the needs identified in Phase 1. Those data might include disability, discomfort, fertility, fitness, morbidity, mortality, and physiological risk factors and their dimensions (distribution, duration, functional level, incidence, intensity, longevity, and prevalence). It is important to note that ranking the health problems in this phase is critical, because there are rarely, if ever, enough resources to deal with all or multiple problems. Also, this phase of the model is used to plan health programs. "A general community development program might apply this model to other problems or social goals identified in Phase 1, skipping Phase 2" (Green & Kreuter, 1999, p. 38).

Phase 3, **behavioral and environmental assessment,** involves determining and prioritizing the behavioral and environmental risk factors or determinants that might be linked to the health problems selected in Phase 2. Depending on health concerns noted in Phase 2, the behavioral factors could be the behavior or actions of individuals, groups, or communities. Behavioral indicators include such things as compliance, consumption patterns, coping, preventive actions, selfcare, and utilization. These indicators can be expressed in the dimensions of frequency, persistence, promptness, quality, and range (Green & Kreuter, 1999). "Environmental factors are those determinants outside an individual that can be modified to support behavior, health, and quality of life" (Green & Kreuter, 1999, p. 40). Examples of environmental indicators include economic, physical, services, and social, and their dimensions (access, affordability, and equity) (Green & Kreuter, 1999). Note that in Figure 2.2, arrows connect both of the boxes in Phase 3 with Phases 1 and 2. The arrows from Phase 3 to Phase 1 represent the skipping of Phase 2 if the model is applied to something other than a health problem.

Once identified, the risk factors and/or determinants need to be prioritized. This can be accomplished by first ranking the factors/conditions by importance and changeability and then using the 2 × 2 matrix presented in Figure 2.3.

Phase 4, **educational and ecological assessment,** identifies and classifies the many factors that have the potential to influence a given behavior into three categories: predisposing, reinforcing, and enabling. **Predisposing factors** include knowledge and many affective traits such as a person's attitude, values, beliefs, and perceptions. These factors can facilitate or hinder a person's motivation to change and can be altered through *direct* communication. Barriers or vehicles created mainly by societal forces or systems make up **enabling factors,** which include access to health care facilities, availability of resources, referrals to appropriate providers, enactment of rules or laws, and the development of skills. **Reinforcing factors** comprise the different types of feedback and rewards that those in the priority population receive after behavior change, which may either encourage or discourage the continuation of the behavior. Reinforcing behaviors can be delivered by, but not limited to, family, friends, peers, teachers, self, and others who control rewards. "Social benefits—such

	More important	Less important
More changeable	High priority for program focus (Quadrant 1)	Low priority except to demonstrate change for political purposes (Quadrant 3)
Less changeable	Priority for innovative program; evaluation crucial (Quadrant 2)	No program (Quadrant 4)

Figure 2.3 Prioritization matrix

Source: From *Health Promotion Planning: An Educational and Ecological Approach, Third Edition* by Lawrence W. Green and Marshall W. Kreuter. Copyright © 1999 by Mayfield Publishing Company. Reprinted by permission of the publisher.

as recognition; physical benefits such as convenience, comfort, relief of discomfort, or pain; tangible rewards such as economic benefits or avoidance of cost; imagined or vicarious rewards such as improved appearance, self-respect, or association with an admired person who demonstrates the behavior—all reinforce behavior" (Green & Kreuter, 1999, p. 171). As with the previous phases, planners must set priorities. The prioritized factors identified in this phase become the focus of the intervention that will be planned (Green & Kreuter, 1999).

Phase 5 consists of an **administrative and policy assessment,** in which planners determine if the capabilities and resources are available to develop and implement the program. It is between Phases 5 and 6 that PRECEDE (the assessment portion of the model) ends and PROCEED (implementation and evaluation) begins. However, there is not a distinct break between the two phases; they really run together, and planners can move back and forth between them.

The four final phases of the model—Phases 6, 7, 8, and 9—make up the PROCEED portion. In Phase 6—**implementation**—with appropriate resources in hand, planners select the methods and strategies of the intervention, and implementation begins. Phases 7, 8, and 9 focus on the **process, impact, outcome evaluation,** respectively, and are based on the earlier phases of the model, when objectives were outlined in the assessment process. Whether all three of these final phases are used depends on the evaluation requirements of the program. Usually, the resources needed to conduct evaluations of impact (Phase 8) and outcome (Phase 9) are much greater than those needed to conduct process evaluation (Phase 7). (See Chapter 6 for a discussion on the relationship of objectives to evaluation.)

Applying PRECEDE-PROCEED

To assist you in understanding how PRECEDE-PROCEED is used, consider the following hypothetical example using a worksite setting. Remember Phase 1 of the model, social assessment, seeks to define the quality of life of the priority population so that the desired outcomes can be identified. This is best done by including those in the priority population. Thus, in a worksite, planners need to involve both the employer and the employees in the process of assessing needs. So, having representation from the various groups within the priority population (labor, management, clerical, etc.) on a planning committee, and letting this committee coordinate a self-study of the priority population would be important. In a worksite setting, it would not be surprising to find such an assessment identifying that employers are concerned with economic outcomes of the company—or turning a profit. Employees may also be concerned about economic outcomes—their own salary or wages—but also about working conditions. Social indicators that may reflect these desired outcomes include production rates, absenteeism for all reasons (use of personal days, vacation days, and sick days), aesthetics of the work environment, morale of the workers, lack of quality leisure time, and low self-worth as an employee of this company.

In Phase 2 of the model, epidemiological assessment, planners use data to identify and rank health goals or problems that are associated with the economic concerns and working conditions that were discovered in Phase 1. Therefore, planners would want to collect and analyze data that reflect the health status of the workforce. Such sources of data could include reviewing the reasons for the use of sick days, reviewing company safety records, providing health screenings for all employees so that physiological risk factors can be identified, and analyzing the health and disability insurance claims of the company. Once identified, planners need to rank those health concerns as they relate to the quality-of-life issues identified in Phase 1. Common occupational diseases and disorders that arise in work settings include musculoskeletal conditions (e.g., back injuries), dermatological conditions resulting from exposure to chemical or other agents, and lung diseases resulting from the inhalation of toxic substances (McKenzie, Pinger, & Kotecki, 2002). For the purpose of this example, let's assume that back injuries received the highest priority in the epidemiological assessment. Employees with back injuries have both an impact on the economic outcome of the company via lost productivity and on the quality of life of the employee who is off the job.

Having prioritized back injuries as the health concern, planners move to Phase 3, behavioral and environmental assessment. In this phase, they want to determine what risk factors or determinants contribute to the back injuries. Is lifting a significant part of the employees' work? If so, are they using good lifting techniques? Are they lifting more weight than they should? Is the work environment conducive to the work the employees are asked to do? Is the work area set up in an ergonomically correct way? Have the workers been provided with appropriate back supports? Answers to these questions will provide the planners with the information they need to conduct the educational and ecological assessment, Phase 4.

The educational and ecological assessment may include (1) surveying the employees to find out what they know about lifting, (2) surveying the employer to find out what kind of training and equipment are provided for new employees and determining what policies are in place to reward injury-free work days, and (3) observing the workers to determine if they are using good lifting techniques. From this assessment, it might be found that the workers know little about appropriate lifting techniques (predisposing factor), they have not been taught any skills for proper lifting, nor have they been provided with back supports (enabling factors), and they are not rewarded for injury-free days (reinforcing factor). Thus, planners decide that an appropriate health promotion intervention would be comprised of an education component to increase knowledge and skills, and the implementation of new corporate polices that require the use of back braces and financial bonuses for a certain number of injury-free work hours.

Through the administrative and policy assessment (Phase 5), planners must determine what organizational and administrative support and resources are available to carry out the health promotion intervention. Will the educational component of the intervention be conducted on company time, employee time, or a combination of the two? Can the educational component of the intervention be conducted by a current employee or will a consultant have to be hired? Are there financial resources to buy every employee a back brace or will braces have to be shared between workers on the different shifts?

Once the availability of program resources is determined, Phase 6, implementation, can begin. The evaluation components (Phases 7, 8, and 9) of this program will be based on the objectives that were created during assessment phases. As each of the objectives were written, it would be important to ensure that criteria (standards of acceptability) noted in each objective were clear. For example, in Phase 7 (process evaluation), planners may be concerned with determining the availability of the educational component of the intervention for each employee. In Phase 8 (impact evaluation), planners would be interested in evaluating changes in the behavior of the employees (e.g., proper lifting technique) and the work environment (e.g., availability of back braces for employees). As for outcome evaluation, Phase 9, planners may be looking for a reduction in the incidence and prevalence of back injuries, or an increase in productivity.

MATCH

MATCH is an acronym for Multilevel Approach to Community Health. This planning model (see Figure 2.4) was developed in the late 1980s (Simons-Morton et al., 1988). Like the PRECEDE-PROCEED model, MATCH has also been used in a variety of settings, including the development of several intervention handbooks created by the Centers for Disease Control and Prevention (Simons-Morton et al., 1995). MATCH is an ecological planning perspective that recognizes that intervention approaches can and should be aimed at a variety of objectives and individuals (B. Simons-Morton, personal communication, October 10, 1999). This is represented in Figure 2.4 by the various levels of influence. The MATCH framework is recognized for emphasizing program implementation (Simons-Morton et al., 1995). "MATCH is designed to be applied when behavioral and environmental risk and protective factors for disease or injury are generally known and when general priorities for action have been determined, thus providing a convenient way to turn the corner from needs assessment and priority setting to the development of effective programs" (Simons-Morton et al., 1995, p. 155).

The Phases and Steps of MATCH

As can be seen in Box 2.1, MATCH is comprised of five phases and several steps within each phase. Phase I of MATCH is *goals selection*. In this phase of MATCH, planners select health-status goals based on several different factors, including the prevalence of the

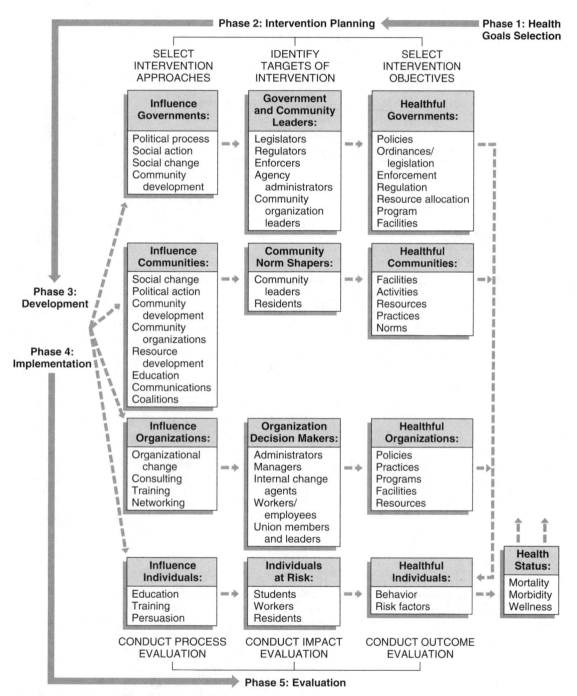

Figure 2.4 MATCH: multilevel approach to community health

Source: Reprinted by permission of Waveland Press, Inc. from B. G. Simons-Morton, W. H. Greene, and N. H. Gottlieb, *Introduction to Health Education and Health Promotion* (2nd ed.). Prospect Heights, IL: Waveland Press, Inc., 1995. All rights reserved.

Box 2.1 MATCH Phases and Steps

Phase 1:   Goals Selection

Step 1: Select health-status goals
Step 2: Select high-priority population(s)
Step 3: Identify health behavior goals
Step 4: Identify environmental factor goals

Phase 2:   Intervention Planning

Step 1: Identify the targets of the intervention
Step 2: Select intervention objectives
Step 3: Identify mediators of the intervention objectives
Step 4: Select intervention approaches

Phase 3:   Program Development

Step 1: Create program units or components
Step 2: Select or develop curricula and create intervention guides
Step 3: Develop session plans
Step 4: Create or acquire instructional materials, products, and resources

Phase 4:   Implementation Preparations

Step 1: Facilitate adoption, implementation, and maintenance
Step 2: Select and train implementors

Phase 5:   Evaluation

Step 1: Conduct process evaluation
Step 2: Measure impact
Step 3: Monitor outcomes

Source: Reprinted by permission of Waveland Press, Inc. from B.G. Simons-Morton, W.H. Greene, and N.H. Gottlieb, *Introduction to Health Education and Health Promotions* (2nd ed.). Prospect Heights, IL: Waveland Press, Inc., 1995. All rights reserved.

---

health problem, the relative significance of the health problem, the changeability of the problem, and other considerations unique to the setting. Also in this phase, planners need to select the priority population, identify the health behaviors most associated with the health-status goals in order to create health behavior goals, and identify the environmental factors—such as access, availability of resources, enabling practices, and barriers—so that environmental goals can be created (Simons-Morton et al., 1995).

In Phase II of MATCH, *intervention planning*, the planner "matches intervention objectives with the intervention targets and intervention actions" (Simons-Morton et al., 1995, p. 163). This begins with identifying the targets of the intervention actions (TIAs). TIAs are those individuals that exert influence or control over the personal or environmental conditions that are related to the target health and behavior goals (i.e., the level of society at which the intervention will be aimed). The levels include (1) individual level (e.g., persons in the priority population); (2) interpersonal level (e.g., family members, coworkers, friends, teachers, and others close to those in the priority population); (3) organizational level (e.g., a decision maker in an organization); (4) societal level (e.g., community leaders); and (5) governmental level. After identifying the TIAs, they are matched with the health behavioral and environmental factors identified in Phase I. Once this match is made, the planner selects an intervention action(s) to be used. Intervention actions commonly used by health educators include teaching, training, counseling, policy advocacy, consulting, community organization, social marketing, and social action. If the TIAs are individuals, planners need to consider those mediating factors causally associated with target behaviors, such as knowledge, attitudes, skills, experiences, and reinforcements (Simons-Morton et al., 1995).

The third phase of MATCH is *program development* and begins with the creation of the program units or components. Components are frequently organized according to a priority population subgroup (e.g., males, females, minority or age groups), proposed objectives (e.g., smoking, diet, physical activity), intervention target and level, setting and structural unit (e.g., classroom, food service, health services), or intervention approach or channel (e.g., interpersonal, media) (Simons-Morton et al., 1995,). After the creation of the program components, planners either select from already developed curricula or develop their own guides. This would include the development of individual session or lesson plans, and the acquisition or creation of instructional materials, products, and resources (Simons-Morton et al., 1995).

In Phase IV, *implementation preparations,* planners prepare for implementation and conduct the interventions. To achieve effective implementation, planners must (1) develop a specific proposal and advocate for the adoption of change; (2) develop the need, readiness, and environmental supports for change; (3) provide evidence that the intervention works; (4) identify and select change agents and opinion leaders and sell them on the need for change; and (5) establish good working relationships with the decision makers (Simons-Morton et al., 1995). In addition, depending on who will implement the program, there may be a need to select, train, support, and monitor those who do the implementation (Simons-Morton et al., 1995).

Phase V of MATCH is *evaluation.* Like the PRECEDE-PROCEED model, MATCH's evaluation also includes process, impact, and outcome components. "Process evaluation is concerned with the utility of the implementation plan and procedures, the extent and quality of implementation, and the effects of implementation on immediate learning outcomes" (Simons-Morton et al., 1995, p. 183). Impact evaluation is concerned with measuring the targeted mediators (usually knowledge, attitudes, and practices), health behaviors, and environmental factors (Simons-Morton et al., 1995). Outcome evaluation is typically focused on health behaviors but may also monitor long-term maintenance of changes in behavior or environmental factors. However, because of the time it takes for some outcomes to develop, there are often occasions in program planning when there is not enough time or resources to do outcome evaluation (Simons-Morton et al., 1995).

Applying MATCH

To help you understand the phases and steps of MATCH, consider this implementation example. As you read through this example, it will help if you refer to a diagram of the model in Figure 2.4. As is common when using MATCH, let's assume that the needs assessment is complete and that heart disease is the focus of the program we are planning. The behavioral risk factors that are apparent are lack of exercise and poor eating habits, and the environmental risk factors we are concerned with are the lack of exercise facilities in the community and meals served in the school lunch program. See Table 2.1 for a presentation of the program focus.

We begin our planning with goals selection (Phase I). Based on the epidemiological data available to us, it is obvious that heart disease is the leading cause of death in our community and that the heart disease death rate is much greater than the national average. We also know that several of the behaviors associated with the disease are changeable. Therefore, our health-status goal will be to reduce the prevalence of heart disease. We have decided to focus on elementary school children for the program because they are accessible, they possess a number of the behavioral risks, and the school administration is interested in seeing such a program in the school. The health behavior goals chosen will be to decrease sedentary lifestyle and to improve eating habits. These were chosen because of their prevalence in the children, their association with heart disease, and their changeability. Environmental goals will focus on available exercise facilities, the school's curriculum with regard to physical activity and nutrition, and school policies that can influence physical activity and eating habits.

For Phase II, intervention planning, we need to identify the levels of society at which we plan to intervene, what our intervention objectives will be, the mediators with which we will be concerned, and what intervention approaches we will take (see Table 2.2). It is decided that we will intervene at the (1) individual level, with the fifth- and sixth-graders, to influence their exercise and eating behaviors with an educational approach aimed at knowledge, attitudes, skills, and behaviors; (2) organizational level, with the members of the board of education, school administrators, teachers, and school cafeteria workers, to change the physical education and nutrition curricula and policies related to the creation of school lunch menus via organization change and training approaches; and (3) governmental level, with the city parks and recreation division, to lobby for enhanced resources by better equipping the recreational areas within the city.

Phase III, program development, will focus on several program components, including (1) the training of teachers for classroom instruction for the fifth and sixth-graders in physical activity and nutrition, (2) the training of cafeteria workers to create healthier school lunches, and (3) lobbying the city parks and recreation board for better equipped parks. The training for the teachers will include the selection or development of a curriculum, scheduled in-service sessions, and the acquisition of the materials to support the curriculum development. A similar approach will be taken with the cafeteria workers by conducting in-service sessions aimed at planning and preparing nutritious meals. In preparation for the lobbying, policy advocacy, and interest-group pressure of city council and the parks and recreation board, sessions will need to be planned with appropriate resources to training advocates in political action techniques.

With the program components in place, Phase IV, implementation preparations, can begin. Planners will next facilitate the adoption, implementation, and mainte-

Table 2.1 Behavioral and environmental risk factors for MATCH example

Health Problem	Behavioral Risk Factors	Environmental Risk Factors
Heart disease	1. Lack of exercise 2. Poor eating habits	1. Lack of exercise facilities 2. School lunch program

Table 2.2 MATCH Phase II—objectives, mediators, intervention approaches by societal level

Step 1 Focus of the Intervention	Step 2 Objectives	Step 3 Mediators	Step 4 Intervention Approaches
Individual Students • 5th-graders • 6th-graders	Health behaviors • Exercise • Eating habits	Knowledge Attitudes Skills Behavior	*Educational* • Teaching • Positive reinforcement
Organizational Board of education School administrators Teachers School cafeteria workers	Programs Practices Policies Resources	Knowledge Attitudes Skills Behavior	*Organizational Change* • Curricula change • School lunch menu policy • In-service training
Governmental City council City parks and recreation board City parks and recreation workers	Programs Practices Policies Resources	Knowledge Attitudes Skills Behavior	*Political Action* • Lobbying • Policy advocacy • Interest-group pressure

nance of their program components by preparing those impacted by the program for change. This will mean selling them on the need for change. This can be done by showing those who are affected the possible consequences of no change, that many of the opinion leaders in the community support the change, and that similar programs have been successful in other communities. Of course, with implementation, planners will need to select and, if necessary, train the implementors so they can conduct the in-service sessions for the teachers and cafeteria workers, and prepare those who will be lobbying the city parks and recreation board.

Finally, the planners will need to plan for program evaluation (Phase V). Process evaluation will examine the success of the implementation of the various program components. How was the quality of the in-service sessions? What was good about them? How could they be improved? What were the immediate learning outcomes for the teachers, cafeteria workers, and those learning lobbying skills? What was the quality of the curriculum offered for the fifth- and sixth-graders? How did the implementation go with the school lunches using the new menu? The impact evaluation will measure the knowledge, attitudes, and health practices of the fifth- and sixth-graders with regard to physical activity and nutrition. It will also include an examination of changes that may have occurred at the city parks. Since the health goal of the program was to reduce the prevalence of heart disease in the community and aimed at students in grades 5 and 6, the resources would not be available to track these students for a long period of time. Thus, outcome evaluation would not be conducted.

Consumer-Based Planning

PRECEDE-PROCEED and MATCH are examples of time-honored models that have been used successfully in many health promotion settings. It is important for planners to understand and be able to apply these models. Although these and other planning models presented in this chapter (referred to by some as *practitioner-driven models*) use data from the consumer (priority population) in the planning process, in *consumer-based planning*, all program decisions are based on consumer input and made with consumers in mind. In other words, consumer-based planning includes consumers throughout the entire planning process. Data are collected to understand the wants, needs, and preferences of consumers themselves, then used to continually test all aspects of intervention and communication strategies. There is some evidence to suggest that this planning approach is more effective than practitioner-driven approaches (Neiger & Thackeray, 2002).

Two methodologies that generally apply a consumer-based planning strategy are health communication and social marketing. Social marketing, in particular, is defined and characterized by its consumer orientation. Though they are generally considered distinct approaches, they both craft communication strategies, develop interventions, and perform evaluations to improve programs, only after they identify who their consumers are, what they need, how they will respond and change most effectively.

Health Communication

Health communication is the use of strategies to inform and influence individual and community decisions to enhance health (NCI, 2002). It is also commonly defined by the form it takes in health promotion programs (i.e., mass media, media advocacy, risk communication, public relations, entertainment education, print material, electronic communication). The effective use of health communication principles can be used narrowly to design an intervention such as a brochure or website, or it can be used broadly to design a complete communication campaign (NCI, 2002).

The sophistication with which health information is communicated has changed dramatically over the last few decades (USDHHS, 2000). The private sector, in particular, has been successful in designing communication and marketing campaigns that combine cutting-edge technology with segmentation approaches and tailored messages. This level of expertise and detail must be matched by planners if we are to compete for attention and active participation among consumers. For example, research indicates that effective health communication campaigns adapt audience-centered approaches (USDHHS, 2000). This requires that planners understand consumer tendencies, needs, and preferences before designing campaigns and messages.

Planners must also avoid attaching unrealistic expectations to their health communication campaigns. For example, health communication alone is rarely sufficient to change behavior and reduce the risk of disease. It can, however, influence attitudes, perceptions, awareness, knowledge, and social norms, which all tend to act as precursors to behavior change. A one-dimensional approach to health promotion that relies solely on mass media without proper program support strategies or interventions has been shown to be insufficient (USDHHS, 2000).

Planners must also be able to communicate with multiple audiences using multiple channels. In addition to the primary population of interest, secondary and tertiary audiences such as health promotion partners, health care providers, the news media, and policymakers, must receive appropriate health communication to support the basic objectives of a campaign (Nelson, Brownson, Remington, & Parvanta 2002).

Channels in health communication include interpersonal, small group, organizational, community, and mass media.

Today, with the Internet and digital technology, we find ourselves in a new age of communication that holds the potential to drive a health revolution (Ratzan, 1999). At the same time, we know that transmission of information or mere data do not equal effective communication (Ratzan, 1999). To the contrary, driving a health revolution will require that those who perform health communication use strategic approaches based on established communication and behavioral theories, and incorporate consumer feedback to create targeted interventions and messages.

Social Marketing

Social marketing has been defined as a program-planning process designed to influence the voluntary behavior of a specific audience segment to achieve a social rather than a financial objective. Borrowing from commercial marketing principles, the process offers benefits the audience wants, reduces barriers the audience faces, and uses persuasion to influence intentions to act favorably (Albrecht, 1997).

A frequent misinterpretation of social marketing is that it is limited to narrow interventions, such as communication or advertising strategies. Used correctly, social marketing is best viewed as a planning framework that positions consumers at the core of all activity. Although it is not necessarily a complicated process, it can represent a time-consuming and resource-intense process.

Social marketing strategies have been used in varying degrees for over 30 years in international and domestic settings, with the primary intent to improve health conditions and quality of life in general. Early international social marketing interventions focused primarily on immunizations, family planning, agricultural reforms, and nutrition (Walsh et al., 1993). Social marketing activity in the United States has focused on diverse issues, including the prevention of AIDS and cardiovascular disease, low-fat eating, the Five-a-Day Campaign, prevention and treatment of drug use, and breast cancer screening (Neiger et al., 2001).

Based on the results of a Delphi survey conducted among leading social marketing authorities (Maibach, Shenker, & Singer, 1997), ten key elements displayed in Box 2.2 best characterize social marketing. What becomes readily apparent is that social marketing attempts to strategically understand the consumer and ensure that interventions are not only based on consumer input but also tested with consumers before being implemented. This is significantly different from traditional health promotion practice. In fact, the hallmark of social marketing is a continual focus on the consumers who will eventually participate in the health promotion program. Therefore, consumers should be placed at the center of all program planning and implementation by addressing not only their wants and needs, but also their concerns. The most critical responsibility of social marketers is an assurance that what is finally offered in the form of an intervention satisfies consumer wants and needs.

Two models that capture the critical characteristics of health communication and social marketing are CDCynergy and SMART, respectively. They both focus on priority audiences, rely heavily on consumer data for decision making, and attempt to continually return to the consumer for feedback and program improvement.

Box 2.2 Key Elements That Best Characterize the Practice of Social Marketing

- Audience-centered program development
- Promotion of voluntary behavior change
- Audience segmentation and profiling
- Formative research to develop and test programs
- A range of product development based on audience research
- Product distribution based on audience research
- Program promotion through channels identified in audience research
- Process evaluation
- Outcome evaluation
- Audience and community involvement in the planning process

Source: Maibach, Shenker, and Singer (1997).

CDCynergy

Perhaps the most comprehensive and theoretically based health communication planning model is *CDCynergy,* or *Cynergy* for short, developed by the Office of Communication at the Centers for Disease Control and Prevention (CDC) in the mid 1990s. Although it is an interactive CD-ROM tool, its contents resemble most planning models and contain the basic components outlined in the generalized model (see Figure 2.1), and included in both the PRECEDE-PROCEED and MATCH models. However, it does pay closer attention to audience analysis and feedback, segmentation principles, and targeted communication strategies.

CDCynergy was developed primarily for public health professionals at the CDC with responsibilities for health communication. However, because of widespread interest in the model, CDC made it available to other health professionals who found the model useful for health promotion in community, worksite, school, and health care (including managed care) settings. Although it is considered public domain (meaning restrictions are not placed on copying or general use), CDC currently requires training before releasing a copy of the CD-ROM.

The basic edition of CDCynergy presents a general methodology for health communication planning, a step-by-step guide, a reference library and links to templates that allow tailored plans to be created (CDC, 2003). In addition, CDC and its partners have produced content specific editions of Cynergy to meet the specific needs of planners addressing various health problems. These editions include: cardiovascular disease, immunizations, micronutrients, diabetes, tobacco prevention and control, emergency risk communication and social marketing. CDC has also produced an abbreviated edition of the model entitled *CDCynergy Lite* (see Box 2.3) to help practitioners expedite the health communication planning process when necessary.

The Phases of CDCynergy

Cynergy uses six phases involving multiple steps to help planners acquire a thorough understanding of a health problem and who it affects; explore a wide range of possible strategies for influencing the problem; systematically select the strategies that show the most promise; understand the role communication can play in planning, implementing, and evaluating selected strategies; and develop a comprehensive communication plan (CDC, 2003). Box 2.3 displays the six sequential yet interrelated phases, which are designed to build on the previous phases and prepare program planners for subsequent phases.

Box 2.3 CDCynergy Lite—*An Abridged Version of the CDCynergy Health Communication Model*

Phase 1:   Describe Problem

- Identify and define health problems that may be addressed by your program interventions.
- Examine and/or conduct necessary research to describe the problems.
- Assess factors and variables that can affect the project's direction, including strengths, weaknesses, opportunities, and threats (SWOT).

Phase 2:   Analyze Problem

- List causes of each problem you plan to address.
- Develop goals for each problem.
- Consider strengths, weaknesses, opportunities, threats, and ethics of health 1) engineering, 2) communication/education, 3) policy/enforcement, and 4) community service intervention options.
- Select the types of intervention(s) that should be used to address the problem(s).

Phase 3:   Plan Intervention

- Decide whether communication is needed as a dominant intervention and/or as support for other intervention(s).
  - If communication is used as a dominant intervention, list possible audiences.
  - If communication is to be used to support Community Services, Engineering, and/or Policy/Enforcement interventions, list possible audiences to be reached in support of each selected intervention.
- Conduct necessary audience research to segment intended audiences.
- Select audience segment(s) and write communication objectives for each audience segment.
- Write a creative brief to provide guidance in selecting appropriate concepts/messages, settings, activities, and materials.

Phase 4:   Develop Intervention

- Develop and test concepts, messages, settings, channel-specific activities, and materials with intended audiences.
- Finalize and briefly summarize a communication implementation plan. The plan should include:
  - Background and justification, including SWOT and ethics analyses

(Box 2.3 *continues*)

(Box 2.3 *continued*)

- Audiences
- Communication objectives
- Messages
- Settings and channels for conveying your messages
- Activities (including tactics, materials, and other methods)
- Available partners and resources
- Tasks and timeline (including persons responsible for each task, date for completion of each task, resources required to deliver each task, and points at which progress will be checked)
- Internal and external communication plan
- Budget
  - Produce materials for dissemination.

Phase 5:   Plan Evaluation

- Determine stakeholder information needs.
  - Decide which types of evaluation (e.g., implementation, reach, effects) are needed to satisfy stakeholder information needs.
  - Identify sources of information and select data collection methods.
  - Formulate an evaluation design that illustrates how methods will be applied to gather credible information.
  - Develop a data analysis and reporting plan.
    - Finalize and briefly summarize an evaluation implementation plan. The plan should include:
    - Stakeholder questions
    - Intervention Standards
    - Evaluation methods and design
    - Data analysis and reporting
    - Tasks and timeline (including persons responsible for each task, date for completion of each task, resources required to deliver each task, and points at which progress will be checked)
    - Internal and external communication plan
    - Budget

Phase 6:   Implement Plan

- Integrate, execute, and manage communication and evaluation plans.
- Document feedback and lessons learned.
- Modify program components based on feedback.
- Disseminate lessons learned and evaluation findings.

Source: Centers for Disease Control and Prevention. (2003).

The first phase of CDCynergy is called *Describe Problem*. Like other planning models, CDCynergy initially relies on good epidemiologic data and professional expertise to identify a primary health problem or contributing factor that merits attention and resources. Although programs and interventions are not generally implemented in a consumer-based model before obtaining adequate consumer input, an initial focus based on epidemiology or other good information is important to set the planning process in the right direction. Phase 1 requires the planner to state the problem and determine if the organization has the authority, capacity, and justification to address the problem (CDC, 2003).

A short written problem statement assesses the difference between what is occurring and what should occur in relation to the identified health problem. Using epidemiologic data, the problem is described in terms of who is affected and to what extent, where the problem exists geographically, when it occurs, and any related trends that may be evident. The problem statement also determines and describes distinct subgroups affected by the health problem.

In addition to describing the scope and magnitude of the problem, Phase 1 examines whether the organization is in a good position to address the problem. To help make this determination, Cynergy walks planners through several questions related to current strengths, weaknesses, opportunities, and threats.

Finally, the organization assesses whether it has the capacity to address the problem. It does this by analyzing things such as human resources, including knowledge and expertise, technology resources, and the political climate in general. If the organization cannot adequately respond to these questions, it is important to stop the Cynergy planning process and either identify a more appropriate problem or use a more appropriate planning approach.

At the conclusion of Phase 1, program planners end up with a brief description of the problem, a rationale for why the organization is addressing the problem, and a list of factors that justify the organization's involvement with the problem (CDC, 1999a). This problem definition and description can then provide a rationale to justify a program to supervisors, funding agencies, decision makers, the public, the press, constituents, or program partners. It gives program planners confidence in decision making and provides a clear direction and foundation for subsequent phases.

Whereas Phase 1 identifies the problem and provides a rationale for why an organization is doing something about the problem, Phase 2, *Analyze Problem*, guides program planners in describing the problem in more detail. The first task in this phase is identification of factors that directly or indirectly contribute to the problem, including biology, behavior, the environment, policies (or lack of policies), other barriers, and resources. A thorough understanding of contributing factors allows the planners to more effectively identify appropriate interventions.

For example, let's assume that the problem statement in Phase 1 pertained to a lack of physical activity among older adults. Contributing factors could include a lack of awareness among older adults of the relationship between physical activity and chronic diseases. Perhaps older adults experience discomfort during and after exercise, or maybe adequate walking paths or other resources do not exist for physical activity.

A direct cause is a factor representing an immediate cause of the health problem whereas an indirect cause is something that exerts an effect on the direct cause (CDC, 2003). Following the example of lack of physical activity among older adults, a direct cause may be lack of safe and convenient walking paths. An indirect cause may be unwillingness by political leaders to spend public funds to provide these walking paths. In this sense, Cynergy helps planners step back from the primary cause and address secondary causes as well.

During Phase 2, planners also prioritize the importance of sub-problems. In part, priority setting will be influenced by the complexity or difficulty of the direct and indirect causes leading to the health problem. Other criteria for priority setting may include: size and seriousness of the problem, effectiveness of interventions, community concern and lost productivity. This process of setting priorities helps planners avoid overcommitting scarce resources by addressing too many subgroups and too many problems. Stakeholders will ultimately decide how much time, money, personnel, and energy can be devoted to multiple populations and problems. Generally though, it is best to do fewer things well.

Once a manageable number of sub-problems have been selected, goals are developed for each. These goals will merely identify general outcomes and time frames to help planners further examine relevant theories and possible interventions. Program planners consider strengths, weaknesses, opportunities, and threats (SWOT), as well as ethics related to each of the potential interventions. Phase 2 then requires planners to actually select the intervention(s) that will be implemented for each sub-problem and develop a corresponding logic model which displays a sequence of all relevant steps in the implementation process. Finally, given the selection of interventions, Phase 2 examines the need for new partners and resources and pursues appropriate funding.

Phase 3 is titled *Plan Intervention*. In this phase, planners must determine whether communication will play a dominant or supportive role for each intervention. For example, a dominant role might involve a community wide media campaign that includes television and radio spots and paid advertising in newspapers to promote physical activity among older adults. A supportive communication role may be interpersonal communications with city planners to create more opportunities for physical activity in the community.

In order to identify actual audiences for interventions, segmentation is performed. This process narrows a large population to a more manageable size based on common characteristics. To do so, Cynergy recommends that the audience segment, at a minimum, be large enough and unique enough to justify a separate communication intervention (CDC, 2003). Planners decide which segments are appropriate for interventions based on these criteria and how they intend to reach and influence these audiences with communication efforts. As in Phase 2, goals are developed, but these pertain only to communication. Relevant communication theories are considered to gain insight into ways to reach communication goals and direction to perform formative research (CDC, 2003).

In general, formative research is the sum of all preparation activities that occur before a program is implemented. It includes literature reviews and other research needed to develop and achieve communication and program goals. Most significantly, formative research involves research with intended audiences to understand wants, needs, and preferences before interventions are developed and implemented. This information can be collected through surveys, focus groups, in-depth interviews, public hearings and community forums. After formative research is completed, planners should be able to develop profiles for each of the subgroups or audiences previously identified. These profiles include relevant theories and models pertaining to the audience, key data, or information on the audience that relate to its preferences, and preliminary ideas for communication concepts, messages, settings, channels, and support materials (CDC, 2003).

With the completion of audience profiles, Phase 3 requires planners to transform communication goals into specific and measurable communication objectives that specify what measurable impact and change will be experienced within the audience segments. Accompanying the communication objectives are creative briefs which are two to four page summaries used to guide the process of developing, testing, and tailoring communication components (i.e., messages, channel-specific activities, materials, settings) of the communication interventions produced in Phase 4 (CDC, 2003). Finally, plans are confirmed with stakeholders and partners discuss evaluation of all significant program components.

Phase 4, *Develop Intervention,* guides planners to test all concepts in the creative briefs with the intended audiences. Most often, this means holding focus groups or performing theatre testing with members of the audience segment to assess their reactions, likes and dislikes. Theater testing involves large groups providing feedback on messages or audiovisual materials either electronically or via questionnaires (NCI, 2002). Adjustments are then made before production and implementation occur.

In Phase 4, planners must also decide upon settings (where the audience segment will receive or be exposed to the communication messages and interventions). Identifying an appropriate setting requires planners to determine where and when the audience is most receptive to communication. Examples include a worksite where employees might see a poster; schools where public announcements may be broadcast; or homes where television may be viewed (CDC, 2003). Other important communication variables addressed in Phase 4 include exploring possible channels and tactics. A channel is the route of message delivery (i.e., interpersonal, small group, organizational, community, mass media). An activity is used within a channel to deliver a message (e.g., holding training classes to help older adults start their own walking clubs). Once activities are identified, planners must also develop necessary supporting materials (i.e., print material, curriculum, posters, public service announcements).

Before communication messages, activities and materials are implemented within appropriate channels, they are pretested (i.e., surveys, interviews, focus groups) with the audience segment. After appropriate feedback is received, communication materials are produced for dissemination.

Phase 5, *Plan Evaluation,* follows CDC's *Framework for Program Evaluation in Public Health* (CDC, 1999c). This model, a six-step approach includes: 1) engaging stakeholders; 2) describing the program; 3) focusing the evaluation design; 4) gathering credible evidence; 5) justifying conclusions; and 6) ensuring use and sharing lessons learned (see Chapter 14 for more on this framework). Planners develop a data analysis and reporting plan, formalize agreements, develop internal and external communication plans with staff and partners, and create timetables and a budget (CDC, 2003).

In specific terms, Phase 5 addresses both formative and summative evaluation (see Chapter 13 for more information on both types of evaluation). This means that those who perform evaluation are examining how well the program is being implemented and how well the consumers are responding to the communication strategies. Evaluators also determine whether changes in direct and indirect causes are being made as a result of accomplishing the communication objectives. Phase 5 includes measurements of the reach and exposure of communications, cost analysis, and relevance of theories that are linked with the communication strategies.

The final phase in Cynergy, Phase 6, is *Implement Plan*. The important components of this phase involve working with partners to: a) integrate, execute, and manage communication and evaluation plans, b) document feedback, and c) modify program components based on feedback. This phase also addresses issues such as lessons learned during the course of program implementation and delivery, how these lessons can be shared with others, and how this new discovery can be directed back to the program. This includes the creation of a dissemination plan for key findings.

Careful observance and completion of all steps and phases in the Cynergy model will result in a strategic communication plan that is science and audience based. This will increase the likelihood of achieving program goals and objectives and, more importantly, reducing the related health problems.

SMART

Although social marketing has been used to improve health for over 30 years, relatively few social marketing planning frameworks exist. Bryant (1998) and Andreason (1995) have outlined sequential processes to facilitate social marketing activity. An attempt has also been made to synthesize existing social marketing frameworks into a standardized sequence of phases or steps (Walsh et al., 1993). **SMART (Social Marketing Assessment and Response Tool)** (Neiger, 1998), influenced primarily by Walsh and colleagues (1993), is also a composite of these planning frameworks but differs in sequence of steps, certain content areas, and consistency with models most often used in health promotion settings. Unlike other models, SMART has been used from start to finish on multiple occasions in successful social marketing interventions (Neiger & Thackeray, 2002). A careful review of the model provides an excellent overview of social marketing in general.

As displayed in Box 2.4, SMART is composed of seven phases. Like other social marketing planning models, the central focus of SMART is consumers. The heart of this model, composed of Phases 2 through 4, pertains to acquiring a broad understanding of

---

Box 2.4 The SMART Model

Phase 1:   Preliminary Planning

- Identify a health problem and name it in terms of behavior.
- Develop general goals.
- Outline preliminary plans for evaluation.
- Project program costs.

Phase 2:   Consumer Analysis

- Segment and identify the priority population.
- Identify formative research methods.
- Identify consumer wants, needs, and preferences.
- Develop preliminary ideas for preferred interventions and communication strategies.

(Box 2.4 *continues*)

(Box 2.4 *continued*)

Phase 3:   Market Analysis

- Establish and define the market mix (4Ps).
- Assess the market to identify competitors (behaviors, messages, programs, etc.), allies (support systems, resources, etc.), and partners.

Phase 4:   Channel Analysis

- Identify appropriate communication channels.
- Assess options for program distribution. Determine how channels should be used.
- Assess options for program distribution.
- Identify communication roles for program partners.

Phase 5:   Develop Interventions, Materials, and Pretest

- Develop program interventions and materials using information collected in consumer, market, and channel analyses.
- Interpret the marketing mix into a strategy that represents exchange and societal good.
- Pretest and refine the program.

Phase 6:   Implementation

- Communicate with partners and clarify involvement.
- Activate communication and distribution strategies.
- Document procedures and compare progress to time lines.
- Refine the program.

Phase 7:   Evaluation

- Assess the degree to which the priority population is receiving the program.
- Assess the immediate impact on the priority population and refine the program as necessary.
- Ensure that program delivery is consistent with established protocol.
- Analyze changes in the priority population.

Source: Adapted from Walsh et al., (1993) by Neiger (1998).

the consumers who will be the recipients of a program and its interventions. These three phases seek to understand consumers before interventions are even developed or implemented. Social marketing represents an honest attempt to respond directly to consumer feedback.

The Phases of SMART *Preliminary Planning* is critical for any type of health promotion program. It is also the first phase of SMART. Preliminary planning allows program planners to objectively assess all health problems and determine which one is most appropriate to address. This is most often accomplished through analysis of epidemiologic data, including various mortality and morbidity rates and associated risk factor data. It also includes objective priority setting with predetermined criteria. Sometimes planners do not undergo a process to select a priority health problem because the decision has already been made or the organization is dedicated to a specific health problem (e.g., the American Heart Association). Once a single health problem is determined, it is defined in terms of behaviors. Risk factors, or contributing factors, then become the focus of the social marketing process. This is similar to most health promotion programs.

Although goals are outlined in Phase 1, objectives are not. This makes sense from a social marketing perspective, since consumer research has not yet been performed. The goals are general statements of intent or direction, but they do not specify program components or direct the planner into specific courses of action.

Another task in Phase 1 is to develop preliminary plans for evaluation. Theoretically, it will make sense to most planners to consider evaluation early in the planning process. In reality, evaluation is too often an afterthought. Preliminary decisions regarding evaluation outcomes must be made up front in order to account for personnel, time, and budget requirements. Therefore, it is also important to determine how preprogram (pretest or baseline) and postprogram (posttest) data will be collected and to identify valid survey or data collection instruments. Planners can also control for various kinds of bias or error in data collection if these basic evaluation concepts are considered before the program is implemented.

Finally, program costs need to be projected before the social marketing project begins. Social marketing can be an expensive proposition in terms of staff costs and direct expenses. When performed correctly, a social marketing project can easily take a year before implementation even begins. Program planners and organizations must decide if they are ready to make these kinds of time and financial commitments. Planning for both cost-benefit and cost-effectiveness analyses, outlined in Chapter 14, are appropriate in this phase.

At the end of Phase 1, the social marketing planners have (1) identified the focus of interest in terms of modifiable behaviors, (2) developed goals that provide general direction, (3) outlined preliminary plans for evaluation, and (4) estimated total project costs. Based on this information, the planners and organizations can make an educated decision about the potential costs and benefits of the project.

Phase 2 of SMART is *Consumer Analysis*. In social marketing language, the process of performing consumer analysis is formative research. **Formative research,** as defined in social marketing, is a process that identifies differences among subgroups within a population, identifies a subgroup, determines the wants and needs of the subgroup, and identifies factors that influence its behavior, including benefits, barriers, and readiness to change (Bryant, 1998).

As discussed in CDCynergy, it is important to narrow a large and perhaps unwieldy population into smaller segments that make a project more manageable. Segmentation also allows a planner to focus on a subpopulation that is either at highest risk or, for other important reasons, is the most appropriate focus for social marketing interventions. At times, and perhaps too often, health promotion programs are distributed and implemented to anyone and everyone in the population. Dismal results are then discouraging and perplexing. In contrast, programs that segment populations based on factors such as readiness to change, interest, learning style, support, self-efficacy, and locus of control hold more promise for successful outcomes (Albrecht & Bryant, 1996).

Segmentation can be performed with demographic, psychographic, attitudinal, or behavioral methods. Attitudinal variables involve judgments about products and services, benefits sought, and readiness to change. Behavioral variables include rationale for purchase decisions, product use, user status, and loyalty level (Albrecht & Bryant, 1996). (See Chapter 11 for more information on segmentation.)

Once a priority audience has been segmented, and only after segmentation has occurred, does the bulk of formative research occur—that is, actually talking to consumers in the priority population about their wants, needs, and preferences. A commonly used method is focus groups. In-depth interviews, key informant interviews, public hearings, opinion polls, and a variety of other survey techniques can also be used to collect information about the priority population. The purpose of these techniques is to find out what consumers think about the health problem that has been identified as well as its related behaviors or contributing factors. (See Chapter 5 for different techniques of data collection.)

It is important to remember that no single type of data collection technique is necessarily best in performing formative research. To the contrary, it is helpful to use multiple methods to gain a better perspective of the priority population. It is a mistake for those who engage in social marketing to perform one or two focus groups in the name of consumer analysis and allege they understand their consumers. In fact, Beckwith (1997) criticized focus groups, claiming dominant people control discussions and that they reveal more about group dynamics than market dynamics.

At the conclusion of Phase 2, a priority population is identified. Adequate formative research has been performed yielding data about major themes, directions, and consumer preferences related to interventions and communication messages. Although Phases 2 through 4 are often performed simultaneously, information collected in Phase 2 can provide context for the other two phases. For example, knowing about consumer preferences related to some type of behavior change allows planners to more effectively understand consumer preferences related to the market mix and communication strategies.

Phase 3, *Market Analysis,* examines the fit between the focus of interest (desired behavior change) and important market variables within the priority population. *Marketing mix* is a term that is often used in both commercial and social marketing. It is composed of four components, also known as the 4Ps: product, price, place, promotion. (See Chapter 11 for a discussion of the 4Ps.)

All of the factors in the market mix are analyzed in context of the priority population and provide additional issues that should be addressed in the formative research process. Market analysis also analyzes the marketplace to identify competitors and allies. For example, a competitor in social marketing may be anything that vies for the necessary resources to engage in the behavior as prescribed. If the product is an exercise program that combines strength training and cardiovascular endurance, a competitor may be a toning program that focuses on different outcomes. A busy schedule may be a competitor. An ally may be a supportive workplace that encourages and even promotes exercise behavior.

At the conclusion of this phase, consumer analysis is enriched by a better understanding of important market variables that influence consumers. Combined with consumer analysis and channel analysis, market analysis provides a powerful combination of useful information about consumers, the environment they live in, and strengths and weakness associated with potential social marketing interventions.

The fourth phase of SMART is *Channel Analysis*. Since preliminary message design is addressed through formative research in Phase 2, what remains is consumer feedback on channel selection. Although communication may not be the focal point of a social marketing campaign, it will play a secondary role in communicating important messages about the product. Formative research includes specific questions about the type of communication channels consumers believe are most appropriate for the behavior change in question. As described in CDCynergy, communication channels include interpersonal, small group, organizational, community, and mass media channels. Channels also relate to place in the market mix or how the product is accessed. In other words, the channel must be appropriate for the way the product is distributed. For example, if the product is increased vegetable consumption and the place is the worksite cafeteria, an appropriate channel might be an organizational newsletter.

In most cases, the use of multiple channels increases the likelihood that the messages will be heard and acted upon. However, if the message is not consumer oriented and is not adequately supported by an effective market mix, the channel itself is relatively unimportant. That is why all these factors are planned in unison.

Finally, Phase 4 considers which potential partners, if any, might collaborate in sharing the burden of communication. For example, if mass media is an appropriate channel, and consumer-oriented public service announcements are used in the communication strategy, perhaps television and radio stations would be willing to donate air time. One problem frequently experienced in social marketing is that multiple organizations with similar missions communicate competing, albeit only slightly different messages. In extreme cases, the messages can be nearly polar opposites. For this reason alone, it is important to develop communication partners. At the conclusion of Phase 4, communication channels are identified that are consistent with preliminary messages, and product distribution points and potential communication and intervention partners are identified.

Phase 5 of SMART consists of *Developing Interventions, Materials, and Pretesting*. Once formative research is performed, it is critical that the data are transferred or infused adequately into the design of programs, interventions, and communication strategies. To do this, data must be analyzed and categorized appropriately to assure that planners understand what they have seen, heard, and observed. As planners meet to design programs and materials, they should keep formative research data in front of them and refer to them often. Discussion and decisions should reflect all data and represent a consensus among all planners. In other words, materials and methods should represent what was learned in formative research.

Once a program prototype is developed, it is imperative to return to the priority population and test the concepts before implementing a widespread campaign. In fact, social marketing represents a process of continually returning to the consumers until the program and all its support mechanisms are consistent with their views and preferences. Several mechanisms are available to perform pretesting. One example is a pilot test where the program can be implemented with the priority population on a smaller, less expensive scale. Theater testing or focus groups can also be used to test communication messages, key components of interventions, and program formats and sequences.

Phase 6 of SMART is *Implementation*. Implementation in social marketing is closely related to the implementation factors addressed in CDCynergy. This phase is concerned with clarifying everyone's role, including external partners. This means that procedures are communicated and documented, and that time lines are developed and followed. In this phase, the communication and distribution plans are activated and the actual program and its interventions are offered. In addition, the program is refined continually, based on consumer feedback.

The seventh and final phase of SMART is *Evaluation*. The preliminary evaluation strategies that were identified in Phase 1 now take effect. Evaluation always has at least two major objectives: improve the quality of the program and determine the effectiveness of the program. With respect to quality, program planners assess the degree to which the priority population, within the larger population, is actually receiving the program or interventions. Planners also assess the immediate impact the program is having and whether the interventions and related support strategies are acceptable and motivational to the priority population. Planners also ensure that program delivery is consistent with program protocol or at least consistent with developed time lines.

Ultimately, social marketing, and all its related work, is of little value unless behavior change occurs and health is improved. Evaluation also concerns itself with measuring these outcomes. Effective planners and evaluators also make sure that evaluation results are folded back into the program so that it can be improved before it is too late, and communicate evaluation results effectively to stakeholders.

Other Planning Models

As noted at the beginning of this chapter, there are other planning models available to planners in addition to the PRECEDE-PROCEED, MATCH, CDCynergy and SMART models. Because these models are not currently used as much as those already presented, they are presented here in abbreviated form. If you are interested in learning more about these models, check the original sources provided in the reference section at the back of the book.

A Systematic Approach to Health Promotion (Healthy People 2010)

A Systematic Approach to Health Promotion is the planning model that was used to develop *Healthy People 2010* and is composed of four key elements: 1) goals; 2) objectives; 3) determinants of health; and 4) health status. Whether used for planning activities at the national, state, or local community levels, these four elements remain the same.

As in other planning models, goals provide general direction for this approach and serve to guide the development of objectives which specify outcomes as well as time frames (USDHHS, 2000). The two general goals associated with *Healthy People 2010* are: 1) increasing quality and years of healthy life; and 2) eliminating health disparities.

A total of 467 objectives involving 28 focus areas are included in *Healthy People 2010*. As in other planning initiatives, objectives specify who will be effected, what will change, where it will occur, when change will occur, and how much change will occur (see Chapter 6 for more information on goals and objectives).

The *Healthy People 2010* model does the best job of any planning model in addressing the determinants of health (risk or protective factors that lead to illness or well-being respectively). Determinants in this model include behaviors (i.e., physical activity, wearing safety belts, proper diet), biology (a person's genetic predisposition to health or disease, family history), social environment (i.e., interactions with family, friends, colleagues and others in the community), physical environment (e.g., that which is seen, touched, heard, smelled and tasted), policies and interventions, and access to quality health care. Collectively, these determinants have a profound effect on the health and well-being of individuals, communities and the nation. More importantly, they represent the focus of health promotion interventions identified throughout *Healthy People 2010*. In order to change the health status of a community, planners must ultimately address and modify key determinants.

Finally, health status (i.e., death rates, life expectancy, quality of life, morbidity from specific diseases), a primary standard of success by which health educators can be evaluated, is determined as a baseline measure and later as a measurement of program success. However, health status, often synonymous with leading causes of death, generally results from a combination of determinants such as behaviors, injury, violence, other factors in the environment or a lack of quality health services. Understanding and monitoring these determinants may prove more useful than tracking death rates that reflect the cumulative impact of many factors (USDHHS, 2000).

Mobilizing for Action through Planning and Partnerships (MAPP)

Mobilizing for Action through Planning and Partnerships (MAPP) was developed by the National Association of County and City Health Officials (NACCHO). As such, it represents a planning approach common to city or county health departments (also known as local health departments). The vision for implementing the MAPP approach involves improving health and quality of life through mobilized partnerships and taking strategic action (NACCHO, 2001).

MAPP is composed of multiple steps in six general phases. In the first phase of MAPP, *Organizing for Success and Partnership Development,* core planners assess whether or not the MAPP process is timely, appropriate and even possible. This involves assessing resources, including budgets, the expertise of available personnel, support of key decision makers and other stakeholders, and general interest of community members. If resources are not in place, the process is delayed. If the decision is made to undertake a MAPP process, the following work groups are created: 1) a core support team, which prepares most, if not all of the material needed for the process; 2) the MAPP Committee, composed of key sponsors (usually influential figures from the private sector who lend legitimacy and resources) and stakeholders who guide and oversee the process; and 3) the community itself, which provides input, representation and decision making. This phase answers basic questions about the general feasibility, resources and appropriateness of the MAPP process.

Phase 2 of the MAPP process, *Visioning,* guides the community through a process that results in a shared vision (what the ideal future looks like) and common values (principles and beliefs that will guide the remainder of the planning process) (NACCHO, 2001). Generally, a facilitator conducts the visioning process and involves anywhere from 50–100 participants including the advisory committee, the MAPP committee, and key community leaders.

Phase 3, the *Four MAPP Assessments,* is the strength and defining characteristic of the MAPP model. The four assessments include: 1) the community themes and strengths assessment (community or consumer opinion); 2) the local public health assessment (general capacity of the local health department); 3) the community health status assessment (measurement of the health of the community by use of epidemiologic data), and 4) the forces of change assessment (forces such as legislation, technology, and other environmental or social phenomenon that do or will impact the community). Collectively, the MAPP assessments provide insight on the gaps that exist between current status in the community and what was learned in the visioning phase as well as strategic direction for goals and strategies (NACCHO, 2001).

In Phase 4 of MAPP, *Identify Strategic Issues,* a prioritized list of the most important issues facing the health of the community is developed. Only issues that jeopardize the vision and values of the community are considered. An important task in this phase is consideration of what would happen if certain issues are not addressed, understanding why an issue is strategic, consolidating overlapping issues, and identifying a prioritized list. Phase 5, *Formulate Goals and Strategies,* creates goals related to the vision and priority strategic issues. It also selects and adopts strategies. This phase is not unlike similar phases in the models that have already been discussed in this chapter. Finally, Phase 6, *The Action Cycle,* is similar to implementation and evaluation phases in other planning models. In this phase, implementation details are considered, evaluation plans (gathering credible evidence) are developed, and plans for disseminating results are made (NACCHO, 2001).

Though this model is relatively new compared with models such as PRECEDE-PROCEED or MATCH, it is one model that bridges practitioner-based models with consumer-based models. This means that professionals who are trained to assess health needs and develop appropriate interventions make decisions jointly with the consumers or members of the priority population who will actually receive the interventions. It holds particular promise as a successful planning approach within local health department jurisdictions.

Assessment Protocol for Excellence in Public Health (APEX-PH)

Assessment Protocol for Excellence in Public Health (APEX-PH), a planning and assessment process also developed by NACCHO, was introduced in 1991 after extensive collaboration and testing with many public health partners (NACCHO, 1991). APEX-PH was developed initially to help county or local health departments respond to the Institute of Medicine's (IOM) report "The Future of Public Health," where it was stated that every public health agency should regularly and systematically collect, assemble, and analyze information on community health needs (IOM, 1988). Although APEX-PH has been largely subsumed by the MAPP model, many local health departments still use APEX-PH, particularly because of its first phase, the organizational assessment, which is familiar and flexible to those responsible for planning efforts.

APEX-PH is promoted by NACCHO as a planning model for local health officials to assess the organization and management of the health department, provide a framework for working with community members and other organizations in assessing the health status of the community, and establish a leadership role for the health department in the community. It is considered a flexible tool that can be easily integrated with other planning tools (NACCHO, 1991).

The APEX-PH process involves three steps. The first, *Organizational Capacity Assessment,* requires the local health department to perform an internal assessment of administrative capacity including strengths, weaknesses, resources, and expertise. Because the second step in the APEX-PH process involves a community assessment, health directors and their teams will also need to assess internal capacity to conduct a comprehensive data collection and analysis process.

The second step in APEX-PH is *The Community Process*. During this step, health data are collected and analyzed in addition to community opinion data. One challenge to this approach is finding a balance between data that are often in conflict. For example, epidemiologic data in the United States will most often dictate that chronic diseases such as heart disease, cancer or stroke (or their determinants) be the focus of a program activity. Consumer opinion data, on the other hand, often focus on social or environmental problems such as violence, drug use, teen pregnancy, or neighborhood safety. When both types of data are collected, planners must inevitably compromise and identify multiple priorities using multiple interventions. During this step, problems are analyzed and priorities are developed.

The final step in APEX-PH, *Completing the Cycle*, is similar to the final steps in most planning models. That is, this step guides the development of policies, services, and other interventions, creates an implementation plan and assures that all programs are monitored and evaluated.

APEX-PH has established a track record of success within local health departments. It has also spawned the development of **PACE-EH**, which is a planning protocol used by local health departments for environmental health planning. Lessons learned from APEX-PH have been successfully transferred to the MAPP model, which carries forward the tradition and promise of sequential and meaningful planning efforts within counties and cities across the United States.

SWOT (Strengths, Weaknesses, Opportunities, Threats) Analysis

The **SWOT** analysis has historically been associated with strategic planning efforts in the business and marketing sectors. In simple terms, it is an analysis of an organization's internal strengths and weaknesses, as well as opportunities and threats in the operating environment. Technically, its use should be limited to the preliminary stages of decision making in preparation for more comprehensive strategic planning (Johnson, Scholes, & Sexty, 1989; Bartol & Martin, 1991).

In health promotion practice, SWOT analyses are common among planners who want to minimize planning time and move quickly to action steps. Generally, a facilitator helps a planning group identify issues or problems, set or clarify goals, and create a plan. Common to SWOT analyses is the use of a 2 × 2 matrix that lists strengths and weaknesses along the horizontal axis and opportunities and threats along the vertical axis. The organization can then decide if it prefers to build on strengths or improve upon weaknesses in context of environmental opportunities and threats.

A SWOT analysis requires planners to examine their organization's strengths. This may include an assessment of: what the organization does well or what it does differently or better than similar organizations; existing resources (i.e., funds, equipment, supplies, materials); expertise of personnel; quality of partnerships in the community or track record of successful working relationships. Conversely, the SWOT analysis also examines weaknesses which may pertain to the same factors cited under strengths. In addition, this may involve a poor reputation among stakeholders, including clients. It may involve an inability to address certain health problems or determinants because of codes, regulations, policy, or management decisions that give authority to another entity.

Whereas strengths and weaknesses assessed in a SWOT analysis pertain to the organization's internal environment and opportunities and threats relate to the external environment. Opportunities may involve: unfulfilled consumer needs; loosening or removal of administrative or legislative barriers that finally allow the development of a new program; a new funding stream made available by a government agency or other granting agency; or a newly organized coalition formed to address an emerging health problem. Threats may involve shifts in consumer trends, organizational or ideological competition, or private industry that promotes products or services that are harmful to the health of a community (i.e., the tobacco or alcohol industry, fast food corporations), or changing technology.

The SWOT analysis differs substantially from other models discussed in this chapter. It truly represents rapid internal and external scans that allow planners to implement interventions in a much shorter time frame. Proponents of the SWOT analysis suggest that too much time is spent planning compared to the time delivering actual services. Building upon strengths or addressing specific weaknesses while taking advantage of opportunities in the environment is an advantage of the SWOT analysis. Certainly this approach can lead to challenges if consumer input is not received, if problems are not analyzed thoroughly, if relevant determinants are not addressed, or if interventions are identified and implemented without adequately understanding underlying theory or rationale. In fact, poorly planned programs can be more harmful than no programs at all. However, the SWOT analysis has its place in planning methodology and its simplicity is appealing to many planners.

Healthy Communities

Healthy Communities (or Healthy Cities) is a movement that began in the 1980s in Canada and, with the assistance of the World Health Organization, spread to various locations throughout Europe. As a result, organizations like California Healthy Cities and Indiana Healthy Cities were created in the United States. The movement is characterized by community ownership and empowerment and driven by the values, needs and participation of community members with consultation from health professionals. Another characteristic of Healthy Communities is diverse partnership. It is not uncommon to see partners from business or labor, transportation, recreation, public safety, or politicians participate in the Healthy Communities process. This is not typical of most planning efforts in health promotion.

Although there are various models used in Healthy Communities, the Department of Health and Human Services has produced a guide entitled, *Healthy People in Healthy Communities* (USDHHS, 2001) that provides a five-step framework for the Healthy Communities process in general. Step 1, *Mobilize Key Individuals and Organizations,* identifies and organizes people who care about the health of their community. These people have more than passing interest in their community; they are passionate and willing to work. It does require a process of canvassing the community (e.g., businesses, religious organizations, charities) to find these special people. This step also involves creating a vision for a healthy community among this core group of individuals that reflects their values and personalities. Eventually, this small core group expands into to a larger coalition of individuals and organizations who share in the established vision.

The second step in the process, *Assessing Community Needs, Strengths, and Resources,* involves gathering and evaluating a wide range of data about the community and setting priorities. The third step, *Plan for Action,* requires the coalition to plan an approach to address the priorities that were analyzed earlier. As with other models, this involves creating objectives, identifying appropriate interventions, assigning specific responsibilities to individuals or organizations and developing timelines. Step 4, *Implement the Action Plan,* and Step 5, *Track Progress and Outcomes,* follow patterns associated with planning models discussed earlier in this chapter. Coalition members must understand their roles and responsibilities, communicate effectively, follow up meticulously and track and measure the success of all program components.

While many of the steps associated with Healthy Communities appear quite similar to the Generalized Model, this approach is characterized by community ownership more so than any other planning approach. While organizing community groups and getting people involved requires patience, the model has been implemented widely throughout the world. Lessons learned from Healthy Communities include the idea that the pursuit of shared values in the context of ownership and empowerment is a viable approach to improving health in the community.

The Health Communication Model (National Cancer Institute)

The National Cancer Institute (NCI) has produced a document that is essential to any planner engaged in health communication planning entitled, *Making Health Communications Work* (NCI, 2002). The NCI model for health communication is presented in four phases: 1) Planning and Strategy Development; 2) Developing and Pretesting Concepts, Messages, and Materials; 3) Implementing the Program; and 4) Assessing Effectiveness and Making Refinements.

Planning and Strategy Development involves several steps including: assessing the health issue or problem and identifying potential solutions; defining communication objectives; defining potential audiences and learning about them; investigating appropriate settings, channels and activities best suited for the identified audiences; and developing a communication strategy for each potential audience (NCI, 2002). Like all planning models, the NCI model begins by identifying the most significant health problems facing a community and assessing who in the community may be most vulnerable to the problem, or who, for other reasons, may be the most appropriate audience for communication interventions. Unlike other models, objectives and intervention strategies are developed early in the NCI model. While consumer data are described as one component of assessment, they are not a central or integral component of early decision making in the model.

Developing and Pretesting Concepts, Messages, and Materials direct planners to review existing materials for appropriateness. Often times, print material, public service announcements and other audiovisual resources may be available and appropriate with few, if any, modifications. Still, it may be necessary to create new concepts, messages and materials to meet the needs of a specific audience. In this phase, **message concepts** (messages or visuals in early stages) are developed and tested. These will eventually evolve into messages and materials that become the basis of the communication campaign. In this phase, planners develop and pretest the finished messages and materials in the manner outlined in CDCynergy.

The third phase, *Implementing the Program,* usually begins with a kickoff event that draws positive attention to the campaign and related programs and interventions. This is generally associated with a press conference which brings partners together to formally introduce a new program. Appropriate spokespeople are selected and special attention is given to framing issues to maximize coverage, interest, and participation. Developing strategies for ongoing media relationships and coverage are also designed in this phase. As with other planning models, communication, reinforcement of partnerships, and adherence to planned timelines are characteristics of this phase.

Finally, *Assessing Effectiveness and Making Refinements* involves refining the communication plan as immediate feedback is received through process evaluation and evaluating the effectiveness of the campaign in terms of changes in determinants and health status. Planners must determine what information the evaluation must provide, define the data to collect, decide upon data collection methods, collect and process the data, analyze the data, write an evaluation report, and disseminate the evaluation report (NCI, 2002).

Because health communication is becoming an increasingly important method and discipline within the field of health promotion, use of the NCI model or CDCynergy is imperative if planners are to implement such communication campaigns appropriately. The models themselves share many characteristics. Both have been designed and tested by a range of health professionals in a variety of settings.

Healthy Plan-It (Centers for Disease Control and Prevention)

Healthy Plan-It was developed by the Sustainable Management Development Program at the Centers for Disease Control and Prevention (CDC, 2000) to strengthen in-country management training capacity in the health sector of developing countries. The Health Analysis for Planning Prevention Services (HAPPS), a planning model that was commonly used in the 1980s is the basis for Healthy Plan-It (CDC, 2000). The model itself consists of six steps: 1) priority setting; 2) establishing goals; 3) outcome objectives; 4) strategy; 5) evaluation; and 6) budget.

The first step, *Priority Setting,* involves participatory planning and consensus building, as well as priority setting, using the Basic Priority Rating Process (see Chapter 4). Participatory planning and consensus building requires broad representation from the community, a facilitation process that promotes empowerment, and nurturing respect for all those involved in the planning process. This phase builds a foundation of trust within an atmosphere of flexibility (CDC, 2000). Priority setting examines the size and seriousness of health problems, effectiveness of interventions, and the propriety, economic feasibility, acceptability, resources, and legality associated with all potential health problems. The result is a ranked list of priorities.

The second step, *Establishing Goals,* follows the pattern outlined in previous models. Goals are generalized statements of the result or achievement to which your effort is directed (CDC, 2000). At times funding or other resources for different program emphases become available. Other times, partners may come forward and invite your participation on unrelated initiatives. When these types of opportunities present themselves, goals help planners stay focused on the program emphasis.

The third step in Healthy Plan-It develops *Outcome Objectives.* These are related to the program goal(s), are usually long-term in nature, and are always measurable.

Table 2.3 Summary of health education/promotion planning models (by author and year)

PRECEDE-PROCEED (Green & Kreuter, 1999)	CDCynergy (2003)	SMART (Neiger, 1998)	MATCH (Simons-Morton et al., 1988)	A Systematic Approach to Health Promotion (USDHHS, 2000)
Phase 1 Social assessment	**Phase 1** Describe problem	**Phase 1** Preliminary planning	**Phase 1** Goals selection	**Phase 1** Goals
Phase 2 Epidemiological assessment	**Phase 2** Analyze problem	**Phase 2** Consumer analysis	**Phase 2** Intervention planning	**Phase 2** Objectives
Phase 3 Behavioral and environmental assessment	**Phase 3** Plan intervention	**Phase 3** Market analysis	**Phase 3** Program development	**Phase 3** Determinants of health
Phase 4 Educational and ecological assessment	**Phase 4** Develop intervention	**Phase 4** Channel analysis	**Phase 4** Implementation preparations	**Phase 4** Health Status
Phase 5 Administrative and policy assessment	**Phase 5** Plan evaluation	**Phase 5** Develop interventions, materials, and pretest	**Phase 5** Evaluation	
Phase 6 Implementation	**Phase 6** Implement plan	**Phase 6** Implementation		
Phase 7 Process evaluation		**Phase 7** Evaluation		
Phase 8 Impact evaluation				
Phase 9 Outcome evaluation				

(Table 2.3 *continues*)

(Table 2.3 *continued*)

MAPP (NACCHO, 2001)	APEX-PH (NACCHO, 1991)	SWOT	Healthy Communities (USDHHS, 2001)	NCI Model (NCI, 2002)	Healthy Plan-It (CDC, 2000)
Phase 1 Organizing for success and partnership development	**Phase 1** Organizational capacity assessment	**Phase 1** Strengths	**Phase 1** Mobilize key individuals and organizations	**Phase 1** Planning and strategy development	**Phase 1** Priority setting
Phase 2 Visioning	**Phase 2** Community process	**Phase 2** Weaknesses	**Phase 2** Assessing community needs, strengths, and resources	**Phase 2** Developing and pretesting concepts, messages and materials	**Phase 2** Establishing goals
Phase 3 Four MAPP assessments	**Phase 3** Completing the cycle	**Phase 3** Opportunities	**Phase 3** Plan for action	**Phase 3** Implementing the program	**Phase 3** Outcome objectives
Phase 4 Identify strategic issues		**Phase 4** Threats	**Phase 4** Implement the action plan	**Phase 4** Assessing effectiveness and making refinements	**Phase 4** Strategy
Phase 5 Formulate goals and strategies			**Phase 5** Track progress and outcomes		**Phase 5** Evaluation
Phase 6 The action cycle					**Phase 6** Budget

Outcome objectives also relate to the actual health problem (the specific disease or injury). The basis for the success of planners is generally linked to the degree to which they accomplish program objectives. The fourth step, *Strategy*, involves developing the methods or interventions that will be implemented to accomplish outcome objectives. Strategies are designed to affect the determinants and contributing factors that lead to the health problem and will vary depending upon program goals and objectives.

The final phases, *Evaluation* and *Budget*, identify ways to measure the success of outcome objectives as well as program impacts related to determinants and contributing factors (impact objectives). The process of evaluating program delivery, as well as changes in behaviors and actual health problems, is designed and implemented. Development of program budgets involves planning for physical resources, personnel, facilities, and equipment. While initial budgetary planning may be performed prior to step one to identify planning parameters, actual project costs are analyzed and distributed in the final step.

Still Other Planning Models

The models discussed in this chapter are either some of the more well known models or most widely used models within health promotion. However, still other models are available to planners. These include: The Planning, Program Development, and Evaluation Model (Timmreck, 2003); the Model for Health Education Planning (Ross & Mico, 1980); the Comprehensive Health Education Model (Sullivan, 1973); the Model for Health Education Planning and Resource Development (Bates & Winder, 1984); and the Generic Health/Fitness Delivery System (Patton, Corey, Gettman, & Graff, 1986). These models, all useful and instructive in their own right, share common themes, steps, and phases with the models you have reviewed in this chapter.

What should now be evident is that although various planning models exist, they are more similar than they are different or unique. These models all generally seek to understand and engage community members, assess needs, set goals and objectives, develop an intervention, implement the intervention and evaluate the results as outlined in the Generalized Model. The remainder of the text focuses on the steps outlined in the Generalized Model. As you identify and understand these key steps, planning models and the planning process in general will become much easier to understand and implement.

SUMMARY

A model can provide the framework for planning a health promotion program. Several different planning models have been developed and revised over the years. The planning models for health promotion presented in this chapter are the following:

1. PRECEDE-PROCEED (Predisposing, Reinforcing, and Enabling Constructs in Educational/Environmental Diagnosis and Evaluation; Policy, Regulatory, and Organizational Constructs in Educational and Environmental Development)

2. MATCH (Multilevel Approach To Community Health)

3. CDCynergy

4. SMART (Social Marketing Assessment and Response Tool)

5. A Systematic Approach to Health Promotion (Healthy People 2010)

6. MAPP (Mobilizing for Action Through Planning and Partnerships)
7. APEX-PH (Assessment Protocol for Excellence in Public Health)
8. SWOT (Strengths, Weaknesses, Opportunities, Threats)
9. Healthy Communities
10. The Health Communication Model
11. Healthy Plan-It

To date, probably the best-known model and the one most often used in health promotion is the PRECEDE-PROCEED model. MATCH has also been a time-honored model. The newer models of CDCynergy and SMART are starting to take hold and are being used more and more. And finally, there are several others that have made and continue to make valuable contributions (Table 2.3).

REVIEW QUESTIONS

1. Why is it important to use a model when planning?
2. Name the eleven models presented in this chapter, and list one distinguishing characteristic of each.
3. Of the models presented, which one has been most commonly used? Name the different phases of this model.
4. How are the CDCynergy and SMART models different from the others presented in this chapter?
5. What five or six components seem to be common to all the models? (Note that the names of the components may not be the same, but the concepts are.)

ACTIVITIES

1. After reviewing the models presented in this chapter, create your own model by identifying what you think are the common key components of the models. Provide a rationale for including each component. Then draw a diagram of your model and put it on a transparency so that you can share it with the class. Be prepared to explain your model.
2. In a one-page paper, defend what you believe is the best planning model presented in this chapter.
3. Using a hypothetical health problem for a specific priority population, write a paper explaining the steps/phases for one of the models presented in this chapter.
4. List and describe any potential advantages and disadvantages of using a consumer-based planning model in health promotion. How do these advantages and disadvantages compare with more traditional planning models used in health promotion? Be prepared to discuss your ideas in class.
5. Identify a public service announcement on television or radio, or obtain a copy of one from a nearby health agency. Analyze factors such as messages, settings, and channels. Based on your analysis, was the public service announcement developed appropriately for the intended audience? Summarize your comments in a one-page paper.
6. Using either the CDCynergy or SMART model, identify a relevant health problem or a specific audience, perform or gather appropriate consumer research, and develop ideas for appropriate intervention and communication strategies. Summarize your findings in a three-page paper.

WEBLINKS

1. **http://www.healthypeople.gov/document/**
   Healthy People 2010 (U.S. Department of Health and Human Services)

   At this website, A Systematic Approach to Health Promotion may be viewed in its entirety, including all objectives, focus areas, and leading indicators associated with Healthy People 2010. It is a site with which planners in health promotion must become familiar.

2. **http://www.healthypeople.gov/state/toolkit/default.htm**
   Healthy People 2010 Tool Kit: A Field Guide to Health Planning

   This tool kit provides valuable resources to implement both, A Systematic Approach to Health Promotion (Healthy People 2010) as well as Healthy Communities. The site includes valuable information on: building a leadership structure; identifying and securing resources; identifying and engaging community partners; setting health priorities; obtaining baseline measures, setting targets and measuring progress; managing and sustaining the process; and communicating health goals and objectives.

3. **http://ctb.ku.edu/**
   Community Tool Box

   This website is an indispensable tool for all planners in health promotion. According to the website itself, "the Tool Box involves over 6,000 pages of practical skill-building information on over 250 different topics" related to planning steps and phases discussed in this chapter. "Topic sections include step-by-step instruction, examples, checklists, and related resources."

4. **http://mapp.naccho.org/mapp_introduction.asp**
   National Association of County and City Health Officials

   At this website, the MAPP Model is comprehensively diagrammed and explained. The Four MAPP Assessments are described, including how they are implemented, how to use subcommittees for each assessment, and how to make linkages between assessments.

5. **http://www.hospitalconnect.com/DesktopServlet**
   Association for Community Health Improvement

   This website provides helpful information on the Healthy Communities Initiative including current projects and links.

6. **http://www.cdc.gov/communication/cdcynergy.htm**
   Communication at the Centers for Disease Control and Prevention

   This website provides an overview of CDCynergy, news and updates, information on all editions, current campaigns, practice areas and resources.

7. **http://oc.nci.nih.gov/services/pink-book-2002.pdf**
   Making Health Communications Work (National Cancer Institute, 2002)

   At this website, the entire document (2002 edition) is available, including the Health Communication Model. This is arguably the most comprehensive document available on health communication planning.

CHAPTER 3

Starting the Planning Process

Chapter Objectives

After reading this chapter and answering the questions at the end, you should be able to:

- Explain the importance of gaining the support of decision makers.
- Develop a rationale for planning and implementing a health promotion program.
- Identify the individuals who could make up a planning committee.
- Explain what planning parameters are and the impact they have on program planning.

Key Terms

advisory board	planning committee	steering committee
institutionalized	planning parameters	vendor
organizational culture	program ownership	
pilot program	stakeholders	

Planning a health promotion program is a multi-step process. "To *plan* is to engage in a process or a procedure to develop a method of achieving an end" (Breckon, Harvey, & Lancaster, 1998, p. 145). However, because of the many different variables and circumstances of any one setting, the multi-step process of planning does not always begin the same way. There are times when the need for a program is obvious and that a new program should be put in place. For example, if a community's immunization rate for its children is less than half the national average, a program should be created. There are other times when a program has been successful in the past but needs to be changed or reworked slightly before being implemented again. And, there are situations where planners have been given the autonomy and authority to create the programs needed to achieve better health and quality of life for those in the community they serve. However, when the need is not so obvious, when there has not been success in the past, or when the autonomy is not present, the planning process often begins with the planners working to gain the support of key people in order to obtain the necessary resources to ensure that the planning process and the eventual implementation proceeds as smoothly as possible.

This chapter presents the initial steps of obtaining the support of decision makers creating a program rationale, identifying those who may be interested in helping to plan the program, and establishing the parameters in which the planners must work.

Gaining Support of Decision Makers

No matter what the setting of a health promotion program—whether a business, an industry, the community, a clinic, a hospital, or a school—it is most important that the program have support from the highest level (the administration, chief executive officer, church elders, board of health, or board of directors) (Chapman, 1997; Wolfe, Slack, & Rose-Hearn, 1993) of the "community" for which the program is being planned. It is the individuals in these top-level decision-making positions who are able to provide the necessary resource support for the program.

> "Resources" usually means money, which can be turned into staff, facilities, materials, supplies, utilities, and all the myriad number of things that enable organized activity to take place over time. "Support" usually means a range of things: congruent organizational policies, program and concept visibility, expressions of priority value, personal involvement of key managers, a place at the table of organizational power, organizational credibility, and a role in integrated functioning. (Chapman, 1997, p. 1)

There will be times when the idea for, or the motivating force behind, a program comes from the top-level people. When this happens, it is a real boon for the program planners because they do not have to "sell" the idea to these people to gain their support. However, this scenario does not occur frequently.

Often, the idea or the big push for a health promotion program comes from someone other than one who is part of the top level of the "community." The idea could start with an employee, an interested parent, a health educator within the organization, a member of the parish or congregation, or a concerned individual or group from within the community. The idea might even be generated by an individual outside the "community," such as a **vendor** trying to sell a program to a business. When the scenario begins at a level below the decision makers, those who want to create a program must "sell" it to the decision makers. In other words, in order for resources and support to flow into health promotion programming, decision makers need to clearly perceive a set of values or benefits associated with the proposed program (Chapman, 1997). Without the support of decision makers, it becomes more difficult, if not impossible, to plan and implement a program. Behrens (1983) has stated that health promotion programs in business and industry have a greater chance for success if all levels of management, including the top, are committed and supportive. This is true of health promotion programs in all settings, not just programs in business and industry.

If they need to gain the support of decision makers, program planners should develop a rationale for the program's existence. Why is it necessary to "sell" something that everyone knows is worthwhile? After all, does anyone doubt the value of trying to help people gain and maintain good health? The answer to these and sim-

> ### *Box 3.1 Summary of Information Sources for Building a Rationale*
>
> 1. Needs assessment data
> 2. Epidemiological data about a specific health problem
> 3. Cost-effectiveness data of health promotion programs
> 4. Values and benefits that are important to decision makers
> 5. Data from other successful programs
> 6. Compatibility between the proposed program and the health plan of a state or the nation
> 7. Protecting human resources

ilar questions is that few people are motivated by health concerns alone. Decisions by top-level management to develop new programs are based on a variety of factors, including finances, policies, public image, and politics, to name a few. Thus to "sell" the program to those at the top, planners need to develop a rationale that shows how the new program will help decision makers to meet the organization's goals and, in turn, to carry out its mission. In other words, planners need to position their program rationale politically, in line with the organization. To do this, planners need to amass as many "political data" (data that help to align the program with the organization's mission) as possible; this will enable them to put together a sound rationale to "sell" program development. There are several different sources of information (see Box 3.1) that can be used in developing a rationale. One source would be the results of a needs assessment showing that such a program is needed and wanted. An example of such a situation is the result of a Gallup poll conducted for the American Cancer Society that indicated that there was overwhelming support for comprehensive school health education from adolescent students (ages 12–17), parents, and school administrators (Seffrin, 1994). However, more than likely, a formal needs assessment will not yet have been completed at this point in the planning process. Often, a complete assessment does not take place until permission has been given for planning to begin. However, if an assessment has been completed for this or another related or similar program, data from it can be used to help develop the rationale.

Epidemiological data resulting from "the study of the distribution and determinants of diseases and injuries in human populations" (Mausner & Kramer, 1985, p. 1) is a second source of data that is useful in building a rationale for a program. Epidemiological data are available from a number of different sources and include but are not limited to the: *U.S. Census,* the *Statistical Abstract of the United States,* the *Monthly Vital Statistics Report, Morbidity and Mortality Weekly Report,* the *National Health Interview Survey,* the *National Health and Nutrition Examination Survey,* the *Behavioral Risk Factor Surveillance System (BRFSS),* the *Youth Risk Behavior Surveillance System (YBRFSS),* the *National Hospital Discharge Survey,* and the *National Hospital Ambulatory Medical Care Survey.*

Epidemiological data gain additional significance when it can be shown that the described health problem(s) are the result of modifiable health behaviors and that spending money to promote healthy lifestyles and prevent health problems makes good economic sense. Seffrin (1994, p. 399) presents a good example when he talks about the impact of cigarette smoking on the 48 million smokers in the United States and the United States population in general. He writes, "Not only does tobacco addiction exact an unacceptable burden in health care costs—about $65 billion annually—and a true carnage in human lives—20% of all deaths in 1993—it also strips one-fourth of our population of significant freedom of choice through addiction, and sets an unnecessary and undesirable limit on each smoker's human potential." Examples of another 18 commonly seen health problems (e.g., breast cancer, cervical and colorectal cancer, coronary heart disease, HIV/AIDS transmission, low birth weight, and tuberculosis) in the United States and their related economic impact are presented in a publication titled *An Ounce of Prevention . . . What Are the Returns?* (CDC, 1999a). However, it should be noted that "proving" the economic impact of many health promotion programs is not easy. Research conducted to date, suggest that the economic impact of health promotion programs is modest at best (Golaszewski, 2001). There are a number of reasons for this including the multi-causation of many health problems, the complex interventions needed to deal with them, and the difficulty of carrying out rigorous research studies. Additionally, McGinnis and colleagues (2002) feel that part of the problem is that health promotion programs are held to a different standard than medical treatment programs when cost-effectiveness is being considered.

> "In a vexing example of double standards, public investments in health promotion seem to require evidence that future savings in health and other social costs will off-set the investments in prevention. Medical treatments do not need to measure up to the standard; all that is required here is evidence of safety and effectiveness. The cost-effectiveness challenge often is made tougher by a sense that the benefits need to ac-crue directly and in short term to the payer making investments. Neither of these two conditions applies in many interventions in health promotion" (p. 84).

For those planners interested in using economic impact and cost-effectiveness of health promotion programs as part of a program rationale, we recommend that the work of the following authors be reviewed: Aldana (2001), Chapman (2003), Edington (2001), Golaszewski (2001), and Riedel (1999). For those planners specifically interested in worksite health promotion, a series of articles is presented in the May/June 2001 issue of the *American Journal of Health Promotion* in which ten managers in corporate settings reflect on what matters to them and the decision makers they report to in determining if health promotion is a good investment for their organization.

A fourth source of evidence on which a program rationale can be built is on the values and benefits of such a program to the decision makers. Obviously, these values and benefits vary, depending on the settings and what is important to decision makers. Chapman (1997) outlines the values and benefits associated with health promotion programs in which supporting data and/or documentation exist or can be collected. Further, the values and benefits he presents focus on four different types of programming: for worksites, communities, individuals, and managed care organizations. Chapman's work is presented in Table 3.1

When planners use the value and benefits information associated with the "reduction in health care costs" as part of their rationale, they should do so with caution (Edington & Yen, 1992; Goetzel et al., 1998; Sciacca et al., 1993; Warner, 1987; Warner et al., 1988).

Table 3.1 Values or benefits associated with health promotion programming

Focus	Value or Benefit Statement	Supporting Data and/or Documentation
Worksite	Increased worker morale	Studies using survey instruments that measure employee morale, industry or trade association data, human resource annual surveys with carefully selected questions
	Potentially greater employer loyalty	Survey results and patterns over time, use of loyalty proxy questions, and survey or focus group findings
	Improved employee resiliency and decision making quality	Studies from the psychological and exercise physiology literature
	Positive public and community relations	Recognition awards for local or peer employers, coalition or community consortium activities, industry and trade showcase or write-ups
	Increased worker productivity	Business and industrial management studies, selected studies from the worksite health promotion literature, local or trade data using collective productivity indicators
	Informed, health care cost-conscious workforce	Studies and anecdotal articles about consumer activism, scores from consumer health knowledge surveys, survey results on self-efficacy and consumerism
	Recruitment tool	Social psychology literature and business survey literature, selected labor market survey data
	Retention tool	Social psychology literature and business survey literature, selected labor market survey data
	Opportunity for cost savings via: Reduced sick leave absenteeism	A large number of worksite health promotion studies that address sick leave absenteeism effects, survey data from National Institutes of Occupational Health & Safety (NIOSH) and from trade and industry associations
	Opportunity for cost savings via: Reduced short- and long-term disability claims	A few articles on worksite health promotion programs and their impact on disability days, benefits and business surveys, risk management literature
	Opportunity for cost savings via: Decreased health care utilization	A moderate number of articles on the evaluation of worksite health promotion programs and their impact on health care costs, the medical care research literature and the managed care research literature, which also contain a variety of references; another major set of references are the actuarial studies that have been done on the relationship of health risks to health costs

(Table 3.1 *continues*)

(Table 3.1 *continued*)

Focus	Value or Benefit Statement	Supporting Data and/or Documentation
	Opportunity for cost savings via: Reduced premature retirement	Studies of early medical or disability retirement from the benefits, disability management, and actuarial literature
	Opportunity for cost savings via: Decreased overall health benefit costs	Worksite health promotion evaluation literature, business and benefits management literature, trade or competitor information
	Opportunity for cost savings via: Fewer on-the-job accidents	Worksite health promotion evaluation literature, risk management literature, safety literature, NIOSH publications, publications of the Bureau of Labor Statistics
	Opportunity for cost savings via: Lower casualty insurance costs	Casualty underwriter's publications and risk management literature
	Opportunity for cost savings via: Smaller total workforce	Business literature plus projections at various sick leave and disability reduction levels, review of personal replacement cases that have occurred in the last 2 to 5 years
	Opportunity for cost savings via: Reduced medical leave time	Occupational health literature and payroll system coding data
	Opportunity for cost savings via: Reduced occupational medical costs	Occupational health literature and occupational health unit data
Community	Provides a model for other local organizations	Community health promotion literature and community organization literature plus Robert Wood Johnson Community Snapshots Project
	Contributes to establishing good health as a norm	Community health promotion literature and cultural change literature plus Centers for Disease Control and Prevention publications
	Complements and reinforces national and local public health initiatives	Office of Disease Prevention and Health Promotion publications and Objectives for the Nation: 2000 plus local public health reports and plans
	Improves quality of life of citizenry	Community Health Care Forum materials and National League of Cities publications
	Helps control (and possibly reduce) the economic and social burden on all taxpayers from premature mortality and morbidity	Compression of morbidity literature and community health promotion literature plus Health Care Financing and Agency for Health Services Research publications and studies
	Helps improve the general economic well-being of communities through the improvement in general health status and productivity	Community health promotion literature and national econometric studies and analyses

(Table 3.1 *continues*)

(Table 3.1 *continued*)

Focus	Value or Benefit Statement	Supporting Data and/or Documentation
Individual	Increased morale via employer's, provider's, or community's interest in their health and well-being	Social psychological and psychological literature
	Increased knowledge about the relationship between lifestyle and health	Attitude and correlated research within the health promotion and health education literature
	Increased opportunity to take control of their health and medical treatment	Consumer satisfaction surveys and national market research studies plus self-efficacy literature
	Improved health and quality of life through reduction of risk factors	Literature surrounding the use of SF12 and SF36 and self-reported perception of health status
	Increased opportunity for support from co-workers and environment	Social psychological literature, health education research literature, and cultural change literature
	Reduced work absences	Attitude and correlated research within the health promotion and health education literature
	Reduced out-of-pocket and premium costs for medical care	Attitude and correlated research within the health promotion and health education literature plus Bureau of Commerce and Census publications
	Reduced pain and suffering from illness and accidents	Attitude and correlated research within the health promotion and health education literature
Managed Care Organizations	Greater member satisfaction	Perceived value of health benefit literature, Health Plan Employer Data Information Set (HEDIS) literature
	Increased market share through differentiation	Managed care marketing literature and strategic planning literature for the managed care industry
	More appropriate utilization by consumers and patients	Medical self-care literature, case management literature, medical care literature, and demand management literature
	Reduced utilization and cost through improvements in morbidity	Compression of morbidity literature, epidemiology literature, managed care and demand management literature
	Improved price competitiveness	Managed care literature, financial analysis of managed care industry literature, and benefit survey literature
	Improved HEDIS performance	National Committee on Quality Assurance publications and particularly HEDIS Version 3.0

Source: Chapman (1997), pp. 4–5. Reprinted by permission.

> To establish a cost-based, as well as a health-based, reason for performing more prevention and health promotion, several types of empirical evidence must be gathered and broadly communicated to clinicians, health plan managers, employers, and consumers. First, researchers must demonstrate that poor health habits and modifiable risk factors impose a financial burden, ie [sic], that individuals possessing these risk factors cost more than those without these risks, even in the short run. Second, researchers need to demonstrate that improvements in risk factors result in a reduction in cost. Third, researchers need to demonstrate that health habits can be changed and that the resultant lower risk can be maintained over time. Finally, researchers need to demonstrate that the benefits of changing habits and lowering health risk out-weigh the costs. This involves conducting cost-effective and cost-benefit studies that demonstrate the relative value of prevention activities when compared with the costs of illness treatment or doing nothing. Consequently, the challenges associated with documenting a financial payback for prevention and health promotion are significant. (Goetzel et al., 1998, pp. 843–844)

The first step in this process of establishing the relationship between the presence of modifiable risk factors and increased medical expenditures has been presented (Goetzel et al., 1998). However more research in this area is needed before planners can use "the reduction in health care costs" argument with absolute assurance in their rationale for a health promotion program.

A fifth source of data is other successful programs that have been conducted in similar settings. For example, planners may know of other successful programs in surrounding communities, companies, churches, or schools; the people associated with those programs may be able to provide data they generated or may be willing to share their thoughts on how they "sold" their program to the decision makers. Of course, planners can always refer to successes reported in the professional literature.

A sixth source of information for a rationale is a comparison between the proposed program and the health plan for the nation or a state. Comparing the health needs of the priority population with those of other citizens of the state or of all Americans, as outlined in the goals and objectives of the nation (USDHHS, 2000), should enable planners to show the compatibility between the goals of the proposed program and those of the nation's health plan. A discussion of these national health goals and objectives is presented in Chapter 6.

Finally, when preparing a rationale to gain the support of decision makers, planners should not overlook the most important resource of any community—the people who make up the community. Promoting, maintaining, and in some cases restoring human health should be at the core of any health promotion program. Whatever the setting, better health of those in the priority population provides for a better quality of life. For those planners who end up practicing in a worksite setting, the importance of protecting the health of employees (i.e., protecting human resources) should be noted in developing a rationale. People are a company's single biggest asset (Brennan as cited in Novelli & Ziska, 1982). "Fit and healthy people are more productive, are better able to meet extraordinary demands and deal with stress, are absent less, reflect better on the company or community as exemplars, and so forth" (Chapman, 1997, p. 6).

Creating a Rationale

Planners must realize that gaining the support of decision makers is one of the most important steps in the planning process and it should not be taken lightly. Many pro-

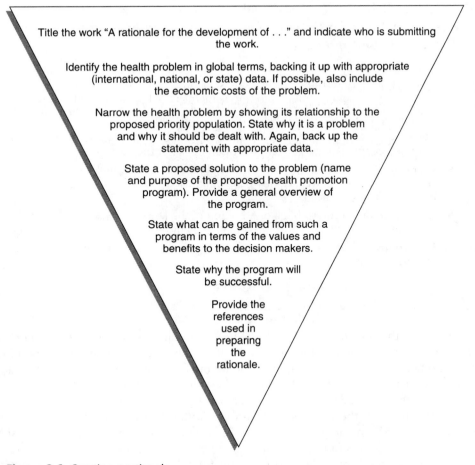

Title the work "A rationale for the development of . . ." and indicate who is submitting the work.

Identify the health problem in global terms, backing it up with appropriate (international, national, or state) data. If possible, also include the economic costs of the problem.

Narrow the health problem by showing its relationship to the proposed priority population. State why it is a problem and why it should be dealt with. Again, back up the statement with appropriate data.

State a proposed solution to the problem (name and purpose of the proposed health promotion program). Provide a general overview of the program.

State what can be gained from such a program in terms of the values and benefits to the decision makers.

State why the program will be successful.

Provide the references used in preparing the rationale.

Figure 3.1 Creating a rationale

gram ideas have died at this stage because the planners were not well prepared. Before making an appeal to decision makers, planners need to be thoroughly prepared. "The 'selling job' should be backed by a soundly researched idea" (McKenzie, 1988, p. 149). By a soundly researched idea, we mean that the planners thoroughly understand the health problem of concern, have engaged the members of the community with whom they plan to work, have an understanding of the needs and wants of the priority population, and are informed, in general terms, about how such a problem can be resolved. There is no formula or recipe for writing a rationale, but through experience, the authors have found a logical format for putting ideas together (see Figure 3.1). Begin the rationale by titling it and indicating who contributed to its authorship. The first paragraph or two of the rationale should identify the health problem in global terms. This is where epidemiological and other needs assessment data can be used. If possible, also include the economic costs of such a problem; it will strengthen the rationale. Most local health problems are also present on the international, national, and/or state levels. Presenting the problem at these higher levels shows decision makers that dealing with the health problem is consistent with the concerns of others.

> ### Box 3.2 Methods for Determining the Values and Benefits That Should Be Emphasized
>
> 1. Examine recent or past meeting minutes, decisions, or comments that are relevant to the value placed on health and prevention.
> 2. Find out from the individuals in a position to know, why past decisions related to budget or employee benefits were made by the managers involved.
> 3. Review past formal reports or evaluations of health programs and benefits that have been commissioned or carried out on behalf of the decision makers.
> 4. Conduct an informal survey of the most influential decision makers to get some sense of their own as well as their perception of the value priorities of the other decision makers involved.
> 5. Conduct a formal survey of all or a portion of the key decision makers involved to determine what is the most important to them.
> 6. Analyze the implementation questions that have been raised in the past on similar programs or topics.
>
> *Source:* Chapman (1997), p. 2. Reprinted by permission.

Showing the relationship of the local health problem to the "bigger problem" at the international, national, and/or state levels is the next logical step in presenting the rationale. Thus the next portion of the rationale should identify the local health problem and state *why* it is a problem and *why* it should be dealt with. If the information is available, include the needs and wants of the priority population.

At this point in the rationale, propose a solution to the problem. The solution should include the name and purpose of the proposed health promotion program, and a general overview of what the program may include. Since the writing of a program rationale often precedes much of the formal planning process, the general overview of the program is often based upon the "best guess" of those creating the rationale. For example, if the purpose of a program is to improve the immunization rate of children in the community, a "best guess" of the eventual program might include interventions to increase awareness and knowledge about immunizations, and the reduction of the barriers that limit access to receiving immunizations. Following such an overview, include statements indicating what can be gained from the program. The benefits of the program should be given in terms that are meaningful to the decision makers. (See Box 3.2 for methods to determine the values and benefits that should be emphasized in your rationale.) This can be done by:

1. Identifying what the program will do for those in the priority population
2. Comparing the proposed program with other successful programs
3. Stating the values and benefits (see Table 3.1) that are important to the decision makers
4. Stating that the program will protect human resources

Next, state why this program will be successful. It can be helpful to point out the similarity of the priority population to others with which similar programs have been successful. Using the argument that the "timing is right" for the program can also be useful. By this we mean that there is no better time than now to work to solve the problem facing the priority population.

Finally, make sure to include a list of the references used to prepare the rationale. This shows decision makers that you have researched your idea. (See the examples of rationales presented in the Activities section at the end of the chapter.)

Identifying a Planning Committee

The number of people involved in the planning process is determined by resources and circumstances of a particular situation. "One very helpful method to develop a clearer and more comprehensive planning approach is to establish a committee" (Gilmore & Campbell, 1996, p. 16). Identifying individuals who would be willing to serve as members of the **planning committee** (sometimes referred to as a **steering committee** or **advisory board**) becomes one of the planner's first tasks. The number of individuals on a planning committee can differ depending on the setting for the program and the size of the priority population. For example, the size of a planning committee for a safety belt program in a community of 50,000 people would probably be larger than that of a committee planning a similar program for a business with 50 employees. There is no ideal size for a planning committee, but the following guidelines, which have been presented earlier (McKenzie, 1988) and are given here in a modified form, should be helpful in setting up a committee.

1. The committee should be comprised of individuals who represent a variety of subgroups within the priority population. To the extent possible, the committee should have representation from all segments of the priority population (e.g., administrators/students/teachers, age groups, health behavior participants/non-participants, labor/management, race/ethnic groups, different sexes, socioeconomic groups, union/nonunion members, etc.). The greater the number of individuals who are represented by committee members, the greater the chance of the priority population's developing a feeling of **program ownership.** With program ownership there will be better planned programs, greater support for the programs, and people who will be willing to help "sell" the program to others because they feel it is theirs (Strycker et al., 1997).

2. The committee should be comprised of willing individuals who are interested in seeing the program succeed. Select a combination of "doers" and "influencers." Doers are people who will be willing to roll up their sleeves and do the physical work needed to see that the program is planned and implemented properly. Influencers are those who with a single phone call or signature on a form will enlist other people to participate or will help provide the resources to facilitate the program. Both doers and influencers are important to the planning process.

3. The committee should include an individual who has a key role within the organization sponsoring the program—someone whose support would be most important to ensure a successful program and institutionalization.

4. The committee should include representatives of other **stakeholders** (people who have a stake in the program being planned) not represented in the priority

population. For example, if health care providers are needed to implement a health promotion program they need to be represented on the planning committee.

5. The committee membership should be reevaluated regularly to ensure that the composition lends itself to fulfilling program goals and objectives.

6. If the planning committee will be in place for a long period of time, new individuals should be added periodically to generate new ideas and enthusiasm. It may be helpful to set a term of office for committee members. If terms of office are used, it is advisable to stagger the length of terms so that there is always a combination of new and experienced members on the committee.

7. Be aware of the "politics" that are always present in an organization or priority population. There are always some people who bring their own agendas to committee work.

8. Make sure the committee is large enough to accomplish the work, but small enough to be able to make decisions and reach consensus. If necessary, subcommittees can be formed to handle specific tasks.

The actual means by which the committee members are chosen varies according to the setting. Commonly used techniques include:

1. Asking for volunteers by word of mouth, a newsletter, a needs assessment, or some other widely distributed publication

2. Holding an election, either throughout the community or by subdivisions of the community

3. Inviting people to serve

4. Having members appointed by a governing group or individual

Once the planning committee has been formed, someone must be designated to lead it. This is an important step (Strycker et al., 1997). The leader (chairperson) "should be interested and knowledgeable about health education programs, and be organized, enthusiastic, and creative" (McKenzie, 1988, p. 149). One might think that most planners, especially health educators would be perfect for the committee chairperson's job. However, sometimes it is preferable to have someone other than the program planners serve in the leadership capacity. For one thing, it helps to spread out the workload of the committee. Planners who are not good at delegating responsibility may end up with a lot of extra work when they serve as the leaders. Second, having someone else serve as the leader allows the planners to remain objective about the program. And third, the planning committee can serve in an advisory capacity to the planners, if this is considered desirable. Figure 3.2 illustrates the composition of a balanced planning committee.

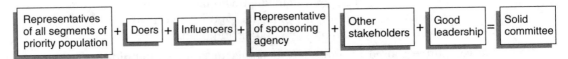

Figure 3.2 Make-up of a solid planning/steering committee

Parameters for Planning

Once the support of the decision makers has been gained and a planning committee formed, the committee members must identify the **planning parameters** within which they must work. There are several questions to which the committee members should have answers before they become too deeply involved in the planning process. In an earlier work (McKenzie, 1988), six such questions were presented, using the example of school-site health promotion programs. The six questions are modified for presentation here. It should be noted, however, that not all of the questions would be appropriate for every program because of the different circumstances of each setting.

1. What is the decision makers' philosophical perspective on health promotion programs? What are the values and benefits of the programs to the decision makers? (Chapman, 1997). Do they see the programs as something important or as "extras"?

2. What type of commitment to the program are the decision makers willing to make? Are they interested in the program becoming **institutionalized?** That is, are they interested in seeing that the "program becomes imbedded within the host organization, so that the program becomes sustained and durable" (Goodman et al., 1993, p. 163)? Or are they more interested in providing a one-time or **pilot program?** (*Note:* Goodman and colleagues [1993] have developed a scale for measuring institutionalization.)

3. What type of financial support are the decision makers willing to provide? Does it include personnel for leadership and clerical duties? Released/assigned time for managing the program and participation? Space? Equipment? Materials?

4. Are the decision makers willing to consider changing the **organizational culture?** For example, are they interested in "well" days instead of sick days? Would they like to create employee nonsmoking and safety belt policies? Change vending machine selections to more nutritious foods? Set aside an employee room for meditation? Develop a health promotion corner in the organization's library?

5. Will all individuals in the priority population have an opportunity to take advantage of the program, or will it only be available to certain subgroups?

6. What is the authority of the planning committee? Will it be an advisory group or a programmatic decision-making group? What will be the chain-of-command for program approval?

After the planning parameters have been defined, the planning committee should understand how the decision makers view the program, and should know what type and amount of resources and support to expect. Identifying the parameters early will save the planning committee a great deal of effort and energy throughout the planning process.

SUMMARY

Gaining the support of the decision makers is an important initial step in program planning. Planners should take great care in developing a rationale for "selling" the program idea to these important people. A planning committee can be most useful in helping with some of the planning activities and in helping to "sell" the program to the priority population. Therefore the committee should be composed of interested individuals, "doers" and "influencers," who are representative of the priority population. If the planning committee is to be effective, it will need to know the planning parameters set for the program by the decision makers.

REVIEW QUESTIONS

1. Why is the support of the decision makers important in planning a program?
2. What kinds of reasons should be included in a rationale for planning and implementing a health promotion program?
3. How important is "selling" the idea of a program to decision makers?
4. What items should be addressed when creating a program rationale?
5. Who should be selected as the members of a planning committee?
6. What are *planning parameters?* Give a few examples.
7. Why is it important to know the planning parameters at the beginning of the planning process?

ACTIVITIES

1. Write a two-page rationale for "selling" a program you are planning to decision makers, using the guidelines presented in this chapter.
2. Write a two-page rationale for beginning an exercise program for a company with 200 employees. A needs assessment of this priority population indicates that the number one cause of lost work time of this cohort is back problems and the number one cause of premature death is heart disease.
3. For a program you are planning, write a two-page description of the individuals (by position/ job title, not name) who will be asked to serve on the planning committee, and provide a rationale for asking each to serve.
4. Provide a list (by position/job title, not name) and a rationale for each of the ten individuals you would ask to serve on a communitywide safety belt program. Use the town or city in which your college/university is located as the community.
5. Following are two program rationales written by former students at Ball State University. Read each of the rationales and then select one to critique using the guidelines presented in this chapter. Critique by describing the following: (a) the strengths of the rationale, (b) the weaknesses, and (c) how you would change the rationale to make it stronger. Be critical! Closely examine the content, reasoning, and references.

Example 1

A rationale for "No Butts About It": A campaign to create a smoke-free ordinance in the restaurants of Delaware County, Indiana.*

The global tobacco use pandemic is responsible for 4.9 million deaths a year worldwide (WHO, 1998). The United States ranks as the second highest consumer of cigarettes in the world with 451 billion consumed each year (WHO, 1998). Tobacco use has been la-

*This rationale was written by Peggy Chute, Fariba Mirzaei, and Joe Turner while they were graduate students at Ball State University, Muncie, IN. Reprinted with permission.

beled the single most important preventable cause of death and disease in the United States, causing more than 440,000 deaths and resulting in more than $75 billion in direct medical costs annually. Nationally, smoking results in more than 5.6 million years of potential life lost each year.

In the United States, approximately 80% of adult smokers started smoking before the age of 18. That means that each day nearly 5,000 young people under the age of 18 try their first cigarette (USDHHS, 2000). It is clear that years of cigarette smoking vastly increase the risk of developing several fatal conditions. Cigarette smoking is responsible for one third of all cancers. It is the leading cause of lung cancer contributing to 90% of all lung cancers. It is also associated with cancers of the mouth, pharynx, larynx, esophagus, stomach, pancreas, uteri cervix, kidney, bladder, and colon (USDHHS, 1994). Smoking also increases the risk of cardiovascular disease including stroke, heart attack, vascular disease, and aneurysm (USDHHS, 1994).

Environmental tobacco smoke (ETS) is a mixture of the smoke given off by the burning end of a cigarette (sidestream smoke) and the smoke emitted at the mouthpiece and exhaled from the lungs of smokers (main stream smoke). ETS, also known as second hand smoke, is a major source of indoor air pollution. In the United States, approximately 38,000 deaths are attributable to ETS exposure each year (NCI, 2000). When a cigarette is smoked, only 15% of the smoke is inhaled by the smoker, the other 85% goes directly into the air. Cigarette smoke contains more than 4,000 substances, and 40 of these are classified as carcinogens (cancer causing agents). Nearly nine out of ten nonsmoking Americans are exposed to ETS, as measured by the levels of cotinine, a chemical the body metabolizes from nicotine, in their blood. Eighty-eight percent of all nontobacco users had measurable levels of cotinine in their blood according to a study conducted by the CDC. The presence of cotinine is documentation that a person has been exposed to ETS. Serum cotinine levels can be used to estimate nicotine exposure over the last two to three days.

ETS is estimated to cause approximately 3,000 lung cancer deaths per year among nonsmokers and contribute to 40,000 deaths related to cardiovascular disease (USDHHS, 1994). These deaths are all due to breathing the smoke of others' cigarettes and make ETS the third leading preventable cause of death in the United States. Some of the highest reported exposures to concentrations of ETS are found in food service establishments (EPA, 1992).

Approximately, one out of every four adults in Indiana smokes making it the fourth highest in the nation (27% compared to the U.S. median of 23.3%) (CDC, 2002). The number of adults between ages 18 to 24 who smoke has risen due to the tobacco companies targeting that age group since 1996 (SFI, 2003). The results of the Indiana Youth Tobacco Survey show that 9.8% of middle school students and 31.6% of high school students are current cigarette smokers (SFI, 2000). The smoking attributable mortality rate (SAM) in Indiana is also higher (341.4/100,000) compared to the median for the United States (295.5/100,000) (CDC, 2002).

The five leading causes of death in Delaware County are cardiovascular disease, malignant neoplasm, chronic obstructive pulmonary disease, and unintentional injuries (Synergy, 1998). Lung and bronchial cancer had higher incidence of death when compared to other cancers. "Residents of Delaware County are clearly at risk for cigarette smoking, with 3 in 10 claiming to smoke and having smoked 100 or more cigarettes in their entire lives" (Synergy, 1998, p. 17). Delaware County residents were significantly higher when compared to the national average and the percentage of smokers increased from 1989 (27%) to 1998 (30%). Currently, Delaware County has no ordinance to prohibit smoking in public, including restaurants. This allows ETS to have effects on their nonsmoking clients, smoking clients, and workers of the restaurants.

One of the national health objectives for 2010 is to reduce public exposure to ETS (USDHHS, 2000). Objective 27-13c is specifically related to laws on smokefree air in restaurants. The base line measure for this objective was only 3 states and the target for 2010 is 51 states (50 states and the District of Columbia).

To reduce public exposure to ETS, the Centers for Disease Control and Prevention recommends smoking bans and restrictions in public places to reduce exposure to second-hand smoke. The Task Force on Community Prevention Services, a nonfederal public health panel, which conducted in-depth systematic reviews on selected tobacco interventions concluded that smoking bans and restrictions are the most effective measures to reduce exposure to second-hand smoke (CDC, 2002).

Local ordinances requiring restaurants to be smokefree have spread rapidly. Over 230 U.S. municipalities in different states, among these states Massachusetts, Texas, Colorado, Wisconsin, New York, Oregon, North Carolina, and Arizona, have smokefree ordinances in some of their cities. Fort Wayne is a good example in the state of Indiana, where a smokefree ordinance was passed in 1998. Additionally, the states of California, Maine, Maryland, Vermont, and Utah have smokefree restaurant laws. Several Canadian jurisdictions also have restaurant smoking bans.

Contrary to popular belief, restaurants that implement smokefree policies do not see a decline in profits. Studies in cities that have implemented such policies have shown sales to remain constant and in some cases sales have increased (Americans for Nonsmokers' Rights, 2002).

In addition to stable economic conditions, health care costs decline due to a decrease in worker's compensation claims, decrease in absenteeism, and an increase in worker productivity (CDC, 2002).

After reviewing national, state and local data it is clear that there is a significant health problem in regards to ETS in Delaware County. It is important to "think globally and act locally." This community problem provides a need for action at the local level. In order to succeed in a local campaign to prohibit smoking in restaurants it is important to mobilize grassroots activities. Educating the citizens regarding the health risks of ETS, and mobilizing local advocates will empower the Tobacco Free Coalition of Delaware County's activities in executing a smokefree ordinance campaign. A significant and active grassroots base of support is the most potent weapon to counter the relentless and well-funded opposition from the tobacco industry. Tobacco control advocates have the expertise to draft sound smokefree policies based on successes and lessons learned from other clean indoor air campaigns across the country, while policymakers often lack tobacco control knowledge or expertise.

The above rationale adds up to the conclusion that the Tobacco Free Coalition of Delaware County can succeed in advocating for and passing a smokefree ordinance in Delaware County if it obtains active grassroots support from the community. Passage of an ordinance in turn will decrease the dangers of ETS exposure in Delaware County. Therefore the *No Butts About It* program can be a means to achieving these goals.

References

Americans for Nonsmoker's Rights Foundation (2002). *Smokefree advertising examples*. Retrieved March 25, 2003, from http://www.no-smoke.org/ads.html

Centers for Disease Control and Prevention (CDC). (2002). Strategies for reducing exposure to environmental tobacco smoke: Increasing tobacco-use cessation, and reducing initiation in communities and health care systems. *Morbidity and Mortality Weekly Report, 49* (RR-12). Retrieved April 6, 2003, from http://www.cdc.gov/mmwr/preview/mmwrhtml/rr4912a1.htm

Centers for Disease Control and Prevention (CDC). (2001). *Clean Indoor Air Regulations, Fact Sheet*. Retrieved March 26, 2003, from http://www.cdc.gov/tobacco/sgr/sgr_2000/factsheets/factsheet_2002clean.htm

Centers for Disease Control and Prevention (CDC). (2002). *Indiana Highlights.* Retrieved April 15, 2003, from http://www.cdc.gov/tobacco/statehi/html_2002/indiana.htm

National Cancer Institute (NCI). (2000). *Cancer Facts, Environmental Tobacco Smoke.* Retrieved April 5, 2003, from http://cis.nci.nih.gov/fact/3_9.htm

Smokefree Indiana (SFI). (2000). *Indiana Youth Tobacco Survey Report.* Retrieved April 5, 2003 from http://www.smokefreeindiana.org/pdf/IYTSExecSumm.pdf

Smokefree Indiana (SFI). (2003, March 3). Indiana smoking rate ranks high. *The Sublink.* Indianapolis, IN: Author.

Synergy. (1998). *Let's Talk Health '98.* Indianapolis, IN: Synergy.

U.S. Department of Health and Human Services (USDHHS). (2000). *Healthy People 2010 (CD-ROM Version).* Washington, DC: Author.

United States Department of Health and Human Services (USDHHS). (1994). *Preventing tobacco use among young people: A report of the Surgeon General.* Atlanta, GA: Author.

World Health Organization (WHO). (1998). *Tobacco Free Initiative.* Retrieved March 26, 2003 from http://www.who.int/tobacco/repsitory/stp84/30%20Map%206%20Cig.%20Consumption.pdf

Example 2

A Rationale for "Mind, Body, and Soul": A Health Education Program at First Presbyterian Church, Muncie, IN*

The health status of Americans has improved greatly in the last 50 years as evidenced by the decrease in the number of cases of communicable disease, increased life expectancy, and the declining death rates (NCHS, 1997). However, the health status of Americans could be further improved if Americans were willing to make additional changes. We now know that better control of behavioral risk factors alone—such as lack of exercise, poor diet, use of tobacco and other drugs, and alcohol abuse—could prevent between 40 and 70% of all mature deaths, one-third of all acute disabilities, and two-thirds of chronic disabilities (USDHHS, 1990).

Closer to home, recent data also indicate that the health status of Hoosiers has improved but they too could do more to improve their health. In 1996, 32% of the adults (>17 years of age) in Indiana were overweight, 29% were current smokers, and 66% were classified as having a sedentary lifestyle (ISDH, 1998). The data from Indiana are also consistent with the data that were collected from the members of the adult education class, the Mariners, at First Presbyterian Church in Muncie, IN. The data collected using a health risk appraisal (HRA) (Healthier People Software, no date) and a health and spirituality questionnaire (developed by health science students from Ball State University) indicated that the Mariners were interested in educational programs on faith and its relationship to health, humor and healing, and stress management (including prayer as a means of stress reduction). In addition, there appears to be a need for or an interest in programs associated with aging (including Alzheimer's disease), the family, nutrition, weight control, and exercise.

It seems logical to try to address some of the health needs and interests of those in the Mariners class through the Christian Education program of the church. For a long time, religious organizations have functioned as "healing" institutions as evidenced by the mental health issues addressed through pastoral counseling (Ransdell & Rehling, 1996). The idea of addressing the health needs and interests of a target population in combination with

*This rationale was written by the undergraduate students enrolled in the program planning classes at Ball State University, Muncie, Indiana.

spiritual practices has been encouraged. "In recent years, both the validity of spiritual and religious practices as well as the potential to the overall health and well-being have not only been acknowledged by modern medicine, but encouraged as mechanisms for health enhancement" (Droege, 1996, p. 7). And further, it makes good sense to offer health related programs at church since the Bible "provides a very powerful foundation for the development of health programs within the spiritual framework of the church" (Jackson, 1991, pp. 8–9). In a more practical sense, religious organizations have a number of important potential advantages for involvement in health education/promotion programs because religious organizations: 1) tend to involve large numbers of entire families, 2) are often the center of the neighborhood and a natural gathering place, 3) have a long history of outreach and helping others, 4) often have a talented and multi-disciplinary membership, 5) have been found to be receptive to the efforts of primary prevention, and 6) have the facilities to accommodate such programs (Lasater, Carleton, & Wells, 1991). In addition, religious organizations are good settings for health education/promotion programs because when people attend they do so with the expectation of learning; religious organizations are accepted as educational institutions (Lasater, Carleton, & Wells, 1991). Consequently, the church is a natural community arena for health education/promotion programs that focus on behaviors which are then reinforced by the social support and social networks that exist in churches (Levin, Larson, & Puchalski, 1997; Thomas, Quinn, Billingsley, & Caldwell, 1994).

There are several benefits that can be anticipated from the Mind, Body, and Soul program offered at First Presbyterian Church. First and foremost, it should be expected that the Mariners class members will increase their knowledge about the topics presented. Such knowledge will be beneficial to both the Mariners class members and the people—family and friends— with whom they come in contact. Second, such a program will introduce participants to topics that have not been addressed before in the class. Third, the program will provide participants with an opportunity to apply spiritual and religious concepts to everyday living. And fourth, such a program may attract other members of the congregation to the Mariners class that have not attended in the past.

The Mind, Body, and Soul program for the First Presbyterian Church Mariners class has great potential for being successful for several reasons. First as noted earlier, the Bible provides a solid base on which to build a health education/promotion program (Jackson, 1991). A number of the scriptures support the healing power of faith (Lloyd, 1994). Class members are interested in learning more about the Bible. Second, the majority of similar other church-based health promotion programs have been highly successful (Cook, 1993). And finally, the program will be well planned and will meet the needs and interests of the class members. Ransdell and Rehling (1996) have indicated that such programs have a better chance of being successful.

References

Cook, D. A. (1993). Research in African American churches: A mental health imperative. *Journal of Mental Health Counseling, 17:* 320–333.

Droege, T. (1996). Spirituality and healing. *Faith and Health,* Summer: 7.

Healthier People Software. (no date). *Healthier People: Health Risk Appraisal Program.* Memphis, TN: Author.

Indiana State Department of Health (ISDH). (1998). *Indiana Health Behavior Risk Factors.* Indianapolis, IN: Author.

Jackson, C. (1991). Healthy spirits, souls, and bodies. *Spirit of Truth,* June: 8–9.

Lasater, T. M., Carleton, R. A., & Wells, B. L. (1991). Religious organizations and large-scale health related lifestyle change programs. *Journal of Health Education, 22:* 233–239.

Levin, J. S., Larson, D. B., & Puchalski, C. M. (1997). Religion and spirituality in medicine: Research and Education. *The Journal of the American Medical Association, 278:* 792–793.

Lloyd, J. J. (1994). Collaborative health education training for African American health ministers and providers of community services. *Educational Gerontology, 20:* 265–276.

National Center for Health Statistics (NCHS). (1997). *Health, United States, 1996–97 and Injury Chartbook* (DHHS pub. no. PHS 97–1232). Hyattsville, MD: Author.

Ransdell, L. B., & Rehling, S. L. (1996). Church-based health promotion: A review of the current literature. *American Journal of Health Behavior, 20*(4): 195–207.

Thomas, S. B., Quinn, S. C., Billingsley, A., & Caldwell, C. (1994). The characteristics of northern black churches with community outreach programs. *American Journal of Public Health, 84:* 575–579.

U.S. Department of Health and Human Services (USDHHS). (1990). *Prevention '89/'90.* Washington, D.C.: U.S. Government Printing Office.

WEBLINKS

1. http://www.healthfinder.gov/
U.S. Department of Health and Human Services (USDHHS)

This page at the USDHHS website is the home to healthfinder®. Since 1997, healthfinder® has been recognized as a key resource for finding the best government and nonprofit health and human services information on the Internet. The healthfinder® site provides definitions and background information on health problems that will be useful in writing a program rationale.

2. http://www.astho.org
Association of State and Territorial Health Officials (ASTHO)

This is the website for the ASTHO. ASTHO is the national nonprofit organization representing the state and territorial public health agencies of the United States, the U.S. Territories, and the District of Columbia. This website has links to all the state and territorial health departments. If you are planning a program for the community setting, this site contains a lot of information that could help you develop a rationale for your program.

3. http://www.census.gov/statab/www/
The U.S. Census Bureau

This page at the U.S. Census Bureau website provides information about the national data book called *Statistical Abstract of the United States*. The data book contains a collection of statistics on social and economic conditions in the United States. Selected international data are also included. The *Abstract* is also your Guide to Sources of other data from the Census Bureau, other Federal agencies, and private organizations.

4. http://www.welcoa.org/
The Wellness Councils of America (WELCOA)

This is the website for the WELCOA. WELCOA was founded in 1987 as a national nonprofit membership organization dedicated to promoting healthier life styles for all Americans, especially through health promotion initiatives at the worksite. If you are planning a program for the worksite setting, this site contains a lot of information that could help you develop a rationale for your program.

CHAPTER 4

Assessing Needs

Chapter Objectives

After reading this chapter and answering the questions at the end, you should be able to:

- Define needs assessment.
- Explain why a needs assessment must be completed.
- Differentiate between primary and secondary data sources.
- Locate secondary data sources that are in print and on the World Wide Web.
- Explain how a needs assessment can be completed.
- Conduct a needs assessment within a given population.

Key Terms

action research	health assessment	secondary data
assessment	key informants	self-assessments
basic priority rating	needs assessment	service demands
categorical funding	networking	service needs
community analysis/	nominal group process	significant others
community diagnosis	opinion leaders	standard measures
community empowerment	participatory research	subject archive
Delphi technique	primary data	valid
eyeballing data	priority population	website
focus group	search engine	World Wide Web (WWW)

Once the planning committee is in place, the next step in the planning process is to identify the need(s) or problem(s) of those to be served—the **priority population.** Assessing the needs of the priority population may be the most critical step in the planning process because it "provides objective data to define important health problems, set priorities for program implementation, and establish a baseline for evaluating program impact" (Grunbaum et al., 1995, p. 54). Without determining and prioritizing needs, resources can be wasted on unsubstantiated programing.

More significantly, failure to perform a needs assessment may lead to a program focus that prevents or delays adequate attention directed to a more important health problem. For example, a health problem that tends to create a high emotional response, particularly among parents, is head trauma associated with bicycle injuries. Of course, it is a tragedy when a child is presented in an emergency room with a head injury that could have been prevented by using a bicycle helmet. In fact, an estimated 140,000 children are treated annually in the United States in emergency departments for head injuries sustained while bicycling (CDC, 2001).

On face value, this statistic is alarming and quite compelling. But an even more significant determinant of childhood injury and death in the United States is the inadequate use of safety belts or car seats involved with motor vehicle crashes. In fact, motor vehicle injuries are the leading cause of death among children at every age after their first birthday and are the greatest public health threat to children in the United States today (CDC, 2001). A needs assessment will lead planners to determine in most locations, in most instances, that restraining children in motor vehicles with safety belts or approved car seats is an even more important problem.

What Is a Needs Assessment?

To this point, we have used the term **needs assessment** several different times, without defining it. Now, let's take a closer look at the term and what it means. First, it should be noted that other terms have been used in a similar context. Dignan and Carr (1992) used the terms **community analysis/community diagnosis,** whereas Green and Kreuter (1999) used the term **assessment** with the first five phases of the PRECEDE-PROCEED model. The term "community assessment" is used increasingly in health promotion settings. All these terms are used to describe the process by which those who are planning programs can determine what health problems might exist in any given group of people.

Altschuld and Witkin (2000) have defined needs assessment as "the process of determining, analyzing and prioritizing needs, and in turn, identifying and implementing solution strategies to resolve high-priority needs" (p. 253). Petersen and Alexander (2001) suggested that a needs assessment should answer the following questions:

1. Who is the priority population?
2. What are the needs of the priority population?
3. Which subgroups within the priority population have the greatest need?
4. Where are these subgroups located geographically?
5. What is currently being done to resolve identified needs?
6. How well have the identified needs been addressed in the past? (p.17)

A needs assessment can also help identify the most significant health problem within a population, an organization's internal capacity to address specific health problems, the most promising interventions related to identified health problems, and strengths, resources, and assets within the community. In some instances, all of these factors are addressed. In other circumstances, perhaps one or only a few factors are addressed. No matter how needs assessment is defined, the concept is the same:

identifying the needs of the priority population and determining the degree to which these needs are being met.

Acquiring Needs Assessment Data

Two types of data are generally associated with a needs assessment: **primary data** and **secondary data.** Primary data are those data you collect yourself (e.g., a survey, a focus group, in-depth interviews, etc.) which answer unique questions related to your specific needs assessment. Secondary data are those data already collected by somebody else and available for your immediate use. The advantages of using secondary data are that (1) they already exist, and thus collection time is minimal, and (2) they are usually fairly inexpensive to access. Both of these advantages are important to planners because programs are often planned when both time and money are limited. However, a drawback of using secondary data is that the information might not identify the true needs of the priority population—perhaps because of how the data were collected, when they were collected, what variables were considered, or from whom the data were collected. A good rule is to move cautiously and make sure the secondary data are applicable to the immediate situation before using them.

Primary data have the advantage of directly answering the questions planners want answered by those in the priority population. However, collecting primary data can be expensive and when done correctly, take a great deal of time.

An overview of the means of acquiring primary and secondary data are presented in the following pages.

Sources of Primary Data

Primary data can be collected using a variety of methods. Those most commonly used in planning health promotion programs are presented below.

Single-Step or Cross-Sectional Surveys   Single-step surveys, or as they are often called, *cross-sectional surveys*, are a means of gathering primary data in which the data collectors gather the data from the priority population with a single contact—thus, the term *single-step*. Such surveys usually take the form of written questionnaires, telephone interviews, face-to-face interviews, or electronic interviews (see Chapter 5 for information about conducting such surveys). The resulting data are useful for identifying a priority health problem, planning an appropriate program, and providing insight into how best to implement a program (if the surveys include marketing questions, as well). For example, these surveys might include questions that address the best location for a program, the best time of day to offer a program, and how much participants would be willing to pay to take part in the program.

In addition to surveying the priority population, there are other groups of individuals who are commonly asked to respond to single-step surveys for the purpose of collecting primary needs assessment data. They include significant others of the priority population, community opinion leaders, and key informants. **Significant others** may include family members and friends. Collecting data from the significant others of a group of heart disease patients is a good example. Program planners might find it difficult to persuade the heart disease patients themselves to share information about their outlook on life and living with heart disease. A survey of spouses or other family

Data collection method

Total number of people interviewed

Number of interviewers

From: _____ To: _____

Date Collected _____

Rank	Health Problem	Number of Persons Identifying Problem	Percentage of Persons Identifying Problem
1.			
2.			
3.			
4.			
5.			
6.			
7.			
8.			
9.			
10.			

Source:

Source: U.S. Department of Health and Human Services, Centers for Disease Control and Prevention (no date), p. A3-12.

Figure 4.1 Form to tally opinion leader survey data

members might help elicit this information so that the program planners could best meet the needs of the heart disease patients.

Opinion leaders are individuals who are well respected in a community and who can accurately represent the views of the priority population. These leaders are:

1. Discriminating users of the media

2. Demographically similar to the priority group

3. Knowledgeable about community issues and concerns

4. Early adopters of innovative behavior (see Chapter 11 for an explanation of these terms)

5. Active in persuading others to become involved in innovative behavior

Opinion leaders include political figures, chief executive officers (CEOs) of companies, union leaders, administrators of local school districts, and other highly visible and respected individuals. (See Figure 4.1 for a form for tallying opinion leader survey data.) In essence, they are health experts (Altschuld & Witkin, 2000).

➤ **Key informants** are strategically placed individuals who have knowledge and ability to report on the needs of those in the priority population. They may or may not be in positions with formal authority, but they are often respected by others in the community and thus possess informal authority. Because they may be biased, planners need to be careful not to base an entire needs assessment on the data generated from a key informant survey.

Multistep Survey   As its title might suggest, a multistep survey is one in which those collecting the data contact those who will provide the data on more than one occasion. The technique that uses this process is called the **Delphi technique.** It is a process that generates consensus through a series of questionnaires, which are usually administered via the mail or electronic mail. The process begins with those collecting the data asking the priority population to respond to one or two broad questions. The responses are analyzed, and a second questionnaire, with more specific questions, is developed and sent to the priority population. The answers to these more specific questions are analyzed again, and a new questionnaire is sent out, requesting additional information. If consensus is reached, the process may end here; if not, it may continue for another round or two (Gilmore & Campbell, 1996). Most often, this process continues for five or fewer rounds.

Community Forum   The community forum approach brings together people from the priority population to discuss what they see as their group's problems/needs. It is not uncommon for a community forum to be organized by a group representing the priority population, in conjunction with the program planners. Such groups include labor, civic, religious, or service organizations, or groups such as the Parent Teacher Association (PTA). Once people have arrived, a moderator explains the purpose of the meeting and then asks those from the priority population to share their concerns. One or several individuals from the organizing group, called *recorders,* are usually given the responsibility for taking notes or taping the session to ensure that the responses are recorded accurately. However, when moderating a community forum, it is important to be aware that the silent majority may not speak out and/or a vocal minority may speak too loudly. For example, an individual parent's view may be wrongly interpreted to be the view of all parents.

At a community forum, participants may also be asked to respond in writing (1) by answering specific questions or (2) by completing some type of instrument. Figure 4.2 is an example of an instrument that could be used to collect data from participants in a community forum.

Focus Group   The **focus group** is a form of qualitative research that grew out of group therapy. Focus groups are used to obtain information about the feelings, opinions, perceptions, insights, beliefs, misconceptions, attitudes, and receptivity of a group of people concerning an idea or issue. Focus groups are rather small, compared to community forums, and usually include only 8 to 12 people. If possible, it is best to have a group of people who do not know each other so that their responses are not inhibited by acquaintance. Participation in the group is by invitation. People are invited about one to three weeks in advance of the session. At the time of the invitation, they receive general information about the session but are not given any specifics. This precaution helps ensure that responses will be spontaneous yet accurate.

Once assembled, the group is led by a skilled moderator who has the task of obtaining candid responses from the group to a set of predetermined questions. In addi-

Directions: Please rank the need for each program in the community by placing a number in the space to the left of the programs. Use 1 to rank the program of greatest need, 2 for the next greatest need, and so forth, until you have ranked all seven programs. The program with the highest number next to it should be the one that, in your opinion, is least needed. If you feel that a program should not be considered for implementation in our community, please place an X in the space to the left of the program instead of a number. Please note that the number you place next to each program represents its need in the community, not necessarily your desire to participate in it. After ranking the program, place an X to the right of the program in the column(s) that represent the age group(s) to which you feel the program should be targeted.

Program	All ages	Children 5–12	Teens 13–19	Adults 20–64	Older adults 65+
_____ Alcohol education:	_____	_____	_____	_____	_____
_____ Exercise/fitness:	_____	_____	_____	_____	_____
_____ Nutrition education:	_____	_____	_____	_____	_____
_____ Safety belt use:	_____	_____	_____	_____	_____
_____ Smoking cessation:	_____	_____	_____	_____	_____
_____ Smoking education:	_____	_____	_____	_____	_____
_____ Weight loss:	_____	_____	_____	_____	_____

Source: Modified from a form developed by Amy L. Bernard, Ph.D., CHES; Assistant Professor, University of Cincinnati. Adapted by permission.

Figure 4.2 Instrument for ranking program need

tion to eliciting responses to the questions, the moderator may ask the group to prioritize the different responses. As in a community forum, the answers to the questions are recorded through either written notes and/or audio or video recordings, so that at a later date the interested parties can review and interpret the results.

Focus groups are not easy to conduct. Special care must be given to developing the questions that will be asked. Poorly written questions will yield information that is less than useful. In addition, the moderator should be one who is skilled in leading a group. As might be surmised, the level of skill needed to conduct a focus group increases as the topic of discussion becomes more controversial.

Although focus groups have been shown to be an effective way of gathering data, they do have one major limitation. Participants in the groups are usually not selected through a random-sampling process. They are generally selected because they possess certain attributes (e.g., individuals of low income, city dwellers, parents of disabled children, or chief executive officers of major corporations). Participants may not be representative of the priority population. Therefore, the results of the focus group are not generalizable. "Findings [of focus groups] should be interpreted as suggestive and directional rather than as definitive" (Schechter, Vanchieri, & Crofton, 1990, p. 254).

Nominal Group Process   The **nominal group process** is a highly structured process in which a few knowledgeable representatives of the priority population (five to seven people) are asked to qualify and quantify specific needs. Those invited to participate are asked to record their responses to a question without discussing it among themselves. Once all have recorded a response, participants share their responses in a round-robin fashion. While this is occurring, the facilitator is recording the responses on a chalkboard or notepad for all to see. The responses are clarified through a discussion. After the discussion, the participants are asked to rank-order the responses by importance to the priority population. This ranking may be considered either a preliminary or a final vote. If it is preliminary, it is followed with more discussion and a final vote.

Observation   Gathering primary needs assessment data via observation can be accomplished in several different ways. It can be done by the planners or their partners, who can become integrated into the environment where the health problems may occur, so that they can observe the actions of the priority population. Examples of such fieldwork may include watching the eating patterns of children in a school lunchroom, observing workers on an assembly line to see if they are wearing their protective glasses, checking the smoking behavior of employees on break, and observing community members for safety belt use. (See Chapter 5 for more information on observation.)

Self-Assessments   Data can also be collected by those in the priority population through **self-assessments.** "A majority of these approaches address primary prevention issues, such as the assessment of risk factors in one's lifestyle pattern and the secondary prevention process of the early detection of disease symptoms" (Gilmore & Campbell, 1996, p. 109). Examples of such assessments include breast self-examination (BSE), testicular self-examination (TSE), self-monitoring for skin cancer, and **health assessments (HAs).** "Health assessments include instruments known as health risk appraisals or health risk assessments (HRAs), health status assessments (HSAs), various lifestyle-specific (e.g., nutrition, stress, and physical activity) assessment instruments, wellness and behavioral/habit inventories" (SPM Board of Directors, 1999, p. xxiii), and disease/condition status assessments (e.g., chances of getting heart disease or diabetes).

Of the different self-assessments, it is the HAs that have been most useful in the needs assessment process, because from such assessments planners can obtain "group data which summarize major health problems and risk factors" (Alexander, 1999, p. 5). And of the HAs, it is the HRAs that are most often included in the needs assessment process. HRAs are instruments that estimate "the odds that a person with certain characteristics will die from selected causes within a given time span" (Alexander, 1999, p. 5). Even though HRAs are used as part of needs assessments, this was not their original intent. The original purpose of HRAs was to engage family physicians and their patients in conversation about risks of premature death and preventive health behaviors (Robbins & Hall, 1970).

To use an HRA as part of a needs assessment, planners would have those in the priority population complete a questionnaire. The instruments include questions about health behavior (e.g., smoking, exercise), personal or family health history of diseases (e.g., cancer, heart disease), demographics (e.g., age, sex), and usually some physiological data (e.g., height, weight, blood pressure, cholesterol). The resulting risk appraisals, in most cases, are calculated by computers, but there are some HRAs that are hand-scored by the participant or health professional (Alexander, 1999). Most

HRAs generate both individual and group reports. Thus planners can use the individual reports as part of an educational program for the priority population and use the group reports as another source of primary needs assessment data.

There are many HA instruments on the market. An excellent source for examining the different HAs available is the *SPM Handbook of Health Assessment Tools* (Hyner et al., 1999). This volume not only physically presents many of the HAs available today but it also includes information on (1) theoretical models associated with health assessment; (2) the use and selection of health assessment tools, including ethical considerations; (3) specific applications of health assessments; and (4) information on both the historic and prospective views of health assessment.

Although this discussion has revolved around the use of HRAs as means of providing information for a needs assessment, they have also been used to help motivate people to act on their health, to increase awareness, to serve as cues to action, and to contribute to program evaluation. However, the reliability, validity, and effectiveness in predicting risk and prompting behavior change is questionable (Edington, Yen, & Braunstein, 1999).

The following conclusions relative to HRAs can be made:

1. The reliability of HRA risk scores can vary greatly from one instrument to another.

2. Reliability scores decrease when users calculate their own score, as opposed to computer scoring.

3. There is a great variance in the self-reporting of specific risk factors and clinical physiologic measurements.

4. Only those HRAs for which reliability can be demonstrated should be used for evaluating the effectiveness of health education.

Sources of Secondary Data

Several sources of secondary needs assessment data are available to planners. The main sources include data collected by government agencies at multiple levels (federal, regional, state, or local), data available from nongovernment agencies and organizations, data from existing records, and data or other evidence that are presented in the literature.

Data Collected by Government Agencies Certain government agencies collect data on a regular basis. Some of the data collection is mandated by law (i.e., census, births, deaths, notifiable diseases, etc.), whereas other data are collected voluntarily (i.e., usage rates for safety belts). Since the data are collected by the government, program planners can gain free access to them by contacting the agency that collects the data or by finding them in a library that serves as a United States government depository. Many college and university libraries and large public libraries serve as such depositories. Presented here is information about some of the more useful sources of data collected by government agencies.

U.S. Department of Commerce Within the U.S. Department of Commerce is located the Bureau of Census. The bureau is responsible for taking a census of the United States every 10 years. The first census was ordered by George Washington in 1790 for the purpose of apportioning representation to the House of Representatives. The most recent census, taken in 2000, includes data on number of people, income, employment, family size, education, type of dwelling, and many other social indicators. Census data are important to program planners because they are used in calculating disease and death rates (McKenzie, Pinger, & Kotecki, 2002).

Another Bureau of Census publication is the *Statistical Abstract of the United States (SA)*. This book, published since 1878, provides a summary of statistics on the social, political, and economic organization of the United States, individual states and metropolitan areas, and U.S. counties, including easy access to census data on populations, business and geography. With respect to health data, the SA includes information on health expenditures and health coverage (including Medicare and Medicaid), injuries, diseases, disability status, nutritional intakes and food consumption. An edition of *SA* can be purchased from the U.S. Government Printing Office for approximately $50 and is available on-line at http://www.census.gov/prod/www/statistical-abstract-02.html.

Centers for Disease Control and Prevention (CDC) and the National Center for Health Statistics (NCHS)

The National Center for Health Statistics (NCHS) is one of the major centers of the Centers for Disease Control and Prevention (CDC). As the nation's keeper of health data, the NCHS maintains several ongoing data systems. Though all the data systems are useful, six that have been proven very helpful to health promotion program planners have been vital statistics, the National Health Interview Survey (NHIS), the National Health and Nutrition Examination Survey (NHANES), National Hospital Discharge Survey (NHDS), and the Youth Risk Behavior Surveillance System (YRBSS). Vital statistics are statistical summaries of vital records—that is, records of major life events. Included in the major life events are live births, deaths, marriages, divorces, and infant deaths. These data are published in the National Center for Health Statistic's *National Vital Statistics Reports* and in annual volumes making up the *Vital Statistics of the United States*. These vital statistics are produced and available in both published and electronic form.

The three surveys (NHIS, NHANES, and NHDS) conducted by the National Center for Health Statistics provide a variety of data useful to planners. The NHIS is a telephone-administered survey and the principal source of information on the health of the household population in the United States. It measures basic health and demographics and asks various questions on current health topics. NHANES assesses the health and nutrition status of the general U.S. population. But rather than using a telephone survey as in the NHIS, data are collected using a mobile examination center wherein direct physical examinations and clinical and laboratory testing are performed on a representative group of residents. The other survey performed by NCHS, the National Hospital Discharge Survey, assesses characteristics of inpatients discharged from hospitals in the United States. Data are collected by abstracting hospital records and purchasing automated data tapes. Of special note to planners is the availability of the survey questionnaires used in the NHIS, NHANES, and NHDS. These instruments provide good starting points for planners who need to collect primary needs assessment data. The instruments are available directly from the NCHS (http://www.cdc.gov/nchs/).

The Youth Risk Behavior Surveillance System (YRBSS) can be of special use to those planning programs for adolescents and young adults. The YRBSS monitors six categories of priority health risk behaviors: behaviors that contribute to unintentional and intentional injuries, tobacco use, alcohol and other drug use, sexual behaviors that contribute to unintended pregnancy and sexually transmitted diseases, incuding HIV infection, unhealthy dietary behaviors, and inadequate physical activity (CDC, 2003). The YRBSS is conducted every two years among students in grades 9–12 in all 50 states, several large cities and most U.S. territories. Planners can use YRBSS data to: implement or modify programs to address health needs in their location, monitor progress on goals and objectives, and create awareness of the extent of risk behaviors among adolescents (CDC, 2003a).

Other national data that are of use to planners are those presented in the *Morbidity and Mortality Weekly Report (MMWR)*. Reported cases of specified notifiable diseases are reported weekly in the *MMWR*. The *MMWR* is prepared by the CDC staff, based on reports from state health departments.

As a final note about sources of data available from national-level government agencies, planners should consider contacting the National Health Information Center at http://www.health.gov/nhic/.

State and Local Agencies Although the discussion to this point has centered on national data, similar data are available from state and local government agencies. Planners should consult with their local and state health departments to see what is available to them. Three sources of data collected at the local and/or state levels that have been especially useful to program planners are (1) vital statistics (e.g., birth and death records), (2) *Behavioral Risk Factor Surveillance System (BRFSS)* data, and (3) data generated from the *Mobilizing for Action through Planning and Partnerships* (MAPP) process. The BRFSS data are collected by a branch of CDC via a state-based telephone survey of the civilian, noninstitutional, adult population. The survey seeks to gather information about such high-risk behaviors as excessive alcohol use, tobacco use, physical inactivity, and the lack of preventive care, such as screening for various cancers. The results of the BRFSS are published periodically in *MMWR*. (Review information in Chapter 2 on the MAPP process.)

Data Available from Nongovernment Agencies and Organizations In addition to the data available from government agencies, planners should also consult with nongovernment agencies and groups for data. Included among these are health care systems, voluntary health agencies, and business, civic, and commerce groups. For example, most of the national voluntary health agencies produce yearly "facts and figures" booklets that include a variety of epidemiological data. In addition, local agencies and organizations often have data they have collected for their own use. For example, it is not unusual for a local United Way to have performed a needs assessment in the community before distributing funds.

Data from Existing Records These are health data that are often "collected as a by-product of a service effort, such as managing a clinic, an immunization program, or a water pollution control program" (Pickett & Hanlon, 1990, p. 151). These data can also serve as useful secondary needs assessment data. Clinical indicators—such as blood pressure, height, weight, body composition, or blood analysis—are routinely collected by health care professionals. Also often available are records that deal with the utilization or cost of medical services. These data include such items as health insurance claims paid, hospital utilization rates, visits to a doctor's office, disability benefits and insurance premiums paid, and incidental and disability absenteeism. (See Chapter 5 for more information about data from existing records.)

Data from the Literature Planners might also be able to identify the needs of a priority population by reviewing any available current literature about that priority population. An example would be a planner who is developing a health promotion program for individuals infected by the human immunodeficiency virus (HIV). Because of the seriousness of this disease and the number of people who have studied and written about it, there is a good chance that present literature could reflect the need of a certain priority population.

The best means of accessing data from the literature is by using the available literature databases. Most literature databases today are available in several different forms, including computer databases and the Internet. Computer access depends upon the capacity of the library or unit housing the databases. Depending on the database used, planners can expect to find comprehensive listings of citations for journal articles, book chapters, and books, and, in some databases, abstracts of the literature. Within the listings, most databases cite sources by both author and subject/title. Figure 4.3 provides an example of what planners might find when searching a database.

There are many literature databases available to planners. Next is a short discussion of those databases that have proven helpful to health promotion planners.

PsycINFO PsycINFO is a database produced by the American Psychological Association (APA) that includes journal articles, book chapters, and book citations on literature in psychology and related subjects. The database is divided into several major categories, but two of particular interest to planners are (1) behavioral science and (2) mental health.

Medline Medline, accessed through PubMed (http://www.ncbi.nlm.nih.gov/PubMed/) and created by the National Library of Medicine, provides information on medicine, nursing and health care. It also covers the international literature on biomedicine, including the allied health fields and the biological and physical sciences.

Author Citation

Authors   Article title
↓   ↓

Thackeray, R., & Neiger, B. L., Use of social marketing to develop culturally-innovative diabetes interventions. Diabetes Spectrum. 2003; 16(1), 15–20.

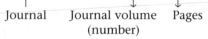

↑   └┬┘   └┬┘
Journal   Journal volume   Pages
(number)

Subject/Title

Article title
↓

Use of social marketing to develop culturally-innovative diabetes interventions. Thackeray, R., & Neiger, B. L., Diabetes Spectrum. 2003; 16(1), 15–20.

Figure 4.3 Sample citations

Information is indexed from approximately 4,600 biomedical journals and selected monographs of congresses and symposia and citations from Index Medicus, International Nursing Index, PREMEDLINE, and AIDSLINE.

Education Resource Information Center (ERIC)   ERIC "is a national information system established in 1966 by the federal government to provide ready access to educational literature by and for educational practitioners and scholars" (Houston, 1987, p. x). Today, it is funded by the Office of Educational Research and Improvement in the U.S. Department of Education. ERIC includes all the information from the printed indexes *Current Index of Journals in Education (CIJE)* and *Resources in Education (RIE)*. ERIC provides full text for approximately 2,200 digests along with references from over 1,000 educational and education-related journals (EBSCO, 2003).

Cumulative Index to Nursing & Allied Health Literature (CINAHL)   The CINAHL grew out of the work of a hospital librarian in the 1940s who created an index for nursing journals. Demand for this work grew over the years until in 1961 the first volume of *Cumulative Index to Nursing Literature (CINL)* was published. "In order to keep pace with the trend toward a multidisciplinary approach to health care, the scope of coverage was expanded in 1977 to include allied health journals. To reflect this change *CINL* changed its title to *CINAHL*" (Marcarin, 1995, p. 3). This database went online in 1984 and today includes references to more than 2,200 journals.

BIOETHICSLINE   BIOETHICSLINE is a database that "covers ethical, legal, and policy issues surrounding health care and biomedical research. Citations come from several different bodies of literature including ethics, health sciences, law, philosophy, religion, social sciences, and the popular media" (Cottrell, Girvan, & McKenzie, 2002, p. 267).

Steps for Conducting a Literature Search

General Search Procedures   The process of searching a database is not difficult, and with the exception of a few individual differences, most indexes are arranged in a similar format. As Figure 4.3 indicated, most indexes include both an author and a subject/title index. An item that is specific to each index is its thesaurus, a listing of the key words the indexes use to index the subject/titles. Planners can find the thesauri in a separate volume with or near the indexes.

Figure 4.4 provides planners with a literature search strategy in the form of a flowchart. The chart begins by identifying the need of the priority population or topic to be searched. At this point, planners can search either by subject/title or by author. If planners know of an author who has done work on their topic, they can search the database using the author's last name. If they do not have information on authors, they will need to match their topic with the key words presented in the thesaurus. Since there are times when a topic is not expressed in the same terms used in the thesaurus, planners will need to look for related terms. Once they have a list of key words, they need to search the database for possible matches. In conducting this search, they need to ensure that they are using the database that covers the years of literature in which they are interested. This search should identify possible sources and citations.

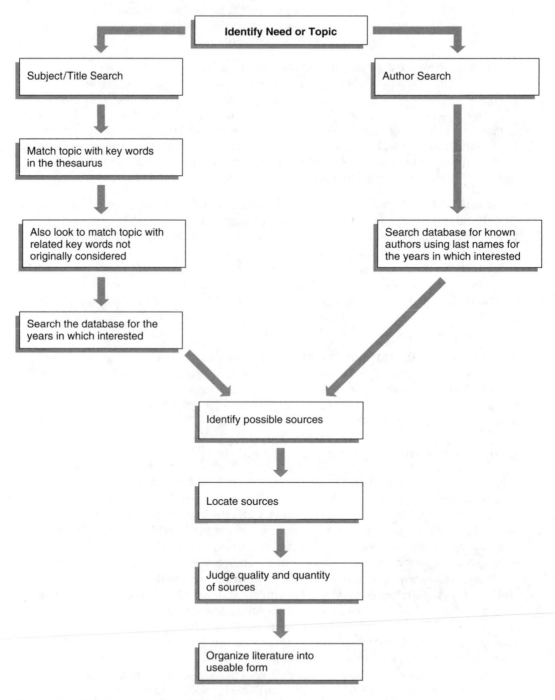

Figure 4.4 Literature search strategy flowchart

Source: Adapted from Deeds (1992) and Macarin (1995).

Once sources are identified, planners may review abstracts (or entire documents) on-line or locate a hard copy of the document. Then, planners must determine the quality and usefulness of the publication in the needs assessment process. One means by which planners can judge the quality of the literature is to examine the references at the end of the publications. First, this reference list may lead planners to other sources not identified in the original search. Second, if the sources found in the database include all those commonly cited in the literature, this can verify the exhaustiveness of the search.

Searching via the World Wide Web   Through the use of the World Wide Web (WWW), planners can obtain access to a variety of needs assessment data rather easily and quickly. The **WWW** "is an interactive information delivery service that includes a repository of resources on almost any subject" (Cottrell et al., 2002, p. 267). The WWW, or "the web," "uses a technology called hypertext. A single hypertext document on the WWW is called a web page. Hypertext is a method of transparently linking one information resource to another" (Kotecki & Siegel, 1997, p.117).

A **website** is a collection of WWW "pages, usually consisting of a home page and several other linked pages" (Olpin & Gotthoffer, 2000, p. 155). To search websites for data, planners can enter the WWW through a web browser, such as Microsoft Internet Explorer or Netscape Communicator. A browser is a special software package that reads the hypertext language and can retrieve documents at multiple sites on the web (Daniel & Balog, 1997). On each browser is a field for users to type in the web address of a site, also known as the Uniform Resource Locator (URL). Entering the specific URL will connect planners with the desired website. Almost all websites contain a home page that "acts as a starting point for information about a person or organization" (Olpin & Gotthoffer, 2000, p. 153) and provides a list of what is available at the site. The home page can be thought of as "a combination of a cover and a table of contents of a book, in that it names the site and directs the user to a list of information options available at the site" (Cottrell et al., 2002, p. 268). Figure 4.5 presents the home page for the Centers for Disease Control and Prevention <http:// www.cdc.gov/>.

If planners do not know the URL of a specific website, they can search for needed information by using a search archive or a search engine. A number of commercial organizations (e.g., Yahoo, Google Groups, etc.) have categorized websites in these two ways. A **subject archive** organizes information by topic and can be found at these commercial sites (see Figure 4.6). The subject archives presented in Figure 4.6 include Business and Economy, Computers and Internet, News and Media, and so on. Choosing one of these subject archives categories presents more subcategories, or links, to Internet resources about the subject. For example, if planners want information on heart disease, they could select the subject archive of "diseases" under "Health" in Figure 4.6. This will bring up an alphabetized list of diseases from which to choose. Planners would then have many sources from which to choose (Kotecki & Siegel, 1997).

Planners can also search the web using a search engine. A **search engine** is unlike a search archive in that the information is not organized into categories. Instead, a search engine indexes the words in web pages on the Internet. The index created by a search engine is called a catalog and users query the catalog for keywords that best describes their topic. When using a search engine, a field for typing in keywords is immediately displayed. After submitting a keyword query, a list of Internet resources is generated. (Kotecki & Siegel, 1997, pp. 118–120)

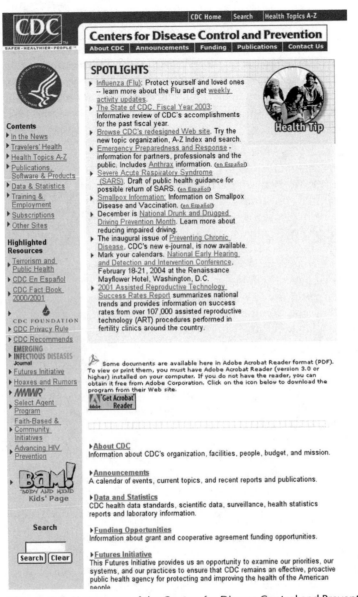

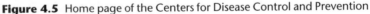

Figure 4.5 Home page of the Centers for Disease Control and Prevention

Popular search engines include Yahoo, Google, Vivisimo, and Ask Jeeves. Planners can experiment with and select the sites that best fit their needs. If planners are using a term that has more than one word (i.e., *heart disease*), it is best to use quotation marks around the term when entering it on the search engine. "This will let the search engine know that all the words are to be included in the term when the search engine is seeking sites that match. If quotation marks are not used, the search engine may seek sites that match only the first word in the multiword term" (Cottrell et al., 2002, p. 270).

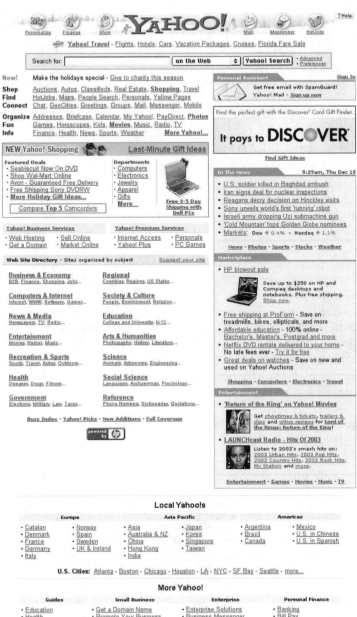

Figure 4.6 Example of a subject archive

As with any data source, planners need to be aware that not all data found via the WWW are valid and reliable. Thus planners need to scrutinize sources just as they would data found in hard copies. Several authors (Jadad & Gagliardi, 1998; Kotecki & Chamness, 1999; Pealer & Dorman, 1997; Silberg, Lundberg, & Musacchio, 1997; Tillman, 1997; Venditto, 1997) have published useful guides for evaluating information obtained via the Internet.

Conducting a Needs Assessment

A number of different approaches can be used to determine the needs of the priority population. "Need assessments range from informal approaches, using educated and informed observations to formal, comprehensive research projects. However, the informal approaches are less reliable than a planned and scientifically developed research approach" (Timmreck, 2003, p. 89). Oftentimes, informal approaches are used because of limited time, personnel, and money. However, as noted in the beginning of this chapter, needs assessment may be the most critical step in the planning process and should not be taken lightly. Resources used on need assessments usually pay dividends many times over. Therefore the authors present a six step process that is more formal in nature: (1) determining purpose and defining the scope of the needs assessment, (2) gathering data, (3) analyzing the data, (4) identifying the factors linked to the health problem, (5) identifying the program focus, and (6) validating the need before continuing on with the planning process. Because the PRECEDE-PROCEED model presents a useful sequence for conducting a needs assessment, it will be presented in parallel with these six steps.

Step 1: Determining the Purpose and Scope of the Needs Assessment

The initial step in the needs assessment process is to determine the purpose and the scope of the needs assessment. In other words, what is the goal of the needs assessment? What does the planning committee hope to gain from the needs assessment? How extensive will the needs assessment be? What kind of resources will be available to conduct the needs assessment? In reality, the first challenge associated with conducting a needs assessment is determining whether an assessment should even be performed, and if so, what type of needs assessment is appropriate. For example, a great deal of health promotion today is driven by what is termed **categorical funding.** This means that the funding that supports programs is earmarked or dedicated to a specific health problem or determinant (i.e., risk factor). If this is the case, planners will not assess needs related to what health problem they should address since this is already predetermined by the funding agency. Likewise, if a planner works for the American Heart Association, he or she will not assess needs to determine a priority health problem—that has already been identified as heart disease.

Even if a health problem is already identified, it may be necessary to identify which determinants are most significant or which intervention strategies demonstrate the most promise in addressing the problem at hand. For example, heart disease may be the priority health problem, but it may be critical to assess the comparative importance of smoking, high blood pressure, and high blood cholesterol to identify appropriate interventions. The extent to which a needs assessment is necessary and appropriate should be determined by stakeholders, including key decision makers.

Some times, it is important to perform a needs assessment even if the health problem or determinant has been identified. For example, if the priority health problem is breast cancer, it is still necessary to collect current information on the degree to which women are either dying or suffering from the disease. It will be important to know how prevalent breast cancer is, where it is most prevalent in the population, high risk subpopulations, economic costs, and general trends over time. Stakeholders will want continual status reports on the extent of the problem.

In other cases, a planner may be found in a situation where a community needs assessment has not been performed for a long period of time or where categorical funding does not dictate what health problem(s) should be addressed. This will require planners and their partners to collect a wide range of data, compare the importance of multiple health problems, and set priorities. In a general sense, this is the process that is often referred to as community assessment. This implies that all significant health problems are examined to assess their relative significance. Stakeholders and planning groups will also usually determine how many health problems will be analyzed in the needs assessment. This will be influenced by how much time, and how many resources can be directed to the needs assessment.

Another important decision that must be made is the extent to which actual consumers or clients will be involved in the needs assessment. The term **action** or **participatory research** has gained popularity in recent years, though it is often misunderstood or used inappropriately. In its truest sense, action research is characterized by at least four factors: 1) **community empowerment** (i.e., community members control decision making); 2) collaboration; 3) acquisition of knowledge through hands-on participation; and 4) a focus on social change. What often results is a scenario where planners invite a few community representatives to participate in assessing needs and setting priorities, but this is rarely representative of the population to be served.

Once the basic purpose and scope of the needs assessment is identified, planners may proceed to data collection. However, planners must not treat this first step too lightly. Although a natural tendency is to move forward quickly, an understanding of why a needs assessment is being performed will give proper direction to all other steps that follow.

Step 2: Gathering Data

The second step in the needs assessment process is gathering data. To do this, planners must consider sources of data that reflect needs from the viewpoint of the planners and also needs perceived by those in the priority population. This usually means both primary and secondary data need to be collected. Because of the cost and availability, data collection should begin with the collection of relevant secondary data. *Relevant* means that the data apply to the situation for which the planning is taking place. If a national program is being planned, then national secondary data should be sought from appropriate national government and nongovernment agencies. If a local program is being planned, then appropriate local data should be sought. When planning a local program, it is not unusual to find that local data do not exist. If that is the case, planners may need to use state, regional or national data (in that order) and apply them to the local area. For example, let's assume diabetes mellitus mortality data are needed for local planning and the only data available are national level data. Planners could use national data (e.g., 24.9 per 100,000 people died of diabetes in 2000) to estimate the number of deaths in a local community. If the population of a local city is 250,000, planners could infer that the number of deaths due to diabetes in the city during 2000 totaled 62 (i.e., 24.9 $\times$ 2.5). If the city's population were older, 62 deaths could be viewed as a low estimate since diabetes deaths are more prevalent in older populations. Conversely, if the population were younger, 62 deaths could be viewed as a high estimate. Obviously, as noted at the beginning of this chapter, there are disadvantages of using secondary data, but good planners use and interpret them in light of their limitations (McDermott & Sarvela, 1999).

Even though primary data will usually take more resources to collect, they provide valuable information about the specific planning situation not available from secondary data and they provide an opportunity to get those in the priority population actively involved in the program planning process. Thus planners need to decide whom to collect the data from and take the necessary steps to collect the data. (The data collection process is presented at length in Chapter 5.)

One particular challenge that will face planners with respect to gathering data is the degree to which needs assessment data will reflect health status as determined by traditional epidemiologic or survey data or whether it will truly represent a consumer orientation as discussed in Chapter 2. At the heart of this challenge is the determination of who will ultimately make decisions in the needs assessment process. Windsor and colleagues (1994) applied marketing vocabulary to the needs assessment process, identifying two types of health needs. The first type is **service needs.** These are the things that health professionals believe should happen with respect to health promotion programming. In truth, planners are trained to collect and analyze data and make programming decisions based on an objective analysis.

The other type of health need consists of things that those in the priority population "say they must have or be able to do in order to resolve a health problem" (Windsor et al., 1994, p.64). These needs are referred to as **service demands.** In fact, people will not likely engage in a program unless it is relevant to them and tailored to meet their needs.

The reality is that both types of needs are important, and if either one is ignored, the actual needs of a priority population may not be addressed. When differences exist (and they usually do) between data related to service needs and service demands, planners still have several options. They can start with consumer preferences, build confidence and trust, and then gradually incorporate some service needs. Another option is to develop an awareness campaign to help potential consumers understand the magnitude of service needs. Still another option is to simultaneously address a service demand and a service need. Perhaps the best approach is to identify health priorities based on service needs, but ensure that all programs and interventions are based on service demands. In this respect, health professionals can make decisions based on objective data, but respond to consumers based on their needs and preferences.

As planners conclude the second step in the needs assessment process, they must remember that each planning situation is different. It is desirable to have both primary and secondary needs assessment data in order to gain a clear picture of both service needs and demands; however, depending on the resources and circumstances, planners may have access to only one or the other. In addition, there is usually a trade-off between quality and quantity of data. Planners must use the best data available under the challenges and constraints facing them.

Step 3: Analyzing the Data

At this point in the needs assessment process, the planners must analyze all the data collected, with the goal of identifying and prioritizing the health problems. The analysis of the data may be formal or informal. The approach used would depend on what data were collected and how objective the planners wanted to be. Formal analysis would consist of some type of statistical analysis. This approach could be used only when appropriate statistical criteria (see any introductory statistics book) have been met. Much of the time, a less formal means of analyzing the data is used. This approach is commonly referred to as **eyeballing data**—that is, looking at the data for obvious differences between current health status and what could be. As Windsor and colleagues (1994, p. 63) have stated, eyeballing the data means looking for differences between "what is and what ought to be."

One strategy that is a mix of formal and informal analyses is the use of **standard measures.** Too often in needs assessments, planners compare apples with oranges. That is to say, they may have mortality data for one health problem, morbidity data for another and perhaps behavioral risk factor data for yet another. Despite the stark differences in data (apples and oranges), planners compare the health problems anyway and make decisions based on obvious inconsistencies. To compare apples with apples as it were, standard measures such as rates or percentages may be a planner's most reasonable option. For example, rates can be standardized per 1,000 or per 100,000 people and compared across health problems. Percentages (i.e., percent of deaths caused by heart disease versus diabetes, or the percent of people who smoke versus the percent of people who are obese) also allows for similar comparisons.

Sometimes this step in the needs assessment process is not very complicated because the problem/need is obvious. For example, breast cancer rates may have risen in a given community, the number of breast screenings may be low, and the consumers may recognize this. Or, in another setting, the planners may find a direct correlation between the health status of a community and the lack of health care. However, not all assessments yield an obvious problem. The data may be mixed or confusing. If planners are working with a multicultural priority population, data analysis may even be more confusing, because health concepts held by one culture may be very different than the health concepts held by the planners. These cultural differences "often involve family, community, and/or supernatural agents in cause and effect, placation, and treatment rituals to prevent, control, or cure illness. A failure to understand and appreciate these 'differences' can have serious implications for success of any health promotion/disease prevention effort" (Kline & Huff, 1999, p. 106). In such cases, it is probably a good idea to see if additional data might be collected for clarification. If obtaining additional data does not help, then relying on those individuals on the planning committee more familiar with the cultural differences or asking more experienced professionals for their opinions may aid in reaching a conclusion.

In completing this step of the needs assessment process, planners will, in essence, be working through the first two phases of the PRECEDE-PROCEED model: social and epidemiological assessment. While analyzing the data, planners may find it helpful to ask the following questions:

1. What is the quality of life of those in the priority population?
2. What are social conditions and perceptions shared by those in the priority population?
3. What are the social indicators (e.g., absenteeism, crime, discrimination, performance, welfare, etc.) in the priority population that reflect the social conditions and perceptions?
4. Can the social conditions and perceptions be linked to health promotion? If so, how?
5. What are the health problems associated with the social problems?
6. Which health problem is most important to change?

The last question in this list is really asking the question, Which health problem/ need should get priority? The health problems/needs must be prioritized not because the lowest-priority problems/needs are not important, but because organizations have limited resources. Thus planners need to see how the health promotion dollars can best be used. Therefore, in setting priorities, the planners should seek answers to these questions:

1. What is the most pressing need?
2. Are there resources adequate to deal with the problem?
3. Can the problem best be solved by a health promotion intervention, or could it be handled better through another means?
4. Are effective intervention strategies available to address the problem?
5. Can the problem be solved in a reasonable amount of time?

After answering these questions, the planners should be able to prioritize the identified problems/needs.

The actual process of setting priorities can take many different forms and range from basic rank ordering by a group of stakeholders, to use of the nominal group process, to a more complex process called the **Basic Priority Rating (BPR) process.** The BPR process was first presented by Hanlon (1974) (it has been more recently presented in Pickett & Hanlon, 1990) and will be discussed here in greater detail because it can greatly help program planners quantify the subjective process of prioritizing. The process requires planners to rate four different components of the identified needs and insert the ratings into a formula in order to determine a rating between 0 and 100. The components and their possible scores (in parenthesis) are:

A. size of the problem (0 to 10)
B. seriousness of the problem (0 to 20)

Table 4.1 Scoring the size of the problem

Incidence or Prevalence per 100,000 Population	Score
50,000 or more	10
5,000 to 49,999	8
500 to 4,999	6
50 to 499	4
5 to 49	2
0.5 to 4.9	0

Source: Public Health Administration and Practice, G. Pickett and J. J. Hanlon, © 1997, McGraw-Hill. Reproduced with permission of The McGraw-Hill Companies.

C. effectiveness of the possible interventions (0 to 10)

D. propriety, economics, acceptability, resources, and legality (PEARL) (0 or 1)

The formula in which the scores are placed is:

$$\text{Basic Priority rating (BPR)} = \frac{(A + B)C}{3} \times D$$

Component *A*, size of the problem, can be scored by using epidemiological rates or determining the percentage of the priority population at risk. The higher the rate or percentage, the greater the score. Pickett and Hanlon (1990) offer the scale noted in Table 4.1 for scoring the size of the problem when using incidence and prevalence rates.

Component *B*, seriousness of the problem, is examined using four factors: economic loss to community, family, or individuals; involvement of other people who were not initially affected by the problem, as with the spread of an infectious disease; the severity of the problem measured in mortality, morbidity, or disability; and the urgency of solving the problem because of additional harm. Because the maximum score for this component is 20, raters can use a 0 to 5 score for each of the four factors.

Component *C*, effectiveness of the interventions, is often the most difficult of the four components to measure. The efficacy of some intervention strategies is known, such as immunizations (close to 100%) and smoking cessation classes (around 30%), but for many, it is not. Planners will need to estimate this score based upon the work of others or their own expert opinions. In scoring this component, planners should consider both the effectiveness of intervention strategies in terms of behavior change, as well as the degree to which the priority population will demonstrate interest in the intervention strategy.

Component *D*, PEARL, consists of several factors that determine whether a particular intervention strategy can be carried out at all. The score is 0 or 1; any need that receives a zero will automatically drop to the bottom of the priority list because a score of zero (a multplier) for this component will yield a total score of zero in the formula. Examples of when a zero may result are if an intervention is economically impossible, unacceptable to the priority population or planners, or illegal. Ideally, some of these assessments will be made before a health problem is considered in the priority setting process.

Once the score for the four components is determined, an overall priority rating for each need can be calculated, and the prioritizing can take place.

Other means of quantifying the prioritization of the needs may include getting the priority population or key people from the community, such as opinion leaders, to rank-order the identified needs.

How will planners know when they have completed Step 3 (Analyzing the Data) of the needs assessment process? Planners should be able to list in rank order the health problems/needs of the priority population.

Step 4: Identifying the Factors Linked to the Health Problem

Step 4 of the needs assessment process is parallel to the third phase of the PRECEDE-PROCEED model: behavioral and environmental assessment. Planners need to identify and prioritize the behavior and environmental risk factors (as well as social factors) that are associated with the health problem. In essence, modifying these factors or determinants is the real work of health promotion. Thus if the health problem is lung cancer, planners should analyze the health behaviors and environment of the priority population for known risk factors of lung cancer. For example, higher than expected smoking behavior may be present in the priority population, and the people may live in a community where smokefree public environments are not valued. Once these risk factors are identified, they too need to be prioritized (see Figure 2.2 for a means of prioritizing these risk factors).

Step 5: Identifying the Program Focus

The fifth step of the needs assessment process is similar to the fourth phase of the PRECEDE-PROCEED model: educational and ecological assessment. With behavioral and environmental risk factors identified and prioritized, planners need to identify those predisposing, enabling, and reinforcing factors that seem to have a direct impact on the targeted risk factors. In the lung cancer example, those in the priority population may not (1) have the skills necessary to stop smoking (predisposing factor), (2) have access to a smoking cessation program (enabling factor), or (3) have people around them who support efforts to stop smoking (reinforcing factor). "Study of the predisposing, enabling, and reinforcing factors automatically helps the planner decide exactly which of the factors making up the three classes deserve the highest priority as the focus of the intervention. The decision is based on their importance and any evidence that change in the factor is possible and cost-effective" (Green & Kreuter, 1999, p. 42)

In addition, when prioritizing needs, planners also need to consider any existing health promotion programs to avoid duplication of efforts. Therefore, program planners should seek to determine the status of existing health promotion programs by trying to answer as many questions as possible from the following list:

1. What health promotion programs are presently available to the priority population?

2. Are the programs being utilized? If not, why not?

3. How effective are the programs? Are they meeting their stated goals and objectives?

4. How were the needs for these programs determined?

5. Are the programs accessible to the priority population? Where are they located? When are they offered? Are there any qualifying criteria that people must meet to enroll? Can the priority population get to the program? Can the priority population afford the programs?

6. Are the needs of the priority population being met? If not, why not?

There are several ways to seek answers to these questions. Probably the most common way is through **networking** with other people working in health promotion and the health care system—that is, communicating with others who may know about existing programs. (See Chapter 9 for a more detailed discussion of networking.) These people may be located in the local or state health department, in voluntary health agencies, or in health care facilities, such as hospitals, clinics, nursing homes, extended care facilities, or managed care organizations.

Planners might also find information about existing programs by checking with someone in an organization that serves as a clearinghouse for health promotion programs or by using a community resource guide. The local or state health department, a local chamber of commerce, a coalition, the local medical/dental societies, a community task force, or a community health center may serve as a clearinghouse or produce such a guide. Another avenue is to talk with people in the priority population. Although they may not know about all existing programs, they may be able to share information on the effectiveness and accessibility of some of the programs. Finally, some of the information could be collected in Step 2 through separate community forums, focus groups, or surveys.

Step 6: Validating the Prioritized Needs

The final step in the needs assessment process is to validate the identified need(s). *Validate* means to confirm that the need that was identified is the need that should be addressed. Obviously, if great care were taken in the needs assessment process, validation should be a perfunctory step. However, there have been times when a need was not properly validated; much energy and many resources have thereby been wasted on unnecessary programs.

Validation amounts to "double checking," or making sure that an identified need is the real need. Any means available can be used, such as (1) rechecking the steps followed in the needs assessment to eliminate any bias, (2) conducting a focus group with some individuals from the priority population to determine their reaction to the identified need (if a focus group was not used earlier to gather the data), and (3) getting a "second opinion" from other health professionals.

Summary

This chapter presented several definitions of needs assessment and a discussion of primary and secondary data. The sources of these data were discussed at length. Also, presented in this chapter was a six-step approach that planners can follow in conducting a needs assessment on a given group of people. It is by no means the only way of conducting an assessment, but it is one viable option.

No matter what procedure is used to conduct a needs assessment, the end result should be the same. Planners should finish with a clearly defined program focus.

REVIEW QUESTIONS

1. What does *needs assessment* mean?

2. Why must a needs assessment be viewed through the eyes of both the planners and the consumers?

3. What is the difference between primary and secondary data?

4. Name several different sources of both primary and secondary data.

5. What advice might you give to someone who is interested in using previously collected data (secondary data) for a needs assessment?

6. What is the difference between a single-step (cross-sectional) and a multistep survey?

7. Explain the difference between a community forum and a focus group.

8. What is a health assessment?

9. What are the six steps in the needs assessment process, as identified in the chapter?

ACTIVITIES

1. Assume that you have been hired by the board of trustees of your college or university to conduct a needs assessment on the student body for the possibility of developing a health promotion program. Assume that there are few secondary data on this group of people, other than national norms for college students. You could conduct a "university forum" or hold a series of focus groups, but instead you have decided to survey a random sample of the population with a paper-and-pencil instrument. Your task now is to develop a needs assessment instrument. When developing the instrument, use questions that will collect data that are reflective of your priority population's awareness of health, attitudes about health, knowledge of health, health behavior, health interests, and demographics, as well as marketing possibilities. After completing the instrument, pilot test it on ten students (for the purposes of this assignment, this does not need to be a random group). Use the results of the pilot test to complete Steps 2, 3, 4, and 5 in the needs assessment process.

2. Develop a needs assessment instrument for a program you will be planning. Collect the same type of data noted in Activity 1, administer the instrument to a small group of people, then complete Steps 2, 3, 4, and 5 in the needs assessment process.

3. Using secondary data provided by your instructor or obtained from the World Wide Web (such as data from a Behavioral Risk Factor Surveillance Survey, state or local secondary data, or data from the National Center for Health Statistics), analyze the data and determine the health problems of the priority population.

4. Administer an HHA/HRA to a group of 25 to 30 people. Using the data generated, identify and prioritize a collective list of health problems of the group.

5. Plan and conduct a focus group on an identified health problem on your campus. Develop a set of questions to be used, identify and invite people to participate in the group, facilitate the process, and then write up a summary of the results based on your written notes and/or an audiotape of the session.

6. Using the data (paper-and-pencil instruments, clinical tests, and health histories) generated from a local health fair, identify and prioritize a collective list of health problems of those who participated.

Weblinks

1. **http://ctb.ku.edu/**
   Community Tool Box

   This site provides excellent resources on community assessment, conducting surveys, identifying problems, and assessing community needs and resources. Topic sections include step-by-step instruction, examples, checklists, and related resources.

2. **http://www.healthypeople.gov/state/toolkit/default.htm**
   Healthy People 2010 Tool Kit: A Field Guide to Health Planning

   This tool kit provides valuable resources for identifying and securing resources, identifying and engaging community partners, and setting health priorities, all important components of conducting an effective needs assessment.

3. **http://mapp.naccho.org/mapp_introduction.asp**
   National Association of County and City Health Officials

   At this website, the MAPP Model is comprehensively diagrammed and explained. The Four MAPP Assessments are described, including how they are implemented, how to use subcommittees for each assessment, and how to make linkages between assessments. A must-have resource for all planners conducting needs assessments.

4. **http://www.cdc.gov/nchs/**
   National Center for Health Statistics

   This website provides statistical information that will guide actions and policies to improve the health of populations in the United States. It includes recent data on vital statistics, NHANES, NHDS, and NHIS.

5. **http://www.statehealthfacts.kff.org/**
   Kaiser Family Foundation State Health Facts Online

   This site contains current state-level data on demographics, health and health policy, including health coverage, access, financing and state legislation. Planners can access information as tables, bar graphs or color-coded maps.

6. **http://www.ebsco.com/home/**
   EBSCO Information Services

   This site provides ready access to many databases described in this chapter.

CHAPTER 5

Measurement, Measures, Data Collection, and Sampling

Chapter Objectives

After reading this chapter and answering the questions at the end, you should be able to:

- Define measurement and quantitative and qualitative measures.
- Briefly describe the four levels of measurement.
- Describe several methods of data collection.
- Discuss the advantages and disadvantages of data collection from self-report (written surveys, telephone interviews, and face-to-face interviews), observation, existing records, and meetings.
- Explain the various types of validity.
- Define *reliability* and explain why it is important.
- Define *bias* in data collection and discuss how it can be reduced.
- Explain why data collection instruments must be culturally appropriate.
- Describe how a sample can be obtained from a population.
- Differentiate between probability and nonprobability samples.
- Describe how a pilot test is used.

Key Terms

anonymous	cultural sensitivity	nominal
bias	discriminant validity	nonprobability sample
census	face validity	nonpropational stratified random sample
cluster sample	field study	
concurrent validity	frame	obtrusive observation
confidential	indirect observation	ordinal
construct validity	internal consistency	parallel forms reliability
content validity	interrater reliability	pilot test
convergent validity	interval	population
criterion-related validity	intrarater reliability	predictive validity
cultural competence	levels of measurement	preliminary review

prepilot	ratio	specificity
probability sample	reliability	strata
proportional stratified random sample	respondents	stratified random sample
proxy measure	sample	survey population
qualitative measure	sampling	systematic sample
quantitative measure	sampling unit	test-retest reliability
random-digit dialing	self-report data	validity
random selection	sensitivity	universe
	simple random sample	unobtrusive observation

I n Chapter 4, we discussed in detail the needs assessment process, emphasizing the importance of collecting and analyzing appropriate needs assessment data. Later, in Chapters 13 through 15, we will again be concerned about data, but then the discussion will revolve around data and its relationship to program evaluation. In this chapter, we will examine the concepts that are considered when trying to determine the quality of data, whether it is for a needs assessment or a program evaluation. Specifically, we will examine the (1) term *measurement,* (2) types of data generated from measurement, (3) levels of measurement, (4) types of measures, (5) desirable characteristics of measures, (6) methods of data collection, (7) sampling, and (8) the importance of pilot testing data collection processes.

Measurement

Measurement is an integral part of program planning and evaluation. It has been defined as the process of assigning numbers or labels to objects, events, or people according to a particular set of rules (Kerlinger, 1986). For example, planners/evaluators can measure the level of fitness of program participants by asking them a question. Using the numbers *1, 2,* and *3,* planners/evaluators can assign the number *1* to those with poor fitness, *2* to those with average fitness, and *3* to those with good fitness. Further, the planners/evaluators need to specify what constitutes poor, average, and good fitness. In other words, measurement means that the program planners/evaluators need to "clearly specify the objects to be measured, the numbers to use, and the rules by which the numbers are assigned to the objects" (Green & Lewis, 1986, p. 58).

The data generated by measurement can be classified into two different categories, depending on the method by which they are collected. **Quantitative measures** "rely on more standardized data collection and reduction techniques, using predetermined questions or observational indicators and established response items" (Green & Lewis, 1986, p. 151). Quantitative data can be transformed into numerical data. Examples of quantitative data would be the number of participants in a smoking cessation program, the ratings on a patient satisfaction survey, and the pretest and posttest scores on a HIV knowledge test. **Qualitative measures** "tend to produce data in the language of the subjects, rarely with numerical values attached to observations" (Green & Lewis, 1986, p. 151). Qualitative data are usually assigned labels or categories (Morreale, no date) and often take the form of narrative (Weiss, 1998). Examples include data generated from case studies, interviews, and descriptions and explanations of observations.

Levels of Measurement

A fundamental question of measurement is deciding how something should be measured (McDermott & Sarvela, 1999). What yardstick should be used to measure the object of interest? For example, consider planners/evaluators who need data on the income levels of their program participants. They could ask the participants income level several different ways:

1. Are you on any type of welfare?
2. What income category best describes your family income? $0 to 10,000, $10,001 to 25,000, $25,001 to 40,000, $40,000+
3. What is your family income? _____

Each of these questions gets at one's income level, but each generates a different form of data. Thus when planners/evaluators begin to think about data collection, they need to consider the form(s) of data they want to use.

There are four **levels of measurement** used to determine how something is to be measured. They are hierarchical in nature, and the form of data collected determines what statistical test can be used to analyze them. The four levels of measurement are (Cottrell & McKenzie, in press):

1. **Nominal** level measures, the lowest level in the measurement hierarchy, enable planners to put data into categories. "The two requirements for nominal measures are that the categories have to be mutually exclusive so that each case fits into one of the categories, and the categories have to be exhaustive so that there is a place for every case" (Weiss, 1998, p. 116). Nominal measures do not convey any value to what is measured but rather just identifies or names it (Dignan, 1995). An example question that would generate nominal data is, "What is your sex?" The possible answers include the categories of "female" and "male." We can then assign numbers to these categories according to a particular rule we create (e.g., 1 = female, 2 = male).

2. **Ordinal** level measures, like nominal level measures, allow planners to put data into categories that are mutually exclusive and exhaustive, but also permits them to rank-order the categories. The different categories represent relatively more or less of something. However, the distance between categories cannot be measured. For example the question "How would you describe your level of satisfaction with your health care? (select one) very satisfied – satisfied – not satisfied" creates categories (very satisfied – satisfied – not satisfied) that are mutually exclusive (the respondent cannot select two categories) and exhaustive (there is a category for all levels of satisfaction), and the categories represent more or less of something (amount of satisfaction). We cannot, however, measure the distance (or difference) between the levels of satisfaction (e.g., what is the difference between very satisfied and satisfied?). Is the distance between very satisfied and satisfied the same distance between satisfied and not satisfied? Ordinal data categories are not an equal distance apart.

3. **Interval** level measures enable planners to put data into categories that are mutually exclusive and exhaustive, and rank-orders the categories. Furthermore, the widths of the categories must all be the same (Hurlburt, 2003) that allows for the distance between the categories to be measured. There is however, no absolute zero value. Thus interval level measures assign numerical values to things according to a particular rule (Dignan, 1995). An example question that generates interval data is: "What was the high temperature today?" We know that a temperature of 70° F is different than a temperature of 80° F, that 80° is warmer than 70°, that there is 10° F difference between the two, and if the temperature drops to 0° F there is still some heat in the air (though not much) because 0° F is warmer than $-10°$ F.

4. **Ratio** level measures, the highest level in the measurement hierarchy, enable planners to do everything with data that can be done with the other three levels of measures, however they are done using a scale with an absolute zero. Example questions that generate interval data include: "What was your score on the test?" How tall are you in inches?" and "During an average week, how many minutes do you exercise aerobically?" An absolute zero "point means that the thing being measured actually vanishes when the scale reads zero" (Hurlburt, 2003, p. 17). For example, when a person has a blood pressure reading of zero over zero, there is in fact no blood pressure.

Because interval and ratio data are continuous and rank-ordered values with equal distance between them, and because most statistical procedures are the same for both types of data (Valente, 2002), some have combined them into a single level of measurement and refer to the resulting data as *numerical data*. However, if given the choice, planners should strive to collect ratio data because it still provides the greatest flexibility in data analysis.

Types of Measures

Many different types of measures are used to conduct needs assessments or evaluate programs. It is important to match the methods of measurement with the focus of the task, whether it be a needs assessments or program evaluation. Typically, health promotion programs focus on one or more of the following types of measures: demographic characteristics, awareness, knowledge, attitudes, motivation, personality traits, skills, behavior, environmental factors or conditions, health status (i.e., health risks, morbidity, or mortality), and quality of life. In the remaining portions of this chapter, we will discuss methods and techniques for collecting data associated with these areas.

Desirable Characteristics of Data

The results of a needs assessment or program evaluation are only as good as the data that are used to gain the results. If a questionnaire was filled with ambiguous questions and the respondents were not sure how to answer, it is highly likely that the data collected would not be reflective of the true knowledge, attitudes, etc., of those responding. Therefore it is of vital importance that planners and evaluators make sure that the data they collect are reliable, valid, unbiased, and culturally appropriate.

Reliability

Reliability refers to consistency in the measurement process. A reliable instrument gives the same (or nearly the same) result every time. However, no instrument will ever provide perfect accuracy in measurement. Green and Lewis (1986) illustrate the theory of reliability with an equation, where total score (obtained score) equals the true score (unobservable) plus an error score. The total score represents the individual's score obtained on the measuring instrument. The true score represents the score for the same individual if all conditions and the measuring instrument were perfect. The error score represents the portion of the total score that is generated from the "imprecision in measurement due to human error, uncontrollable environment occurrences, inappropriateness of measurement instruments, and other unanticipated things" (Dignan, 1995, p. 40). For example, suppose the total score of an individual on a knowledge test was 85 out of a possible 100 points. The question then becomes is the 85% a true indication of the person's knowledge. If the conditions under which the score was generated were perfect and the measurement instrument had perfect reliability the error score would be zero and we could say, "yes the 85% is a true indication of the person's knowledge." However, if the conditions under which the score was generated were *not* perfect (e.g., the person did not have enough time to take the test) and the measurement instrument *did not* have perfect reliability (e.g., it included several poorly worded questions) the error score would *not* be zero and we say, "no the 85% is *not* a true indication of the person's knowledge. This person may really know more, or maybe less, than was indicated by the score." Thus planners need to strive to collect data under the best conditions with the most reliable measurement instruments possible (Cottrell & McKenzie, in press). Several methods of determining reliability are available.

Internal Consistency   **Internal consistency,** which is the most commonly used method of estimating reliability (Windsor et al., 1994), refers to the intercorrelations among the individual items on the instrument, that is, whether all items on the instrument are measuring part of the total area. This can be done by logically examining the instrument to ensure that the items reflect what is to be measured and that the level of difficulty of all items is the same. Statistical methods can also be used to determine internal consistency by correlating the items on the test with the total score.

Test-retest reliability   **Test-retest reliability,** or stability reliability, "is used to generate evidence of stability over a period" (Torabi, 1994, p. 57) of time. To establish this type of reliability the same instrument is used to measure the same group of people under similar, or the same conditions, at two different points in time and the two sets of data generated by the measurement are used to calculate a correlation coefficient (Cottrell & McKenzie, in press). The amount of time between the test and retest may vary from a few hours to a few weeks. A maximum amount of time should be allowed between the test and retest so that individuals are not responding on the basis of remembering responses they made the first time, but it should not be so long that other events could occur in the intervening time to influence their responses. To avoid the problems of retesting, parallel forms (equivalent forms) of the test can be administered to the participants and the results can be correlated.

Rater Reliability   **Rater reliability** focuses on the consistency between individuals who are observing or rating the same event or when one individual is observing or rating a series of events. If two or more raters are involved, it is referred to as **interrater reliability.** If only one individual is observing or rating a series of events, it is referred to as *intrarater reliability.* There are several different ways to calculate rater reliability, but the most common is as a percentage of agreement between/among raters or within an individual rater. An example of interrater reliability would be the percent of agreement between two observers who are observing passing drivers in cars for safety belt use. If ten cars are observed by the raters and they agree eight out of ten times on whether the drivers are wearing their safety belts, the interrater reliability would be 80%. **Intrarater reliability** would be the degree to which one rater agrees with himself or herself on the characteristics of an observation over time. For example, when a rater is evaluating the CPR skills of participants in his or her program, the rater should be consistent while observing and evaluating the skills of the participants.

Parallel Forms Reliability   **Parallel forms reliability,** or equivalent forms or alternate-forms reliability, focuses on whether different forms of the same measurement instrument when measuring the same subjects will produce similar results (means, standard deviations, and item intercorrelations). The usefulness of having measurement instruments that possess parallel forms reliability is being able to test the same subjects on different occasions (e.g., using a pretest posttest evaluation design) without worry that the subjects will score better on the second administration (posttest) because they remember questions from the first administration (pretest) of the instrument. A good example of parallel forms reliability is found in the different versions of the standardized college entrance examinations (Cottrell & McKenzie, in press).

Validity

When designing a data collection instrument, planners/evaluators must ensure that it measures what it is intended to measure. This refers to the **validity** of the measurement—whether it is correctly measuring the concepts under investigation. Using a valid instrument increases the chance that planners/evaluators are measuring what they want to measure, thus ruling out other possible explanations for the results. We will discuss several types of validity.

Face Validity   The lowest level of validity is face validity. A measure is said to have **face validity** if, on the face, the measure appears to measure what it is suppose to measure (McDermott & Sarvela, 1999). It differs from the other forms of validity in that it lacks some form of systematic logical analysis of the content (Hopkins, Stanley, & Hopkins, 1990). An example of face validity might include a planner/evaluator asking a colleague to look over a series of questions to see if the questions seem reasonable to include on a questionnaire about, for example, heart disease. Face validity is a good first step toward creating a valid measurement instrument, but is not a replacement for the other means of establishing validity (Cottrell & McKenzie, in press).

Content Validity   **Content validity** refers to "the degree to which an instrument measures all of the domains that constitute a concept" (Valente, 2002, p. 161). For example, when planning a risk reduction program for cardiovascular disease, the program planner can conduct a review of the literature in the area of cardiovascular risk reduction in order to ensure that all major risk factors, such as smoking, exercise, and diet, are included on a questionnaire.

Content validity is usually established by using a group (jury or panel) of experts to review the instrument. After such a group is identified, they would be asked to review each element of the instrument for its appropriateness to be included. The collective opinion of the experts is then used to determine the content of the instrument. McKenzie and colleagues (1999) present a method of establishing content validity that includes both qualitative and quantitative steps.

Criterion-Related Validity   **Criterion-related validity** refers to the extent to which data generated from a measurement instrument are correlated with data generated from a measure (criterion) of the phenomenon being studied, usually an individual's behavior or performance. Criterion-related validity can be divided into two subtypes: predictive and concurrent validity (McKenzie et al., 1999).

If the measurement used will be correlated with a future measurement of the same phenomenon, as with the use of standardized test scores to predict future college success, the criterion validity is known as **predictive validity. Concurrent validity** is established when a new instrument and an established valid instrument that measure the same characteristics are administered to the same subjects, and the results of the new instrument are compared to the results of the valid instrument. For example, if a planner/evaluator wanted to establish the validity of a new test for breast cancer, he or she administers both the new instrument and another already valid breast cancer instrument to the same subjects and then compares the results. The new instrument would be valid if the results compared favorably with the established instrument. In both subtypes of criterion-related validity, the aim is to legitimize the inferences that can be made by establishing their predictive ability for a related criterion (Borg & Gall, 1989).

Construct Validity   Though criterion-related validity is very useful in establishing validity, there are times when there is not an existing criterion from which to compare, or the phenomenon that planners want to measure is more abstract than concrete, such as the constructs of locus of control, self-efficacy, or subjective norm. In such cases, validity can be established via construct validity (Cottrell & McKenzie, in press). **Construct validity** "is the degree to which a measure correlates with other measures it is theoretically expected to correlate with. Construct validity tests the theoretical framework within which the instrument is expected to perform" (Valente, 2002, p. 161). An instrument that has construct validity will possess both convergent validity and discriminant validity. **Convergent validity** requires that the measurement instrument should correlate with related variables (Bowling, 2002). For example, an instrument that purports to measure a person's self-efficacy for regular exercise should positively correlate with that person's exercise behavior. That is, a person who is self-efficacious with regard to exercise would exercise regularly regardless of the circumstances (i.e., normal day, busy day, inclement weather, while on vacation). **Discriminant validity** requires that the measurement instrument *not* correlate with dissimilar variables (Bowling, 2002). Thus in the exercise example above the self-efficacy instrument would not be expected to correlate positively with a person's inactivity.

Sensitivity and Specificity   When speaking about validity, planners should also be familiar with the terms sensitivity and specificity. These are terms that are used in the health care settings and epidemiology to express the validity of screening and diagnostic tests (Cottrell & McKenzie, in press). **Sensitivity** is defined as the ability of the test to identify correctly those with a disease or condition (Mausner & Kramer, 1985). It is recorded as the proportion of true positive cases correctly identified as positive on the test (Timmreck, 1997). The better the sensitivity the fewer the false positives. **Specificity** is defined as the ability of the test to identify correctly those who do not have a disease or condition (Mausner & Kramer, 1985). It is recorded as the proportion of true negative cases correctly identified as negative on the test (Timmreck, 1997). And the better the specificity the fewer the number of false negatives. "An ideal screening test would be 100% sensitive and 100% specific. In practice this does not occur; sensitivity and specificity are usually inversely related" (Mausner & Kramer, 1985, p. 217).

One final thought before leaving our discussion of validity, the validity of an instrument is thought to be a more important issue than reliability. If an instrument does not measure what is supposed to, then it does not matter if it is reliable (Windsor et al., 1994).

Unbiased

Biased data are those data that have been distorted because of the way they have been collected. In order to effectively plan and evaluate health promotion programs, planners/evaluators must work to eliminate bias. Windsor and colleagues (1994) describe ways in which bias can occur in data collection—for example, when participants do not feel comfortable answering a sensitive question, when participants act differently because they know they are being watched, when certain characteristics of the interviewer influence a response, when participants answer questions in a particular way regardless of the questions being asked, or when a bias sample has been selected from the priority population (see information later in this chapter on sampling). There are a number of steps planners/evaluators can take to limit bias. For example, if data are being collected via observation, the observation should be as unobtrusive as possible. If sensitive questions are being asked of respondents, then those collecting such data need to ensure that the data are being collected in a confidential way (the identity of the respondent can be determined but not released), and consider collecting the data via an anonymous means (there is no way of identifying the respondent). No matter how data are collected, the reduction of bias techniques will increase the accuracy of the results.

Culturally Appropriate

"Culture shapes the way of life shared by members of a population. It is the sociocultural adaptation or design for living that people have worked out (and continue to work out) in the course of their history" (Ogbu, 1987, 156). Therefore, people from different cultures are likely to possess different values, beliefs, traditions, and perceptions. These cultural values, beliefs, traditions, and perceptions affect nearly all activities of individuals, including their health-related behavior (Kline & Huff, 1999) and responding to questions related to health. "As cultures vary, so do notions of what the human body symbolizes, how it should appear, how it functions most appropriately and why, and when and how it should be treated" (AAHE, 1994, p. 5). Thus culture influences program participants' ability to understand, internalize, and exercise positive health practices that will enhance the quality of life. For example, if we examine the diet of individuals from different cultures (i.e., religion, race), it is easy to see the impact of culture on what people eat. Some cultures see some foods as an important part of their diet, while others see the same foods as dirty and not to be consumed. Thus when collecting data from diverse populations, planners/evaluators need to respond appropriately to cultural differences. In other words, planners/evaluators need to be culturally sensitive and work toward being culturally competent. "'**Cultural sensitivity**' implies knowledge that cultural differences (as well as similarities) exist, along with the refusal to assign cultural differences such values as better or worse, more or less intelligent, right or wrong; they are simply differences" (Anderson & Fenichel, 1989, p. 8). **Cultural competence** refers to "a process for effectively working within the cultural context of an individual or community from a diverse cultural or ethnic background" (Campinha-Bacote, 1994, pp. 1–2).

Methods of Data Collection

Self-Report

Written questionnaires, telephone interviews, face-to-face (or in-depth) interviews, and electronic interviews are methods of collecting self-report data. **Self-report data** refers to data that are generated by having individuals (the **respondents**) report about themselves. Thus, respondents are asked to recall ("When was your last visit to your dentist?") and report accurate ("On average, how many calories do you consume a day?") information. Self-report measures are essential for many needs assessments and evaluations because of the need to obtain subjective assessments of experiences (e.g., feelings about available programs, self-assessments of health status, or health behavior, such as eating patterns) (Bowling, 1997). Self-report measures have broad appeal to those who need to collect data, because "they are often quick to administer and involve little interpretation by the investigator" (Bowling, 1997, p. 12). However, planners/evaluators should be aware that self-report data do have limitations. One such limitation is **bias.** (See the previous section of this chapter for a discussion about bias.) To overcome some of these limitations and to maximize the usefulness of self-report, Baranowski (1985, pp. 181–182) has developed eight steps to increase the accuracy of this method of data collection:

1. Select measures that clearly reflect program outcomes.
2. Select measures that have been designed to anticipate response problems and that have been validated.
3. Conduct a pilot study with the target [priority] population.
4. Anticipate and correct major sources of unreliability.
5. Employ quality-control procedures to detect other sources of error.
6. Employ multiple methods.
7. Use multiple measures.
8. Use experimental and control groups with random assignment to control for biases in self-report.

By following these steps, planners/evaluators can enhance the accuracy of self-report, making this a more effective method of data collection.

For a variety of reasons, there are times when those in the priority population cannot respond for themselves or do not want to respond. In such situations, planners will have to collect the data indirectly. Such a method is referred to as a **proxy** (or in-direct) **measure.** A proxy measure is an outcome measure that provides evidence that a behavior has occurred. Or as Dignan (1995) states, "indirect measures are un-mistakable signs that a specific behavior has occurred" (p. 103). Examples of proxy or measures may include: 1) lower blood pressure for the behavior of medication taking, 2) body weight for the behaviors of exercise and dieting, 3) cotinine in the blood for tobacco use, 4) empty alcoholic beverages in the trash for consumption of alcohol, or 5) a spouse reporting on the compliance of his/her partner (Cottrell & McKenzie, in press). Proxy measurements of skills or behavior "usually requires more resources and cooperation than self-report or direct observation" (Dignan, 1995, p. 104). The great-est concern associated with using proxy measures is making sure that the measure is both valid and reliable (Cottrell & McKenzie, in press).

Questions Used in Self-Report   The presentation, wording, and sequence of questions in self-report questionnaires and interviews can be critical in gaining the necessary information. The questionnaire or interview should begin by explaining the purpose of the study and why the individual's responses are important. A cover letter should accompany a mailed questionnaire, explaining the need for the information and including very clear directions for supplying it (see Figure 5.1 for an example of a cover letter). The name, address, and telephone number of the planner/ evaluator or another contact person can also be included in case the respondent needs additional information to complete the questionnaire. A stamped, addressed envelope should be enclosed. Box 5.1 presents a checklist developed by Bourque and Fielder (1995) to use when writing cover letters to potential survey respondents.

With telephone or face-to-face interviews, the interviewer can give information about the study and explain the need for information from the individual contacted. This introduction can be followed by general questions to put the respondent at ease or to develop a rapport between the interviewer and the respondent.

After several general questions come the questions of interest. Any questions that deal with sensitive topics should be posed at the end of the questionnaire or inter-view. Answers to questions about drug use, sexuality, or even demographic informa-tion, such as income level, are more readily answered when the respondents understand the need for the information, are assured of confidentiality or anonymity, and feel comfortable with the interviewer or the questionnaire. If the respondent ends the interview or does not complete the instrument when asked sensitive ques-tions, the other information collected can still be used; this is another advantage of putting these questions at the end.

The actual questions should be clear and unbiased. It is important to avoid ques-tions with a specific direction ("How have you enjoyed the class?") that would guide the respondent's answer. Two-part (double-barreled) questions should also be avoid-ed ("Do you brush and floss your teeth?"). Another problem with question design oc-curs when the question assumes knowledge that individuals may not have or includes terminology that they may not understand ("What cardiovascular benefits do you feel you gain from aerobic exercise?").

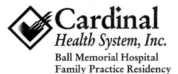

Cardinal
Health System, Inc.
Ball Memorial Hospital
Family Practice Residency

April 1, 2004

Dear Family Physician:

We are conducting a survey to study Indiana family physicians' practices of and preparation for patient education. We respectfully request your response to the enclosed questionnaire at your earliest convenience. The instrument should take you about ten minutes to complete. There are no right or wrong answers. We recognize that some of the questions, by necessity, are quite personal. Be assured that your individual responses will remain anonymous and only summarized group data will be reported. Your participation in the survey is voluntary.

Since the number of questionnaires being sent out is limited, your participation is important for the success of the project. We therefore request that you complete and return the questionnaire in the enclosed, self-addressed, postage-paid reply envelop no later than April 15, 2004. If you have any questions about this survey or want to be sent a copy of the results, please contact Jim McKenzie at 765/285–8345 (voice), 765/285–3210 (fax), or jmckenzie@bsu.edu (email).

Thank you in advance for your assistance in completing the enclosed questionnaire.

Sincerely,

Amy E Banter, M.D.
Associate Director
Family Practice Residency Program
Ball Memorial Hospital

James F. McKenzie, Ph.D., MPH, CHES
Professor
Department of Physiology & Health Science
Ball State University

Encl: Questionnaire
          Self-addressed, postage-paid envelop

Edmund F. Ball medical Education Building
221 N. Celia Ave. • Muncie, IN 47303 • Office: (765) 747-3376 • Toll free: (800) 279-1666
Fax: (765) 741-1983 • E-Mail: jkurtz@cami3.com • Web site: www.ballhospital.org
Cardinal Health System. The System Works. For You.

Figure 5.1 Example cover letter for data collection instrument

---

Box 5.1 Checklist for Cover Letter to Survey Respondents

- Explain the purpose of the study.
- Describe who is sponsoring the study.
- Consider sending an advanced letter.
- Consider using other methods such as newsletters or flyers to publicize the study.
- Include a cover letter with a questionnaire.
  —Use letter head.
  —Date the letter to be consistent with the actual date of the mailing or administration.
  —Provide a name and phone number for the respondent to contact for further information.
  —Personalize the salutation, if feasible.
  —Maximize the attractiveness and readability of the letter.
- Explain how the respondents were chosen and why their participation is important.
- Explain when and how to return the questionnaire.
- Describe incentives, if used.
- Directly or indirectly provide a realistic estimate of the time required by the average respondent to complete the questionnaire.
- Explain how the confidentiality of the respondents' data will be protected.
- Determine whether and how a deadline date will be provided for returning the questionnaires.

Source: Bourque & Fielder (1995), pp.121–122, copyright © by Sage Publications. Reprinted by permission of Sage Publications, Inc.

The way in which data collection questions are worded is extremely important in gaining the needed information. The result of a poorly worded question was evident to one health promotion planner who was planning a smoking cessation program for employees. When asked, "Do you feel we need a smoking cessation program?" most employees said yes. The planner realized later that he should have also asked the question, "If offered, would you attend a smoking cessation program?" since very few employees participated.

If possible, planners/evaluators should use existing questionnaires. This requires gaining permission from the author if the document is not in the public domain. (Documents in the public domain can be freely used without requesting permission but yet giving credit for the work of others.) The advantages to using questionnaires that have been developed by experts include increased credibility, lower cost, less planning time needed, and more documentation of validity and reliability. The major disadvantage—one that prevents the use of existing questionnaires in many cases—is that the items on the existing instrument may not all be relevant or appropriate to the program being planned or evaluated. Adaptations may be needed so that the questionnaire will fit with program objectives or the local target population.

If a questionnaire is not available, one must be developed. When designing a questionnaire (see Box 5.2 for steps to follow when developing a data collection instrument) to collect self-reported data, evaluators/planners can use several types of questions. The most structured or closed types of questions have yes-no or multiple-choice responses, and are most often used for knowledge questions. These types of responses are the easiest to tabulate but do not allow the individual to elaborate on the answers. They may also force a person into a choice because of the limited number of responses to each question. An "other" category, with space to list the exact nature of the "other" response, may serve to give the respondent another option. However, giving the respondents an opportunity to provide their own answers on multiple-choice questions makes it more difficult to categorize responses when the data are analyzed, thus reducing one of the main benefits of such questions. One way to ensure that the most common responses to questions are included in the multiple choices is to involve several individuals (especially those in the priority population) in the formation of the instrument.

Attitude questions generally use less structured forms. Scales, such as Likert or semantic differentials, are often used, with the respondent choosing a response along a

---

Box 5.2 Steps for Creating a Measurement Instrument

Step 0: Be familiar with the related literature.

Step 1: Determine the specific purpose (or goal) and the objectives of the proposed instrument.

Step 2: Who are the individuals who are to be measured?

Step 3: Identify the conceptual theory/model that will provide the foundation for the instrument.

Step 4: Create a table of specifications and specifications for the instrument.

Step 5: Identify items from other existing instruments that could be used.

Step 6: Create new instrument items.

Step 7: Create directions for completing the instrument, and directions and instructions for administering the instrument.

Step 8: Establish procedures for scoring the instrument.

Step 9: Assemble an initial draft of the instrument.

Step 10: Establish face validity for the instrument.

Step 11: Check the readability of the instrument.

Step 12: Establish content validity for the instrument.

Step 13: Pilot-test the instrument.

Step 14: Conduct item analysis, factor analysis, and checks of psychometric qualities.

Step 15: Review, revise, and reassess.

Step 16: Conduct a second pilot-test, if necessary.

Step 17: Determine a cut score.

Step 18: Refine as needed and create the final version.

Source: Cottrell & McKenzie (in press).

continuum, generally ranging from a five- to a seven-point scale. For example, re-sponses to the statement, "I feel that it is important to limit my use of salt," might be rated on a five-point scale ranging from "strongly agree" to "strongly disagree."

Unstructured or open-ended questions—such as essay questions, short-answer questions, journals, or logs—may be used to gain descriptive information about a pro-gram, but are generally not used when collecting quantitative data. Such responses are often difficult to summarize or to code for analysis. Box 5.3 provides examples of structured and unstructured types of questions.

Written Questionnaires   Probably the most often used method of collecting self-reported data is the written questionnaire. It has several advantages, notably the abil-ity to reach a large number of respondents in a short period of time, even if there is a large geographic area to be covered. This method offers low cost with minimum staff time needed. However, it often has the lowest response rate.

With a written questionnaire, each individual receives the same questions and in-structions in the same format, so that the possibility of response bias is lessened. The corresponding disadvantage, however, is the inability to clarify any questions or con-fusion on the part of the respondent.

As mentioned, the response rate for mailed questionnaires tends to be low, but there are several ways to overcome this problem. One way is to include with the questionnaire a postcard that identifies the person in some way (such as by name or identification number). The individual is asked to return the questionnaire in the envelope provided and to send the postcard back separately. Anonymity is thus maintained, but the planner/evaluator knows who returned a questionnaire. The planner/evaluator can then send a follow-up mailing (including a letter indicating the importance of a response and another copy of the questionnaire with a return envelope) to the individuals who did not return a postcard from the first mailing. The use of incentives also can increase the response rate. For example, some hospitals offer free health risk appraisals to those who return a completed needs assessment instrument.

The appearance of the questionnaire is also extremely important when collecting data. It should be attractive, easy to read, and offer ample space for the respondents' answers. It should also be easy to understand and complete, since written question-naires provide no opportunity to clarify a point while the respondent is completing the questionnaire. All mailed questionnaires should be accompanied by a cover letter, as previously discussed.

Short questionnaires that do not take a long time to complete and questionnaires that clearly explain the need for the information are more likely to be returned. Planners/evaluators should give thought to designing a questionnaire that is as easy to complete and return as possible.

Telephone Interviews   Compared to mailed surveys or face-to-face interviews, the telephone interview offers a relatively easy method of collecting self-reported data at a moderate cost. The planner/evaluator must choose a way of selecting individuals to participate in this type of data collection; this method will reach only those individu-als who have access to a telephone. One possibility is to call a randomly selected group of people who have completed a health promotion program. Another method is to se-lect telephone numbers at random from a telephone directory—for example, a local

Box 5.3 Examples of Self-Report Questions

Structured (Closed)

I. *Dichotomous*

  1. What is your sex?
     a. Female   b. Male

  2. A risk factor for heart disease is sedentary lifestyle.
     a. True   b. False

II. *Multiple Choice*

  1. The leading cause of death in the United States for adults is
     a. Cancer   b. Heart disease
     c. Injuries   d. AIDS

  2. What type of computer do you use?
     a. IBM   b. Apple
     c. Gateway   d. Other (please specify): _____

III. *Matching*

  Vitamin deficiencies
  1. Vitamin A   a. Frequent infection
  2. Vitamin C   b. Slow blood clotting
  3. Vitamin D   c. Night blindness
  4. Vitamin K   d. Bone softening

  Grams of saturated fats
  1. Butter, 1 tbsp.   a. 9
  2. Ice cream, 4 oz. b. 7.1
  3. Chicken, 3 oz.   c. 5
  4. One hot dog   d. 1.2

Less Structured (But Still Closed)

I. *Likert*

  1. Women should be able to
     have an abortion if they   *Strongly*   *Strongly*
     choose to do so.   *agree*   *Agree*   *Neutral*   *Disagree*   *disagree*

  2. I feel I can exercise
     regardless of   *Strongly*   *Strongly*
     weather conditions.   *agree*   *Agree*   *Neutral*   *Disagree*   *disagree*

II. *Semantic Differentials*

  1. Smokeless tobacco is   *Good*   __ __ __ __ __   *Bad*
  2. When taking a test, I feel *Nervous* __ __ __ __ __   *Calm*

(Box 5.3 *continues*)

(Box 5.3 *continued*)

III. *Rank Order*

  1. Put the following values in order, from most important in your life to least important:
     a. health   _____
     b. love   _____
     c. friendship _____
     d. emotional security _____
     e. financial security _____

  2. Rank-order the following servings of foods from highest to lowest sources of protein:
     a. tuna   _____
     b. rice   _____
     c. sirloin steak _____
     d. cottage cheese _____
     e. bread   _____
     f. broccoli   _____

Unstructured (Open)

  I. *Completions*

  1. I like to exercise because _____

  2. The types of foods I generally eat are _____

  II. *Short-answer*

  1. List five advantages to conducting a worksite health promotion program.

  2. Describe the correct way to lift a heavy object to avoid straining your back.

  III. *Essay*

  1. Explain the difference between aerobic and anaerobic exercise. Include examples of each type of exercise, and discuss the importance of each in total fitness.

  2. Discuss the incidence of tuberculosis in the world today, including who is at risk and the public health measures to reduce the problem.

telephone book, student directory, church directory, or employee directory. This method will not reach all the population, since some people have unlisted telephone numbers. One way to overcome this problem is a method known as **random-digit dialing,** in which telephone number combinations are chosen at random. This method would include businesses as well as residences and nonworking as well as valid numbers, making it more time consuming. The numbers may be obtained from a table of random numbers or generated by a computer. The advantage of random-digit dialing is that it includes the entire survey population with a telephone in the area, including people with unlisted numbers. Drawbacks to this method include some peoples' resistance to answer questions over the telephone or resentment in being interrupted with an unwanted call. This later reason seems to be more of a problem with the increase in telemarketing. Those conducting the interviews may also have difficulty reaching individuals because of unanswered phones or answering machines.

Telephone interviewing requires trained interviewers; without proper training and use of a standard questionnaire, the interviewer may not be consistent during the interview. Explaining a question or offering additional information can cause a respondent to change an initial response, thus creating a chance for interviewer bias. The interviewer does have the opportunity to clarify questions, which is an advantage over the written questionnaire, but does not have the advantage of visual cues that the face-to-face interview offers.

Face-to-Face Interviews　At times, it is advantageous to administer the instrument to the respondents in a face-to-face interview setting. This method is time consuming, since it may require not only time for the actual interview but also travel time to the interview site and/or waiting time between interviews. As with telephone interviews, the interviewer must be carefully trained to conduct the interview in an unbiased manner. It is important to explain the need for the information in order to conduct the needs assessment/evaluation and to accurately record the responses. Methods of probing, or eliciting additional information about an individual's responses, are used in the face-to-face interview, and the interviewer must be skilled at this technique.

This method of self-report allows the interviewer to develop rapport with the respondent. The flexibility of this method, along with the availability of visual cues, has the advantage of gaining more complete evaluation data from respondents. Smaller numbers of respondents are included in this method, but the rate of participation is generally high. It is important to establish and follow procedures for selecting the respondents. There are also several disadvantages to the face-to-face interview. It is more expensive, requiring more staff time and training of interviewers. Variations in the interviews, as well as differences between interviewers, may influence the results.

Electronic Interviews　With more and more individuals having access to the Internet, email has been explored (Kittleson, 1995, 1997, 2003) as a means of collecting data. Advantages to this type of data collection is that it is low in cost and almost instantaneous (McDermott & Sarvela, 1999). However, it has several drawbacks, including (1) access to a limited population, (2) lack of anonymity for respondents, and (3) easily ignored (McDermott & Sarvela, 1999). Until the drawbacks are overcome, this means of data collection will be used sparingly.

Group Interviews　Interviewing individuals in groups provides for economy of scale. That is, data can be collected from several people in a short period of time. But there are some drawbacks of such data collection that primarily revolve around one or more group members influencing the response of others. A specific form of group interview discussed in the previous chapter is focus groups. Focus groups are useful in collecting information for a needs assessment, but can also be used to determine if programs are being implemented effectively or determine program outcomes.

Observation

Observation, defined as "notice taken of an indicator" (Green & Lewis, 1986, p. 363), can be used to obtain information regarding the behavior of participants in a program. The observation can be direct or indirect. *Direct observation* means actually seeing a situation or behavior. For example, planners/evaluators might observe students in the cafeteria to gain information about actual food choices and consumption. This method is somewhat time consuming, but it seldom encounters the problem of people refusing to participate in the data collection, resulting in a high response rate.

Observation is generally more accurate than self-report, but the presence of the observer may alter the behavior of the people being observed. For example, having someone observe smoking behavior may cause smokers to smoke less out of self-consciousness due to their being under observation, not as a result of the program. When respondents know they are being observed it is referred to as **obtrusive observation. Unobtrusive observation** means just the opposite, persons are being studied not aware they are being measured, assessed, or tested. Typically, unobtrusive observation provides less bias data, but some question whether or not unobtrusive observation is ethical.

Differences among observers may also bias the results, since different observers may not observe and report behaviors in the same manner. Some behaviors, such as safety belt use, are very easy to observe accurately. Others, such as a person's degree of tension, are more difficult to observe. This method of data collection requires a clear definition of the exact behavior to observe and how to record it, in order to avoid subjective observations. Observer bias can be reduced by providing training and by determining rater reliability. If the observers are skilled, observation can provide accurate evaluation data at a moderate cost.

As noted earlier in this chapter, *indirect observation* (or proxy measures) can also be used to determine whether or not a behavior has occurred. This can be completed by either "observing" the outcomes of a behavior or by asking others (e.g., a spouse) to report on such outcomes (see the earlier discussion on proxy measures). In addition, these measures can be used to verify self-reports when observations of the actual changes in behavior cannot be observed.

Existing Records

Using existing records may be an efficient way to obtain the necessary information for a needs assessment or evaluation without the need for additional data collection. The advantages include low cost, minimum staff needed, and ease in randomization. The disadvantages to using this method of data collection include difficulty in gaining access to necessary records and the possible lack of availability of all the information needed for program evaluation.

Examples of the use of existing records include checking medical records to monitor blood pressure and cholesterol levels of participants in an exercise program, reviewing insurance usage of employees enrolled in an employee health promotion program, and comparing the academic records of students engaging in an after-school weight loss program. In these situations, as with all needs assessments or evaluations using existing records, the cooperation of the agencies that hold the records is essential. At times, agencies may be willing to collect additional information to aid in the needs assessment for or an evaluation of a health promotion program. Keepers of records are concerned about confidentiality and the release of private information. The importance of privacy for those planners working in health care settings was further emphasized in April 2003 with the enactment of the *Standards for Privacy of Individually Identifiable Health Information* section (The Privacy Rule) of the Health Insurance Portability and Accountability Act of 1996 (officially known as Public Law 104–191 and referred to as HIPAA). The Rule sets national standards that health plans, health care clearinghouses, and health care providers who conduct certain health care transactions electronically must implement to protect and guard against the misuse of individually identifiable health information. Failure to implement the standards can lead to civil and criminal penalties (USDHHS, 2003). Planners can deal with these privacy issues by getting permission from all participants to use their records or by using only anonymous data.

Meetings

Meetings are a good source of information for a preliminary needs assessment or various aspects of evaluation. For example, if a fitness program is being evaluated, the evaluators, staff, and some participants may meet early in the planning and implementation stages to discuss the status of the program.

The meeting structure can be flexible to avoid limiting the scope of the information gained. The cost of this form of data collection is minimal. Possible biases may occur when meetings are used as the sole source of data collection. Those involved may give "socially acceptable" responses to questions rather than discussing actual concerns. There also may be limited input if relatively few participants are included, or if one or two participants dominate the discussion.

Summarized in Table 5.1 are the advantages and disadvantages of the various methods of data collection. As discussed in Chapter 14, it may be beneficial to combine methods of data collection as well as to incorporate quantitative and qualitative data.

Sampling

The need to select participants from whom data will be collected can occur at several times during the processes of program planning or evaluation. Depending on the size of the priority population, planners/evaluators may want to collect data from all participants **(census)** or from only some of the participants **(sample).** Each of the participants is referred to as a sampling unit. A **sampling unit** is the element or set of elements considered for selection as part of a sample (Babbie, 1992). A sampling unit "may be an individual, an organization, or a geographical area" (Bowling, 2002, p. 166).

Figure 5.2 illustrates the relationship between groups of individuals. All individuals, unspecified by time or place, constitute the **universe**—for example, all U.S. citizens, regardless of where they reside in the world. Within the universe is a **population** of individuals specified by time or place, such as all U.S. residents in the 50 United States on January 1, 2004. Within this population is a **survey population,** composed of all individuals who are accessible to the planners. The key term here is *accessible*. For example, all U.S. citizens who are accessible and can be reached by telephone would be a survey population. Obviously, this would not include those without telephones, such as those who chose not to own them, those institutionalized, and the homeless.

A survey population may still be too large to include in its entirety. For this reason, a sample is chosen from the survey population, a process called **sampling.** These are the individuals who will be included in the data collection process. Using a sample rather than an entire survey population helps contain costs. For example, using a sample reduces the amount of staff time needed to conduct interviews, the cost of postage for written questionnaires, and the time and cost of travel to conduct observations.

Table 5.1 Methods of data collection

Method	Advantages	Disadvantages
SELF-REPORT		
Written questionnaire via mail	Large outreach	Possible low response rate
	No interviewer bias	Possible unrepresentation
	Convenient	No clarification of questions
	Low cost	Need homogeneous group if
	Minimum staff time required	response is low
	Easy to administer	No assurance addressee was
	Quick	respondent
	Standardized	
Telephone interview	Moderate cost	Possible problem of representation
	Relatively easy to administer	Possible interviewer bias
	Permits unlimited callbacks	Requires trained interviewers
	Can cover wide geographic area	
Face-to-face interview	High response rate	Expensive
	Flexibility	Requires trained interviewers
	Gain in-depth data	Possible interviewer bias
	Develop rapport	Limits sample size
		Time consuming
Electronic mail*	Low cost	Must have email access
	Ease and convenience	Self-selection
	Almost instantaneous	Lacks anonymity
		Risk of being "purged"
		Lack of "cueing"
		Must be short
		Noninvasive items only
Group interview	High response rate	May intimidate and suppress
	Efficient and economical	individual differences
	Can stimulate productivity of	Fosters conformity
	others	Group pressure may influence
		responses
OBSERVATION	Accurate behavioral data	Requires trained observers
	Can be unobtrusive	May bias behavior
	Moderate cost	Possible observer bias
		May be time consuming
EXISTING RECORDS	Low cost	May need agency cooperation
	Easy to randomize	Certain data may be unavailable
	Avoid data collection	Often incomplete
	Minimum staff needed	Confidential restrictions
MEETINGS	Good for formative evaluation	Possible result bias
	Low cost	Limited input from participants
	Flexible	

*From McDermott and Sarvela (1999).

How the sample is chosen is critical to the result of the needs assessment or evaluation: Does the information gained from the sample reflect the knowledge, attitudes, and behaviors of the survey population? According to Green and Lewis (1986), the sampling bias is the difference between the sampling estimate and the actual population value. The sampling bias can be controlled by controlling the sampling

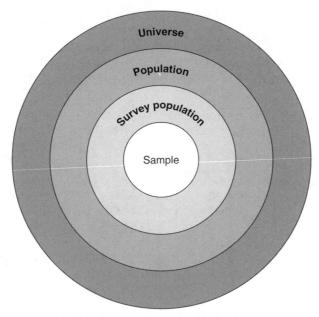

Figure 5.2 Relationship of groups of individuals

procedure—that is, how the sample is chosen. The ability to generalize the results to the survey population is greater when the sampling bias is reduced.

Probability Sample

Increasing the chance that the sample is representative of the survey population is achieved by **random selection.** This assures that each person in the survey population has an equal chance and known probability of being selected, thus creating a **probability sample.**

There are a number of different methods for selecting a probability sample. The most basic of the probability sampling methods is selecting a **simple random sample (SRS).** In order to select a SRS, or for that matter any probability sample, the planner must have a list or "quasi-list" (Babbie, 1992) of all sampling units in the survey population. This list is referred to as the **frame.** Often times sampling frames have the names and contact information for all in the survey population such as with membership lists, patients of a clinic, and parents of children enrolled in a certain school or program. Other times the frame may be just the title of an individual or organization, such as the Director of Environmental Services in the 94 local health departments in Indiana, or a list of all the voluntary health agencies in the county (Cottrell & McKenzie, in press).

Once the sampling frame has been identified, the planner can proceed with the process of selecting a SRS. It begins with assigning a number with an equal number of digits to each sampling unit in the frame. Suppose, for example, we have a frame of 200 individuals. Thus the first person in the frame would be given the number 000. The rest of the individuals in the frame would be assigned consecutive numbers and the last person in the frame would be assigned the number 199. Once it is decid-

Table 5.2 Abbreviated table of random numbers

Row/Column	A	B	C	D	E
1	75 51	02 17	71 04	33 93	36 60
2	42 75	76 22	23 87	56 54	84 68
3	00 47	37 59	08 56	23 81	22 42
4	74 01	23 19	55 59	79 09	69 82
5	66 22	42 40	15 96	74 90	75 89
6	09 24	34 42	00 68	72 10	71 37
7	89 22	10 23	62 65	78 77	47 33
8	51 27	23 02	13 92	44 13	96 51
9	17 18	01 34	10 98	37 48	93 86
10	02 28	54 60	01 11	28 35	54 32

ed how large the sample should be, the sample can be selected. For the purpose of this example let's suppose a sample size of 20 is desired. To select these 20 individuals, a computer could be used to randomly select 20 numbers between 000 and 199, or it could be done manually by using a table of random numbers (see Table 5.2) (Cottrell & McKenzie, in press).

In order to use a table of random numbers, the manner in which the table will be used needs to be set forth. Since these tables are generated randomly (by computer), it really does not matter which way one moves through the table as long as it is done in a consistent manner. For example, the process set forth could be to: 1) use the first three digits in the columns of numbers (because all individuals in the example frame have a three digit number i.e., 000 to 199), 2) proceed down the columns (as opposed to up or across the rows), 3) at the bottom of the column proceed to the top of the next column to the right, and 4) proceed in this same manner until the 20 individuals are selected. To insure that this process is indeed random, the process must begin with a random start. That is, the planner cannot just pick the first number at the top of column one and proceed down through the column because every individual in the survey population would not have an equal chance of being selected. The planner can accomplish the random start by closing his/her eyes and pointing to a place on the table of random numbers then opening his/her eyes and proceeding through the table in the way that was set forth above (Cottrell & McKenzie, in press).

A **systematic sample** also uses a frame and takes every *N*th person (determined by dividing the survey population size by the sample size, *N/n*), beginning with a randomly selected individual. For example, suppose that we want to choose a sample of ten people from a survey population of 100. We start by randomly choosing a number between 001 and 100, such as 026, using a table of random numbers. We then choose every tenth (*N/n* = 100/10 = 10) person (036, 046, 056, 076, 086, 096, 006, 016) until we have the ten subjects for the sample. In this way, everyone in the survey population has an equal chance of being selected. A simple random sample or systematic sample can also be used to select groups instead of individuals. When this occurs, it is called **cluster sampling.**

Table 5.3 Summary of probability sampling procedures

Sample	Primary Descriptive Elements
Simple Random	Each subject has an equal chance of being selected if table of random numbers and random start are used.
"Fishbowl" (or "Out of a Hat")	Approximates simple random sampling, but not as precise. Can be done with or without replacement.
Systematic	Using a list (e.g., membership list or telephone book), subjects are selected at a constant interval (N/n) after a random start.
Nonproportional Stratified	The population is divided into subgroups based on key characteristics (strata), and subjects are selected from the subgroups at random to ensure representation of the characteristic.
Proportional Stratified	Like the stratified random sample, but subjects are selected in proportion to the numerical strength of strata in the population.
Cluster or Area	Random sampling of groups (e.g., teachers' classes) or areas (e.g., city blocks) instead of individuals.
Matrix	The responses of several randomly selected subjects to different items are combined to form the response of one.

Source: Adapted from E. R. Babbie, *The Practice of Social Research,* 6th ed. (Belmont, CA: Wadsworth, 1992); P. C. Cozby, *Methods in Behavioral Research,* 3rd ed. (Palo Alto, CA: Mayfield, 1985); P. D. Leedy, *Practical Research: Planning and Design,* 5th ed. (New York: Macmillan, 1993); and R. J. McDermott and P. D. Sarvela, *Health Education Evaluation and Measurement: A Practitioner's Perspective,* 2nd ed. (New York: McGraw-Hill, 1999).

If it is important that certain groups should be represented in a sample, a **stratified random sample** can be selected. Such a method would be used if the planners felt that a certain variable (i.e., such as size, income, or age) might have an influence on the data collected from the participants. A stratified random sample might also be used if it is believed that because of the small numbers of a certain group in the survey population, representatives from that group may not be selected using a simple random sample. That is, you may have a survey population of 100 participants and in that 100 there are only eight of one group. If you were to select a sample of ten from the 100, there is a good chance that none of the eight from the small group might be selected (Cottrell & McKenzie, in press).

Here is an example of the use of a stratified random sample. To begin with, the planner first must divide the survey population into subgroups (or **strata**) then select a simple random sample from each strata. Suppose we were interested in collecting data from companies within a particular state concerning the number of health education programs offered for employees. Based upon past experience, we suspect the size of the business (i.e., number of employees) would affect the data we wanted to collect. That is, small companies might have fewer health education programs in general than large companies. Also, we know that there are only a couple of companies in the state that have a large number of employees. We could then divide the companies into strata by size, say small (1–100 employees), medium (101–1,000 students), and large (1,001+). Once the planners have decided how many to select from each strata, they have to decide whether to conduct a proportional stratified random sample or nonproportional stratified random sample. A **proportional stratified ran-**

dom sample would be used if the planners wanted the sample to mirror, in proportion, the survey population. That is, draw out the companies in the same proportions that they are represented in the survey population. Say in our example that there are 600 small companies, 350 medium companies, and 50 large companies and the desired sample size is 100. Planners would then select simple random samples of 60 small, 35 medium, and 5 large companies (Cottrell & McKenzie, in press).

A **nonproportional stratified random sample** may be used if the planners want equal representation from the different strata within the survey population. For example, suppose we wanted to collect information about the opinions of college students on a medium-size regional campus (the survey population) about a new alcohol use policy that was put in place by the administration and we wanted to hear equally from the different level of students (freshmen [n = 4,000], sophomores [n = 3,000], juniors [n = 2,000], and seniors [n = 1,000]) because it was thought that the policy would affect each class differently. If a sample size of 200 was desired, we would randomly select (using a simple random sample method) 50 students from each of the classes (Cottrell & McKenzie, in press). (See Table 5.3 for a summary of probability sampling procedures.)

Nonprobability Sample

There are times when a probability sample cannot be obtained or is not needed. In such cases, planners/evaluators can take **nonprobability samples,** samples in which all individuals in the survey population do not have an equal chance and a known probability of being selected to participate in the needs assessment or evaluation. Participants can be included on the basis of convenience (because they have volunteered or because they are available or can be easily contacted) or because they have a certain characteristic.

Nonprobability samples have limitations in the extent to which the results can be generalized to the total survey population. Bias may also occur since those who are

Table 5.4 Summary of nonprobability sampling procedures

Sample	Primary Descriptive Elements
Convenience	Includes any available subject meeting some minimum criterion usually being part of an accessible intact group.
Volunteer	Includes any subject motivated enough to self-select for a study.
Grab	Includes whomever investigators can access through direct contact, usually for interviews.
Homogeneous	Includes individuals chosen because of a unique trait or factor they possess.
Judgmental	Includes subjects whom the investigator judges to be "typical" of individuals possessing a given trait.
Snowball	Includes subjects identified by investigators, and any other persons referred by initial subjects.
Quota	Includes subjects chosen in approximate proportion to the population traits they are to "represent."

Source: R. J. McDermott & P. D. Sarvela, *Health Education Evaluation and Measurement: A Practitioner's Perspective,* 2nd ed. (New York: McGraw-Hill, 1999). Reprinted with permission of The McGraw-Hill Companies.

not included in the sample may differ in some way from those who are included. For example, including only the individuals who complete a health promotion program may bias the results; the findings might be different if all participants, including those who attended but did not complete the program, were surveyed.

Nonprobability samples can be used when planners/evaluators are unable to identify or contact all those in the survey population. These samples can also be used when resources are limited and a probability sample is too costly or time consuming. It is important that planners/evaluators understand the limitations of this type of sample when reporting the results. (See Table 5.4 for a summary of nonprobability sampling procedures.)

Sample Size

An often-asked question associated with sampling is, how many individuals are needed for planners to feel confident that sampling error is within an acceptable range so that reasonable conclusions can be drawn from the data analyzed? There is not an easy answer to this question. Appropriate sample size is determined by both practical and statistical considerations. From a practical standpoint, often the resources (i.e., personnel, financial) available to collect data is the determining factor on how large the sample will be. Asked another way, is the desired sample size affordable?

When analyzing sample size from a statistical standpoint, there are three major theoretical considerations used; central limit theorem (CLT), precision and reliability, and power analysis (Norwood, 2000). The CLT can provide the quickest answer to the sample size question. Mathematically, it has been shown that when a sample size approaches 30 in number, characteristics of that group approach the normal distribution of the group from which it was drawn. Thus a general rule for comparison purposes is, no group should be smaller than 30.

Determining sample size using precision and reliability, and power analysis is much more complicated. There is not enough space in this chapter to provide for the detailed explanations needed. Tables 5.5 and 5.6 are provided as examples of the application of these considerations. Detailed explanations of these concepts are presented in many statistics textbooks.

Table 5.5 Sample sizes for studies describing population proportions when the population size is known

| Population size/ | 95% Confidence Interval | | |
Sample size for precision of	±1	±3	±5
500	*	*	222
1,000	*	*	286
5,000	*	909	370
10,000	5,000	1,000	385
100,000	9,091	1,099	398
→∞	10,000	1,111	400

*=In these cases the assumption of normal approximation is poor, and the formula used to derive them does not apply.

Source: This table is derived from Yamane (1973).

Table 5.6 Sample sizes for the one-sample case for the mean

Directional ("one-tailed") test for numerical (interval or ratio) data

Effect size/Power	alpha = .05		alpha = .01	
	.80	.90	.80	.90
.20	155	215	251	326
.50	27	37	43	55
.80	12	17	19	23

Nondirectional ("two-tailed") test for numerical (interval or ratio) data

Effect size/Power	alpha = .05		alpha = .01	
	.80	90	.80	90
.20	197	263	292	372
.50	34	44	50	63
.80	15	19	22	27

Source: This table is derived from Hinkle, Oliver, & Hinkle (1985).

Pilot Test

A **pilot test** (sometimes referred to as *piloting* or a *pilot study*) is a set of procedures used by planners/evaluators to try out various processes during program development on a small group of subjects prior to actual implementation. In other words, a pilot test can be thought of as a dress rehearsal for planners/evaluators (McDermott & Sarvela, 1999). The purpose of using pilot tests is to identify and, if necessary, correct any problems prior to implementation with the priority population. Thus pilot tests permit a thorough check of all planned processes to help increase the chances of having a successful program. Throughout the program planning process, planners/evaluators may use pilot tests to detect any problems with sampling, data collection instruments, data collection procedures, data analysis procedures, interventions, curricula, and program evaluation (McDermott & Sarvela, 1999). Since this chapter has focused on data collection, the remaining portions of this discussion will focus on the pilot testing of data collection. Pilot testing will also be discussed in Chapter 12, as it relates to the implementation of a program.

Once the data collection method has been determined and the data collection instrument has been selected or created, a trial run of the instrument, data collection procedures, and analyses should be conducted. During the piloting process, it would not be uncommon for the planners/evaluators to find problems, such as ambiguous questions, difficulty with code sheets, and misunderstood directions. Further, the data collected in the pilot test should be statistically analyzed or compiled to make sure that there is no difficulty with this step in the data collection process. Revising the data collection process using the information gained from the pilot test helps ensure that the actual data collection will proceed smoothly.

Several authors (Borg & Gall, 1989; McDermott & Sarvela, 1999; Parkinson and Associates, 1982; Stacy, 1987) have suggested processes for pilot testing. They have been combined here into a single process. Several of the preceding authors have presented hierarchies for pilot testing: preliminary review, prepilot, pilot tests, and field tests. The first, and lowest, level in the piloting hierarchy is a preliminary review. A

preliminary review is conducted when those responsible for the data collection process ask colleagues, not people from the priority population, to review the data collection instrument. At a minimum, all data collection instruments should be subjected to this type of review. Specifically, in a preliminary review, colleagues would be asked to complete the instrument as if they were subjects in hopes of identifying problems, and also respond to several other questions about the instrument, such as the appropriateness of (1) the instrument's title, (2) the introductory statement explaining the purpose of the data collection, (3) the directions, (4) the order or grouping of the questions, (5) the questions (e.g. unclear or too personal), (6) the length of the instrument, and (7) the method of returning the instrument, to name a few. **Prepilots** (or mini-pilots) are used by planners/evaluators with five or six members of the priority population to assess the quality of materials, instruments, and data collection techniques. Methods used to collect this information include observations, interviews, and focus groups. The **pilot test** requires the actual implementation of the instrument. A representative sample of the priority population is used to determine the quality of the instrument. A **field study** is a final pilot test, combining all materials previously tested separately (e.g., instrument, curriculum materials) into a complete program. If enough subjects are used during the field study, it may be possible to check the validity and reliability of the instrument. If at all possible, the use of this sequence of piloting techniques is desirable, but planners/evaluators are often limited by time and resources, and so not all the steps can be completed.

Ethical Issues Associated with Data Collection

Several ethical issues should be considered when collecting data. Weiss (1998) begins a discussion of these issues with the need for voluntary participation by the respondents. Planners/evaluators should make it clear to the respondents that they have the opportunity to decline to participate without penalty. A second issue is that of private and/or sensitive data. If planners/evaluators need to ask questions that reveal private and sensitive data, they need to ensure anonymity or confidentiality (not report results that could identify a given individual). During data collection, planners/evaluators may hear about illegal acts, such as drug use or other crimes, or the data collectors may be provided with access to confidential data. The planners/evaluators must consider the ethical issues and the legal ramifications of such issues. Weiss (1998) advises checking out state and national laws, and discussing these ethical situations with knowledgeable colleagues.

Summary

This chapter focused on helping you understand the terms measurement, measures, data collection, and sampling. A brief overview of measurement and measures was provided, along with the four levels of measurement: nominal, ordinal, interval, and ratio. Several different examples of questions used at each of the levels were also presented. Next, four desirable characteristics of data were discussed, including reliability, validity, unbiased, and culturally appropriate. With this background information, you were introduced to the primary means of data collection, mainly self-report, observation, existing records, and meetings. This was followed by a discussion of techniques used to draw the various probability and nonprobability samples, and when the various sampling techniques might be most useful. The chapter concluded with a short presentations on the importance of using a pilot test and ethical issues associated with data collection.

REVIEW QUESTIONS

1. What is meant by *measurement,* and *qualitative and quantitative measures?*
2. Name and give an example of each of the four levels of measurement.
3. What are the advantages and disadvantages of using an existing data collection instrument?
4. What is validity? What is reliability? Why are they so important?
5. What is bias in data collection? Name three ways in which it can be reduced.
6. Why must data collection instruments be culturally appropriate?
7. Describe each method of data collection (self-report, observation, existing data, and meetings), and list two advantages and disadvantages of each.
8. How does a planner/evaluator determine who will participate in the data collection?
9. Describe three types of probability samples.
10. When, if ever, should nonprobability samples be used?
11. What is the purpose of a preliminary review, a prepilot (or mini-pilot), a pilot test, and a field study? How is each conducted?
12. What ethical issues should be considered when collecting data?

ACTIVITIES

1. Construct a three-page written questionnaire on a health promotion topic of your choice that could be administered to a group of college students.
2. Conduct a prepilot test on your written questionnaire developed in activity number 1 on five or six of your friends, colleagues, or classmates. After the pilot test, identify any flaws you see in the questionnaire or data collection process.
3. Assume that you are charged with the responsibility of collecting data from all the students on your campus who have enrolled in a fitness course. Assume also that this group of students is too large to collect data from everyone. Explain how you would obtain a representative sample from this population.
4. Visit a survey research center on your campus or in your community. Ask about the methods of data collection, and if possible arrange to observe a face-to-face or telephone interview. Write a two-page paper describing your reaction to this experience.
5. Review a needs assessment or evaluation instrument. Identify the level of measurement for the questions, types of measurement, and the types of question.
6. Photocopy a page from a local telephone book. Let's assume that this page represents a sampling frame for your priority population. Go through the frame and divide it into groups of 10 by using the first 10 numbers as group 1, the second 10 as group 2, and so on, until all the numbers are used. Be sure you do not use fax or business numbers. If you have an odd number of telephone numbers (not an even 10), do not use that

group. With this information, explain how you would select a simple random sample of 20 numbers, a systematic sample of 10 numbers, a proportional stratified sample of 40 numbers stratified on the first 3 numbers of the telephone numbers, and a cluster sample of 10 groups, assuming that the groups of 10s you formed are your clusters.

WEBLINKS

1. **http://www.astho.org**
   The Association for State and Territorial Health Officers (ASTHO)

   This is the website for the ASTHO which is the national nonprofit organization representing the state and territorial public health agencies of the United States, the U.S. Territories, and the District of Columbia. Among other items, this site includes links to each of the state and territorial health departments.

2. **http://www.cdc.gov/nchs/default.htm**
   National Center for Health Statistics (NCHS)

   This is the website for the NCHS. It is a rich source of data about America's health and the instruments used to collect the data.

3. **http://www.surveysystem.com/index.html**
   Creative Research Systems

   This is the website for a commercial company called Creative Research Systems. The site includes a lot of information about survey data collection and includes a calculator for determining appropriate sample size.

CHAPTER 6

Mission Statement, Goals, and Objectives

Chapter Objectives

After reading this chapter and answering the questions at the end, you should be able to:

- Explain what is meant by the term *mission statement.*
- Define *goals* and *objectives,* and distinguish between the two.
- Identify the different levels of objectives as presented in the chapter.
- State the necessary elements of an objective as presented in the chapter.
- Specify an appropriate criterion for objectives.
- Write program goals and objectives.
- Describe the use for *Healthy People 2010.*

Key Terms

action/behavioral objectives
attitude objectives
awareness objectives
conditions
criterion
environmental objectives
goal

impact objectives
knowledge objectives
learning objectives
mission statement
objectives
outcome

outcome/program objectives
process/administrative
   objectives
skill development/acquisition
   objectives
SMART

To plan, implement, and evaluate effective health promotion programs, planners must have a solid foundation in place to guide them through their work. The mission statement, goals, and objectives of a program can provide such a foundation. If prepared properly, a mission statement, goals, and objectives should not only give the necessary direction to a program but also provide the groundwork for the eventual program evaluation. There are two old sayings that help express the need for a mission statement, goals, and objectives. The first is: If you do not know where you are going, then any road will do—and you may end up someplace where you do not

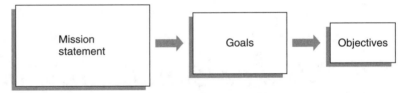

Figure 6.1 Relationship of mission statement, goals, and objectives

want to be, or you may eventually end up where you want to be, but after wasted time and effort. The second is: If you do not know where you are going, how will you know when you have arrived? Without a mission statement, goals, and objectives, a program may lack direction, and at best it will be difficult to evaluate. Figure 6.1 shows the relationship between a mission statement, goals, and objectives. The size of the rectangles presented in Figure 6.1 have special meaning. The rectangle that represents the mission statement is the largest, while the rectangle representing the objectives is the smallest meaning that ideas presented go from broad to narrow in scope.

Mission Statement

Sometimes referred to as a program overview or program aim, a **mission statement** is a short narrative that describes the general focus of the program. The statement not only describes the intent of a program but also may reflect the philosophy behind it. The mission statement also helps to guide planners in the development of program goals and objectives. Box 6.1 presents examples of mission statements for several different settings.

Box 6.1 Examples of Mission Statements

Setting	Mission Statement
Community Setting	The mission of the Walkup Health Promotion Program is to provide a wide variety of primary prevention activities for residents of the community.
Health Care Setting	This program is aimed at helping patients and their families to understand and cope with physical and emotional changes associated with recovery following cancer surgery.
School Setting	School District #77 wants happy and healthy students. To that end, the district's personnel strives, through a coordinated school health program, to provide students with experiences that are designed to motivate and enable them to maintain and improve their health.
Worksite Setting	The purpose of the employee health promotion program is to develop high employee morale. This is to be accomplished by providing employees with a working environment that is conducive to good health and by providing an opportunity for employees and their families to engage in behavior that will improve and maintain good health.

Program Goals

Although some individuals use the terms *goals* and *objectives* synonymously, they are not the same: There are important differences between them. Ross and Mico (1980, p. 219) have stated that "a goal is a future event toward which a committed endeavor is directed; objectives are the steps to be taken in pursuit of a goal." Deeds (1992, p. 36) defined a goal as a "broad timeless statement of a long-range program purpose," whereas Neiger (1998) defined goals as general statements of intent. In comparison to objectives, a **goal** is an expectation that:

1. Is much more encompassing, or global
2. Is written to include all aspects or components of a program
3. Provides overall direction for a program
4. Is more general in nature
5. Usually takes longer to complete
6. Does not have a deadline (CDC, 2003)
7. Usually is not observed, but rather must be inferred because it includes words like *evaluate, know, improve,* and *understand* (Jacobsen, Eggen & Kauchak, 1989)
8. Is often not measurable in exact terms

Program goals are not difficult to write and need not be written as complete sentences. They should, however, be simple and concise, and should include two basic components: who will be affected, and what will change as a result of the program. Goals typically include verbs such as *improve, increase, promote, protect, minimize, prevent,* and *reduce* (CDC, 2003). A program need not have a set number of stated goals. It is not uncommon for some programs to have a single goal while others have several. Box 6.2 presents some examples of goals for health promotion programs.

Box 6.2 Examples of Program Goals

- To reduce the incidence of cardiovascular disease in the employees of the Smith Company.
- All cases of measles in the City of Kenzington will be eliminated.
- To prevent the spread of HIV in the youth of Indiana.
- To reduce the cases of lung cancer caused by exposure to secondhand smoke in Yorktown, IN.
- To reduce the incidence of influenza in the residents of the Delaware County Home.
- The survival rate of breast cancer patients will be increased through the optimal use of community resources.

Objectives

As Ross and Mico (1980) have indicated, **objectives** are more precise and represent smaller steps than program goals—steps that, if completed, will lead to reaching the program goal(s). Stated another way, objectives specify intermediate accomplishments or benchmarks that represent progress toward the goal (CDC, 2003). Objectives outline in measurable terms the specific changes that will occur in the priority population at a given point in time as a result of exposure to the program. "Objectives are crucial. They form a fulcrum, converting diagnostic data into program direction" (Green & Kreuter, 1999, p. 106). Objectives can be thought of as the bridge between needs assessment and a planned intervention. Knowing how to construct objectives for a program is a most important skill for planners.

Different Levels of Objectives

There are several different levels of objectives associated with program planning. The different levels are sequenced or placed in a hierarchical order to allow for more effective planning (Cleary & Neiger, 1998; Deeds, 1992; Parkinson & Associates, 1982). Objectives are created at each level in order to help attain the program goal. The "objectives should also be *coherent* across levels, with objectives becoming successively more refined and more explicit, level by level" (Green & Kreuter, 1999, p. 107). Achievement of the lower-level objectives will contribute to the achievement of the higher-level objectives and goals. Table 6.1 presents the hierarchy of objectives and indicates their relationship to program outcomes and evaluation.

Process/Administrative Objectives The **process/administrative objectives** are the daily tasks, activities, and work plans that lead to the accomplishment of all other levels of objectives (Deeds, 1992). They help shape or form the program and thus focus on all program inputs (all that are needed to carry out a program), implementation activities (actual presentation of the program), and stakeholder reactions. More specifically, these objectives would focus on such things as program resources (materials, funds, space); appropriateness of intervention activities; priority population exposure, attendance, participation, and feedback; feedback from other stakeholders such as the funding and sponsoring agencies; and data collection techniques, to name a few.

Learning Objectives The second level of objectives in the hierarchy comprises **learning objectives.** They are the educational or learning tools that are needed in order to achieve the desired behavior change. They are based upon the analysis of educational and organizational assessment of the PRECEDE-PROCEED model.

Within this level of objectives, there is another hierarchy (Parkinson & Associates, 1982). This hierarchy includes four types of objectives, beginning with the least complex and moving toward the most complex. Complexity is defined in terms of the time, effort, and resources necessary to accomplish the objective. The learning objectives hierarchy begins with **awareness objectives** and moves through **knowledge, attitude,** and **skill development/acquisition objectives.** This hierarchy indicates that if those in the priority population are going to adopt and maintain a health-enhancing behavior to alleviate a health concern or problem, they must first be aware of the health concern. Second, they must expand their knowledge and understanding of

Table 6.1 Hierarchy of objectives and their relation to evaluation

Type of Objective	Program Outcomes	Possible Evaluation Measures	Type of Evaluation
Process/ Administrative Objectives	Activities presented and tasks completed	Number of sessions held, exposure, attendance, participation, staff performance, appropriate materials, adequacy of resources, tasks on schedule	Process (form of formative)
Learning Objectives			Impact (form of summative)
Awareness	Change in awareness	Increase in awareness	
Knowledge	Change in knowledge	Increase in knowledge	
Attitudes	Change in attitude	Improved attitude	
Skills	Change in skills	Skill development or acquisition	
Action/Behavioral Objectives	Change in behavior	Current behavior modified or discontinued, or new behavior adopted	Impact (form of summative)
Environmental Objectives	Change in the environment	Protection added to, or hazards or barriers removed from the environment	Impact (form of summative)
Program Objectives	Change in quality of life (QOL), health status, risk factors, and social benefits	QOL measures, morbidity data, mortality data, measures of risk (i.e., HRA), physiological measures, signs and symptoms	Outcome (form of summative)

Source: Adapted from Deeds (1992) and Cleary and Neiger (1998).

the concern. Third, they must attain and maintain an attitude that enables them to deal with the concern. And fourth, they need to possess the necessary skills to engage in the health-enhancing behavior.

Action/Behavioral Objectives   **Action/behavioral objectives** describe the behaviors or actions in which the priority population will engage that will resolve the health problem and move you toward achieving the program goal (Deeds, 1992). Action/behavioral objectives are commonly written about adherence (e.g., regular exercise), compliance (e.g., taking medication as prescribed), consumption patterns (e.g., diet), coping (e.g., stress-reduction activities), preventive actions (e.g., brushing and flossing teeth), self-care (e.g., first aid), and utilization (e.g, appropriate use of the emergency room).

Environmental Objectives   **Environmental objectives** outline the nonbehavioral causes of a health problem that are present in the social, physical, and/or psychological environments. Environmental objectives are written about such things as the state of the physical environment (e.g., clean air or water), the social environment (e.g., access to health care), or the psychological environment (e.g., the emotional learning climate).

As we leave our discussion of environmental objectives, it should be noted that there are some who group the four types of learning objectives (i.e., awareness, knowledge, attitudes, and skills), action/behavioral objectives, and environmental objectives into a single category known as **impact objectives.** They get this label because they all form the groundwork for impact evaluation. (See the last column in Table 6.1. The term *impact objectives* is a parallel term with the terms *process objectives* and *outcome objectives*.)

Outcome/Program Objectives   **Outcome/Program objectives** are the ultimate objectives of a program and are aimed at changes in health status, social benefits, risk factors or quality of life. "They are outcome or future oriented" (Deeds, 1992, p. 36). If these objectives are achieved, then the program goal will be achieved. These objectives are commonly written in terms of reduction of risk, physiologic indicators, sign and symptoms, morbidity, disability, mortality, or quality of life measures.

Developing Objectives

Does every program require objectives from each of the levels just described? The answer is no! However, too often, health promotion programs have too few objectives, all of which fall into one or two levels. Many planners have developed programs hoping solely to change the health behavior of a priority population. For example, a smoking cessation program may have an objective of getting 30% of the participants to stop smoking. Perhaps this program is offered, and only 10% of the participants quit smoking. Is the program a failure? If the program has a single objective of changing behavior, its sponsors would have a good case for saying that the program was not effective. However, it is quite possible that as a result of participating in the smoking cessation program, the participants increased their awareness of the dangers of smoking. They probably also increased their knowledge, changed their attitudes, and developed skills for quitting or cutting back on the number of cigarettes they smoke each day. These are all very positive outcomes—and they could be overlooked when the program is evaluated, if the planner did not write objectives that cover a variety of levels.

Criteria for Developing Objectives

In addition to making sure that the objectives are written in an appropriate manner, planners also need to be realistic with regard to the other parameters of the program. These are some of the questions that planners should consider when writing objectives:

1. Can the objective be realized during the life of the program or within a reasonable time thereafter? It would be quite realistic to assume that a certain number of people will not be smoking one year after they have completed a smoking cessation program, but it would not be realistic to assume that a group of elementary school students could be followed for life to determine how many of them die prematurely due to inactivity.

2. Can the objective realistically be achieved? It is probably realistic to assume that 30% of any smoking cessation class will stop smoking within one year after the

program has ended, but it is not realistic to assume that 100% of the employees of a company will participate in its fitness program.

3. Does the program have enough resources (personnel, money, and space) to obtain a specific objective? It would be ideal to be able to reach all individuals in the priority population, but generally there are not sufficient resources to do so.

4. Are the objectives consistent with the policies and procedures of the sponsoring agency? It would not be realistic to expect to incorporate a no-smoking policy in a tobacco company.

5. Do the objectives violate any of the rights of those who are involved (participants or planners)? Right-to-know laws make it illegal to withhold information that could cause harm to a priority population.

6. If a program is planned for a particular ethnic/cultural population, do the objectives reflect the relationship between the cultural characteristics of the priority group and the changes sought?

The CDCynergy planning model has created an acronym for the criteria for objectives presented above called SMART. **SMART** stands for **s**pecific, **m**easurable, **a**chievable, **r**ealistic, and **t**ime-phased (CDC, 2003). Every objective planners write for their programs should be SMART!

Elements of an Objective

For an objective to provide direction and to be useful in the evaluation process, it must be written in such a way that it can be clearly understood, states what is to be accomplished, and is measurable. To ensure that an objective is indeed useful, it should include the following elements:

1. The *outcome* to be achieved, or what will change.
2. The *conditions* under which the outcome will be observed, or when the change will occur.
3. The *criterion* for deciding whether the outcome has been achieved, or how much change.
4. The *priority population*, or who will change.

The first element, the **outcome,** is defined as the action, behavior, or something else that will change as a result of the program. In a written objective, the outcome is usually identified as the verb of the sentence. Thus words such as *apply, argue, build, compare, demonstrate, evaluate, exhibit, judge, perform, reduce, spend, state,* and *test* would be considered outcomes (see Box 6.3 for a more comprehensive listing of appropriate outcome words). It should be noted that not all verbs would be considered appropriate outcomes for an objective; the verb must refer to something measurable and observable. Words such as *appreciate, know, internalize,* and *understand* by themselves do not refer to something measurable and observable, and therefore they are not good choices for outcomes.

The second element of an objective is the **conditions** under which the outcome will be observed, or when it will be observed. "Typical" conditions found in objectives might be "upon completion of the exercise class," "as a result of participation," "by the

Box 6.3 Outcome Verbs for Objectives

abstract	copy	gather (information)	organize	seek
accept	count	generalize	pair	select
adjust	create	generate	participate	separate
adopt	criticize	group	partition	share
advocate	deduce	guess	perform	show
analyze	defend	hypothesize	persist	simplicity
annotate	define	identify	plan	simulate
apply	delay (response)	illustrate	practice	solve
approximate	demonstrate	imitate	praise	sort
argue	derive	improve	predict	spend (money)
(a position)	describe	infer	prepare	state
ask	design	initiate	preserve	structure
associate	determine	inquire	produce	submit
attempt	develop	integrate	propose	subscribe
balance	differentiate	interpolate	prove	substitute
build	discover	interpret	qualify	suggest
calculate	discriminate	invent	query	summarize
categorize	dispute	investigate	question	supply
cause	distinguish	join	recall	support
challenge	effect	judge	recite	symbolize
change	eliminate	justify	recognize	synthesize
choose	enumerate	keep	recommend	tabulate
clarify	estimate	label	record	tally
classify	evaluate	list	reduce	test
collect	examine	locate	regulate	theorize
combine	exemplify	manipulate	reject	translate
compare	exhibit	map	relate	try
complete	experiment	match	reorganize	unite
compute	explain	measure	repeat	visit
conceptualize	express	name	replace	volunteer
connect	extend	obey	represent	weigh
construct	extract	object (to an idea)	reproduce	write
consult	extrapolate	observe	restructure	
contrast	find	offer	round	
convert	form	order	score	

year 2010," "after reading the pamphlets and brochures," "orally in class," "when asked to respond by the facilitator," "one year after the program," "by May 15th," or "during the class session."

The third element of an objective is the **criterion** for deciding when the outcome has been achieved, or how much change will occur. The purpose of this element is to provide a standard by which the planners/evaluators can determine if an outcome has been performed in an appropriate and/or successful manner. Examples might include "to no more than 105 per 1,000," "with 100% accuracy," "as presented in the lecture," "300 pamphlets," "according to the criteria developed by the American Heart

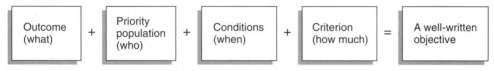

Figure 6.2 Elements of a well-written objective

Association," "95% of the motor vehicle occupants," or "using the technique outlined in the American Cancer Society's pamphlet."

The last element that needs to be included in an objective is mention of the **priority population,** or who will change. Examples are "1,000 teachers," "all employees of the company," and "those residing in the Muncie and Provo areas." Figure 6.2 summarizes the key elements in an objective. (See Box 6.4 for examples of objectives that would include the four primary components.)

Goals and Objectives for the Nation

A chapter on goals and objectives would not be complete without at least a short discussion of the health goals and objectives of the nation. These goals and objectives have been most helpful to planners throughout the United States.

The U.S. government is very interested in improving the health status of Americans. It is concerned about individuals and the population as a whole. The country is facing many problems and issues that revolve around health; the cost of ill health is the most obvious. Therefore for at least some parts of the federal government, there is a goal to improve the health status of the public. Objectives have been developed to guide the work of reaching this goal. Some people have referred to these statements of objectives as the *health plan or agenda or blueprint of health* for the United States.

The first set of objectives was developed by many health professionals throughout the country; it was published in 1980 under the title *Promoting Health/ Preventing Disease: Objectives for the Nation* (USDHHS, 1980). This volume was divided into three main areas: preventive services, health protection, and health promotion. Each of these contained five focus areas, or 15 in all. From these 15 areas came a total of 226 objectives. These objectives, which were based on the data collected for the U.S. Surgeon General's report *Healthy People* (1979), were the basis for health promotion and disease prevention planning during the 1980s.

Data for 1987 provided evidence that nearly half of those objectives had been achieved or were likely to be achieved by 1990, while about a quarter were unlikely to be achieved; the status of the remaining quarter was in doubt because tracking data were not available. Progress was slow for some of the 15 priorities identified in 1980, such as pregnancy and infant health, nutrition, physical fitness and exercise, family planning, sexually transmitted diseases, and occupational safety and health. Substantial progress was made, however, in high blood pressure control, immunization, unintentional injury prevention and control, control of infectious diseases, smoking, and alcohol and drugs (Mason & McGinnis, 1990, p. 442).

As the 1980s came to a close, it was obvious from the evaluation conducted on these national goals and objectives (USDHHS, 1986b) that there was a need to develop new goals and objectives to guide the country through the 1990s. Therefore a second set of goals and objectives called *Healthy People 2000: National Health Promotion*

Box 6.4 Examples of Objectives to Support the Program Goal "To reduce the prevalence of heart disease in the residents of Franklin County"

Process/Administrative Objectives

A. During the next six months, 300 community residents will participate in one of the health department's health promotion activities.

   Outcome (what): Will participate in an activity.

   Priority population (who): Community residents.

   Conditions (when): During the next six months.

   Criterion (how much): 300 residents.

B. By August 4, two different heart disease brochures will be distributed to all residences in the county.

   Outcome (what): Will be distributed.

   Priority population (who): To all residences.

   Conditions (when): By August 4.

   Criterion (how much): Two different.

C. During the pilot testing, the program facilitators will receive a "good" rating from the program participants.

   Outcome (what): Will receive.

   Priority population (who): Program facilitators.

   Conditions (when): During the pilot testing.

   Criterion (how much): "Good" rating.

D. The reading materials will be made available to the program participants 10 days prior to the start of the activity.

   Outcome (what): Materials made available.

   Priority population (who): Program participants.

   Conditions (when): Prior to the start.

   Criterion (how much): 10 days prior.

Learning Objectives

A. Awareness level: After the American Heart Association's pamphlet on cardiovascular health risk factors has been placed in grocery bags, at least 20% of the shoppers will be able to identify two of their own risks.

   Outcome (what): Identify their own risks.

   Priority population (who): Shoppers.

   Conditions (when): After distribution of the pamphlet.

   Criterion (how much): Two risks.

B. Knowledge level: When asked over the telephone, one out of three viewers of the heart special television show will be able to explain the four principles of cardiovascular conditioning.

   Outcome (what): Able to explain.

   Priority population (who): Television viewers.

   Conditions (when): When asked over the telephone.

   Criterion (how much): One out of three.

C. Attitude level: During one of the class sessions, the participants will defend two of their reasons for regular exercise.

   Outcome (what): Defend their reasons.

   Priority population (who): Class participants.

   Conditions (when): During one of the class sessions.

   Criterion (how much): Two of their reasons.

D. Skill development/acquisition level: After viewing the video "How to Exercise," those participating will be able to locate their pulse and count it every time they are asked to do it.

   Outcome (what): Locate their pulse and count it.

   Priority population (who): Those participating.

   Conditions (when): After viewing the video.

   Criterion (how much): Every time.

(Box 6.4 *continues*)

(Box 6.4 *continued*)

Action/Behavioral Objectives

A. One year after the formal exercise classes have been completed, 40% of those who completed 80% of the classes will still be involved in a regular aerobic exercise program.
   Outcome (what): Will still be involved.
   Priority population (who): Those who completed 80% of the classes.
   Conditions (when): One year after the classes.
   Criterion (how much): 40%.

B. During the telephone interview follow-up, 50% of the residents will report having had their blood pressure taken during the previous six months.
   Outcome (what): Will report.
   Priority population (who): Residents.
   Conditions (when): During the telephone interview follow-up.
   Criterion (how much): 50%.

Environment Objectives

A. The percentage of household wells checked by the Franklin County Health Department will increase to 95% by the year 2010.
   Outcome (what): Wells checked.
   Priority population (who): Household wells.
   Conditions (when): By the year 2010.
   Criterion (how much): 95%.

B. By the end of the year, all senior citizens will be provided transportation to the congregate meals.
   Outcome (what): Provided transportation.
   Priority population (who): Senior citizens.
   Conditions (when): By end of year.
   Criterion (how much): All.

Outcome/Program Objectives

A. By the year 2010, heart disease deaths will be reduced to no more than 100 per 100,000 in the residents of Franklin County.
   Outcome (what): Reduce heart disease deaths.
   Priority population (who): Residents of Franklin County.
   Conditions (when): By the year 2010.
   Criterion (how much): To no more than 100 per 100,000.

B. By 2010, increase to at least 25% the proportion of men in Franklin County with hypertension whose blood pressure is under control.
   Outcome (what): Blood pressure under control.
   Priority population (who): Men in Franklin County.
   Conditions (when): By 2010.
   Criterion (how much): To at least 25%.

C. Half of all those in the county who complete a regular, aerobic, 12-month exercise program will reduce their "risk age" on their follow-up health risk appraisal by a minimum of two years compared to their preprogram results.
   Outcome (what): Will reduce their "risk age."
   Priority population (who): Those who complete an exercise program.
   Conditions (when): After the 12-month exercise program.
   Criterion (how much): Half.

D. Those who participate in a formal exercise and fitness program will use 10% fewer sick days during the life of the program than those who do not participate.
   Outcome (what): Use fewer sick days.
   Priority population (who): Those who participate.
   Conditions (when): During the life of the program.
   Criterion (how much): 10% fewer sick days.

and Disease Prevention Objectives was developed (USDHHS, 1990a). That set was much more detailed than the first and was much more useful to all program planners. It included fewer goals and more objectives. In addition, subobjectives were established for people with low incomes, people who are members of some racial and ethnic minority groups, and people with disabilities to help meet their unique needs and health problems (USDHHS, 1994).

Just as the 1990 objectives were not all met, neither were the Healthy People 2000 objectives. In the mid–1990s, the U.S. government published *Healthy People 2000: Midcourse Review and 1995 Revisions* (USDHHS, 1995). That document served as a self-study of progress toward the year 2000 objectives and the beginning point for planning the year 2010 objectives. The context in which the *Healthy People 2010* was framed differed from the 2000 objectives in that planners were working with a broader scientific base, improved surveillance and data systems, and the knowledge that the public had a heightened awareness and demand for preventive services and quality health care (USDHHS, 1997). In January 2000, the latest version of the objectives for the nation, *Healthy People 2010,* was released.

Healthy People 2010 is the most sophisticated Healthy People planning document to date, which is reflective of the effort that went into creating it. The *Healthy People 2010* document is comprised of three parts. *Healthy People 2010: Understanding and Improving Health* is the first of three parts in the Healthy People 2010 series. In addition to providing a history of *Healthy People 2010* and the overall Healthy People initiative, this section presents the Determinants of Health model (see Figure 6.3) on which Healthy People is based, how to use Healthy People as a systematic approach to health improvement, and the Leading Health Indicators (LHIs). The LHIs are new to the Healthy People document and were created to provide a snapshot of the health of the Nation. *Healthy People 2010* identifies ten LHIs (physical activity, overweight and obesity, tobacco use, substance abuse, responsible sexual behavior, mental health, injury and violence, environmental quality, immunization, and access to health care). The LHIs highlight major health priorities for the Nation and include the individual behaviors, physical and social environmental factors, and health system issues that affect the health of individuals and communities. Each of the ten LHIs has one or more Healthy People measures associated with it and will be used to measure progress throughout the decade (USDHHS, 2000).

The second part of the document, *Healthy People 2010: Objectives for Improving Health,* contains the two overarching goals and detailed descriptions of 467 objectives to improve health. The two overarching goals for *Healthy People 2010* are:

—Increase quality and years of healthy life.

—Eliminate health disparities.

The first goal is to help individuals of all ages increase life expectancy and improve their quality of life, while the second goal is to eliminate health disparities among different segments of the population. These two goals are supported by specific objectives in 28 focus areas (see Table 6.2). In the document, each focus area is presented as a chapter. Each chapter contains a concise goal statement that frames the overall purpose of the area, an overview of the health issue that provides the context and background for the objectives, an interim progress report toward the year 2000 objectives, and the 2010 objectives. There are two types of objectives—measurable and developmental. The measurable objectives provide direction for action and include

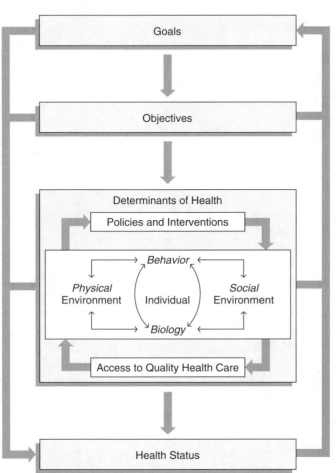

Healthy People in Healthy Communities
A Systematic Approach to Health Improvement

Figure 6.3 Determinants of health
Source: USDHHS (2000).

national baseline data from which the 2010 target was set. The developmental objectives provide a vision for a desired outcome or health status. The purpose of developmental objectives is to identify areas of emerging importance and to drive the development of data systems to measure them. National surveillance systems for tracking these objectives were not available in 2000, but it was expected that such would be in place for most of the objectives by 2004 (USDHHS, 2000).

The third part of the document, *Tracking Healthy People 2010,* provides a comprehensive review of the statistical measures that will be used to evaluate progress. The purpose of this third part is to provide technical information so that others will be able to understand how the data are derived and the major statistical issues affecting the interpretation of the statistics. This is the first set of Healthy People objectives to have such a document (USDHHS, 2000).

Table 6.2 *Healthy People 2010* focus areas

1. Access to Quality Health Services
2. Arthritis, Osteoporosis, and Chronic Back Conditions
3. Cancer
4. Chronic Kidney Disease
5. Diabetes
6. Disability and Secondary Conditions
7. Educational and Community-Based Programs
8. Environmental Health
9. Family Planning
10. Food Safety
11. Health Communication
12. Heart Disease and Stroke
13. HIV
14. Immunization and Infectious Diseases
15. Injury and Violence Prevention
16. Maternal, Infant, and Child Health
17. Medical Product Safety
18. Mental Health and Mental Disorders
19. Nutrition and Overweight
20. Occupational Safety and Health
21. Oral Health
22. Physical Activity and Fitness
23. Public Health Infrastructure
24. Respiratory Diseases
25. Sexually Transmitted Diseases
26. Substance Abuse
27. Tobacco Use
28. Vision and Hearing

Source: USDHHS (2000).

The importance of the Healthy People initiative serving as a blueprint for the Nation's health agenda is evidenced by their widespread use. Since the publication of the first the Healthy People goals and objectives in 1980, there have been a number of other documents created that can help planners develop or adopt appropriate goals and objectives for their programs. A number of states and U.S. territories have taken the national objectives and created similar documents specific to their own residents (USDHHS, 1997). In addition, a number of agencies/organizations have taken similar steps to create documents that could be used by their members and clients in various planning efforts. Examples include the American Association of School Administrators (1990), American College Health Association (2002), American Indian Health Care Association (no date), American Public Health Association (1991), National Dairy Council (1992), and the U.S. Department of Health and Human Services (2001).

The national goals and objectives have been important components in the process of health promotion planning since 1980. It is highly recommended that planners review these objectives before developing goals and objectives for programs. The national objectives may be helpful in providing a rationale for a program and in focusing program goals and objectives toward the areas of greatest need, as planners work toward the year 2010.

SUMMARY

The mission statement provides an overview of a program and is most useful in the development of goals and objectives. The terms *goals* and *objectives* are sometimes used synonymously, but they are quite different. Together, the two provide a foundation for program planning and evaluation. Goals are more global in nature and often are not measurable in exact terms, whereas objectives are more specific and consist of the steps used to reach the program goals. Program objectives can and should be written for several different levels. For objectives to be useful, they should be written so as to be observable and measurable. At a minimum, an objective should include the following elements: a stated outcome (what), conditions under which the outcome will be observed (when), a criterion for considering that the outcome has been achieved (how much), and mention of the priority population (who). As planners develop their goals and objectives for their programs, they should find the *Healthy People 2010* document very useful.

REVIEW QUESTIONS

1. Why is a mission statement important?
2. What is (are) the difference(s) between a goal and an objective?
3. What is the purpose of program goals and objectives?
4. What are the different levels of objectives?
5. What are the necessary elements of an objective?
6. What are the goals and objectives for the nation? How can they be used by program planners?
7. Briefly explain the Healthy People initiative.
8. How can planners use the *Healthy People 2010* goals and objectives in their program planning efforts?

ACTIVITIES

1. Write a mission statement, a goal, and supporting objectives (one at each level) for a program you are planning.
2. Identify which of the following objectives include all four elements necessary for a complete objective; revise those objectives that do not include all the elements:
   a. After the class on objective writing, the students will know the difference between a goal and an objective.
   b. The students know how a skinfold caliper works.
   c. After completing this chapter, the students will be able to write objectives for each of the levels based on the four elements outlined in the chapter.
   d. Given appropriate instruction, the employees will be able to accurately take blood pressure readings of fellow employees.
   e. Program participants will be able to list the reasons why people do not exercise.

3. Write a mission statement, a goal, and supporting objectives (one at each level) for a workshop on responsible use of alcohol by college students.

Weblinks

1. **http://www.healthypeople.gov/**
   Healthy People

   This is the website for the U.S. Government's Healthy People initiative including a complete presentation of the three parts of *Healthy People 2010.*

2. **http://www.cancer.org/**
   American Cancer Society (ACS)

   This is the website for the ACS. In addition to being a great source of cancer information and data, it also includes the mission statement and goals of the ACS.

3. **http://www.americanheart.org**
   American Heart Association (AHA)

   This is the website for the AHA. In addition to being an excellent source of heart health information, it also includes the mission statement of the Association and several other associations and organizations that have an interest in heart health.

CHAPTER 7

Theories and Models Commonly Used for Health Promotion Interventions

Chapter Objectives

After reading this chapter and answering the questions at the end, you should be able to:

- Define *theory, model, constructs, concepts,* and *variables.*
- Explain why health promotion interventions should be planned using theoretical frameworks.
- Briefly explain the theories and models identified in the chapter.

Key Terms

action stage
aversive stimulus
behavior change theories
behavioral capability
behavioral intention
concepts
construct
contemplation stage
continuum theories
decisional balance
direct reinforcement
ecological perspective
efficacy expectations
elaboration
emotional-coping responses
expectancies
expectations
field test
health belief model

lapse
likelihood of action
locus of control
maintenance stage
model
negative punishment
negative reinforcement
outcome expectations
perceived barriers
perceived behavioral control
perceived benefits
perceived seriousness/severity
perceived susceptibility
perceived threat
planning models
positive punishment
positive reinforcement
precontemplation stage
preparation

processes of change
punishment
recidivism
reciprocal determinism
reinforcement
relapse
relapse prevention
self-control
self-efficacy
self-regulation
self-reinforcement
stage
stage theories
subjective norm
termination
theory
variable
vicarious reinforcement

Whenever there is a discussion about the theoretical bases for health education and health promotion, we often find the terms *theory* and *model* used. We begin this chapter with a brief explanation of these terms, to establish a common understanding of their meaning.

One of the most frequently quoted definitions of **theory** is one in which Glanz, Lewis, and Rimer (2002b) modified an earlier definition written by Kerlinger (1986). It states, "A *theory* is a set of interrelated concepts, definitions, and propositions that presents a *systematic* view of events or situations by specifying relations among variables in order to *explain* and *predict* the events of the situations" (p. 25). Green and colleagues (1994, p. 398) have stated, "The role of theory is to untangle and simplify for human comprehension the complexities of nature." In other words, a theory is a systematic arrangement of fundamental principles that provide a basis for explaining certain happenings of life. Hochbaum, Sorenson, and Lorig (1992) defined theories in relationship to health education as "tools to help health educators better understand what influences health—relevant individuals, group, and institutional behaviors—and to thereupon plan effective interventions directed at health-beneficial results" (p. 298).

Nutbeam and Harris (1999) have stated that a fully developed theory would be characterized by three major elements: "It would explain:

- the major factors that influence the phenomena of interest, for example those factors which explain why some people are regularly active and others are not;

- the relationship between these factors, for example the relationship between knowledge, beliefs, social norms and behaviours [sic] such as physical activity; and

- the conditions under which these relationships do or do not occur: the how, when, and why of hypothesised [sic] relationships, for example the time, place and circumstances which, predictably lead to a person being active or inactive" (p. 10).

In comparison, a **model** is a subclass of a theory. Models "are generalized, hypothetical descriptions, often based on an analogy, used to analyze or explain something" (Glanz & Rimer, 1995, p.11). "Models draw on a number of theories to help understand a specific problem in a particular setting or content" (Glanz et al., 2002b, p. 27). Unlike theories, models do "not attempt to explain the processes underlying learning, but only to represent them" (Chaplin & Krawiec, 1979, p. 68).

Though we just went to some effort to make a distinction between words *theory* and *model,* when discussing the terms theory-based endeavors (i.e., *theory-based health education/promotion practice* and *theory-based research*) it is commonly understood in our profession that the word theory is used in a general way to mean either a theory *or* model. Thus as we use the terms *theory* and *theory-based* throughout the remainder of this book, we use them to be inclusive of endeavors based on either a theory *or* a model.

Concepts are the primary elements or the building blocks of a theory (Glanz et al., 2002b). When a concept has been developed, created, or adopted for use with a specific theory, it is referred to as a **construct** (Kerlinger, 1986). "In other words, constructs are synthesized thoughts of key concepts or specific theories" (Cottrell, Girvan, & McKenzie, 2002, p. 100). The operational (practical use) form of a construct is known as a **variable.** Variables "specify how a construct is to be measured in a specific situation" (Glanz et al., 2002b, p. 27).

> Now consider how these terms are used in practical application. A personal belief is a *concept* that has been shown to relate to various health behaviors. Using a *theory* that includes the concept of personal beliefs helps explain why people fear being trapped in a burning vehicle if they use their safety belts. This personal belief of fear acts as a perceived barrier to safety belt use. Perceived barrier is a part of a specific theory and is referred to here as a *construct*. If a health educator develops a program around a theory to help people overcome this barrier and wear their safety belts, then safety belt use is the *variable* being studied. The health educator realizes that this theory, which emphasizes personal beliefs, will not explain all the reasons why people do not wear safety belts. Thus other theories, which emphasize other concepts (i.e., knowledge, environment, incentives, comfort, convenience, etc.) need to be considered.
>
> Eventually, all of these theories may be combined into a *model* that will explain, at least in part, why people wear safety belts. If a model were a perfect model, it would predict with 100% accuracy who would wear safety belts. Unfortunately, behavior is very complex and there are no perfect models in health education. It is therefore important for health educators to keep revising their models to improve their understanding of health behavior. (Cottrell et al., 2002, p. 100)

Based on these descriptions, it seems logical to think of theories as the backbone of the processes used to plan, implement, and evaluate health promotion interventions. "A theory based approach provides direction and justification for program activities and serves as a basis for processes that are to be incorporated into the health promotion program" (Cowdery et al., 1995, p. 248). For example, developmental theories can be used to ensure that the goals and objectives of programs are consistent with the participants' developmental stages and abilities. Theories also can guide program planners in selecting the types of interventions that are needed to accomplish the stated goals and objectives. Appropriate use of learning and behavioral theories can help to ensure congruence between the planned interventions and expected outcomes. Stated a bit differently, "Theories can provide answers to program developers' questions regarding *why* people aren't already engaging in a desirable behavior of interest, *how* to go about changing their behaviors, and *what* factors to look at when evaluating a program's focus" (van Ryn & Heaney, 1992, p. 326). In addition, theoretical frameworks can alert planners to consider important influences outside the teaching-learning process, such as social support and environment, that have an impact on targeted program outcomes (Parcel, 1983).

All health promotion interventions should be planned based upon proven theories. "Theory is not a substitute for professional judgment, but it can assist health educators in professional decision making. Insofar as the application of theory to practice strengthens program justification, promotes the effective and efficient use of resources, and improves accountability, it also assists in establishing professional credibility" (D'Onofrio, 1992, p. 394). However, this is not to say that a theory cannot be modified or expanded to include a logically valid idea or parts of other theories. "In fact, it is well understood that working with a theory has certain disadvantages; one of which is leaving out or ignoring factors that happen not to be theoretically relevant, even though they may be empirically significant" (Jessor & Jessor, 1977).

The importance of theory in planning health promotion interventions is best shown by the large number of health promotion programs that are designed to help facilitate health behavior change in the priority population. Getting people to engage in health behavior change is a complicated process that is very difficult under the best of conditions. Without the direction that theories provide, planners can easily waste valuable resources in trying to achieve the desired behavior change. Therefore, program planners should ground their planning process in the theories that have been the foundation of other successful health promotion efforts. An article by Shea and Basch (1990) provides a good review and rationale of the theories used in some of the most successful health promotion programs: the North Karelia Project, the Stanford Three Community Study, the Stanford Five-City Project, the Minnesota Heart Health Program, and the Pawtucket Heart Health Program. Table 7.1 summarizes the theories and models used in these programs, based on the information provided by Shea and Basch (1990). As can be seen by the information presented in the table, each of these programs is well grounded in theory.

Essentially, the principles and practices of health education are "derived from the egalitarian spirit and progressive theories of education and the fundamental theories of the behavioral sciences" (National Task Force, 1985, p. vii). The remaining sections of this chapter present an overview of the theories that are most often used in creating health promotion interventions. As you read about and study the various theories, you will find that some express the same general ideas, but employ "a unique vocabulary to articulate the specific factors considered to be important" (Glanz et al., 2002b, p. 26). Also, beware that the presentation of theories that follows is by no means comprehensive in nature. For those readers who would like to examine these

Table 7.1 Theories used in five community-based cardiovascular disease prevention programs

Program	Year Begun	Theories Used
Minnesota Heart Health Program	1980	• Social learning theory[a] • Communication-persuasion model[b] • Model of innovation diffusion[d] • Community development[c] • Problem-behavior theory
North Karelia Project	Late 1950s	• Social learning theory[a] • Theory of reasoned action[a] • Communication-persuasion model[b] • Model of innovation diffusion[d] • Community organization model[c]
Pawtucket Heart Health Program	1980	• Community organization model[c] • Social behavioral community psychology theory
Stanford Five-City Project	1978	• Social learning theory[a] • Theory of reasoned action[a] • Communication-persuasion model[b] • Model of innovation diffusion[d]
Stanford Three Community Study	1972	• Social learning theory[a]

[a] = Discussed in Chapter 7.
[b] = Discussed in Chapter 8.
[c] = Discussed in Chapter 9.
[d] = Discussed in Chapter 11.

and other theories in more depth, we would recommend two books: *Health Behavior and Health Education: Theory, Research and Practice* (Glanz, Rimer, & Lewis, 2002a) and *Emerging Theories in Health Promotion Practice and Research: Strategies for Improving Public Health* (DiClemente, Crosby, & Kegler, 2002).

Types of Theories and Models

There are several ways of categorizing the theories and models associated with health education/promotion practice. One way of doing so is to divide them into two groups. The first group includes those theories and models used for planning, implementing, and evaluating health promotion programs. This group has been called **planning models** (or *theories/models of implementation*). The planning models were presented in Chapter 2 of this book. The second group is referred to as **behavior change theories** (or *change process theories*). Behavior change theories "specify the relationships among causal processes operating both within and across levels of analysis" (McLeroy, Steckler, Goodman, & Burdine, 1992, p. 3). In other words, they help explain how change takes place.

Behavior Change Theories

Stimulus Response (SR) Theory

One of the theories used to explain and modify behavior is the stimulus response, or SR, theory (Thorndike, 1898; Watson, 1925; Hall, 1943). This theory reflects the combination of classical conditioning (Pavlov, 1927) and instrumental conditioning (Thorndike, 1898) theories. These early conditioning theories explain learning based on the associations among stimulus, response, and reinforcement (Parcel & Baranowski, 1981; Parcel, 1983). "In simplest terms, the SR theorists believe that learning results from events (termed 'reinforcements') which reduce physiological drives that activate behavior" (Rosenstock, Strecher, & Becker, 1988, p. 175). The behaviorist B. F. Skinner believed that the frequency of a behavior was determined by the reinforcements that followed that behavior.

In Skinner's view, the mere temporal association between a behavior and an immediately following reward is sufficient to increase the probability that the behavior will be repeated. Such behaviors are called *operants;* they operate on the environment to bring about changes resulting in reward or reinforcement (Rosenstock et al., 1988, p. 176). Stated another way, operant behaviors are behaviors that act on the environment to produce consequences. These consequences, in turn, either reinforce or do not reinforce the behavior that preceded.

The consequences of a behavior can come as either **reinforcement** or **punishment.** Individuals can learn from both. Reinforcement has been defined by Skinner (1953) as any event that follows a behavior, which in turn increases the probability that the same behavior will be repeated in the future. Stated differently, reinforcement has "a *strengthening effect* that occurs when operant behaviors have certain consequences" (Nye, 1992, p. 16). Behavior has a greater probability of occurring in the future (1) if reinforcement is frequent and (2) if reinforcement is provided soon after the desired behavior. This immediacy clarifies the relationship between the reinforcement and appropriate behavior (Skinner, 1953). If a behavior is complex in nature, smaller steps working toward the desired behavior with appropriate reinforcement will help to shape the desired behavior. This was found to be true in getting pigeons to play Ping-Pong, and it can be useful in trying to change a complex health behavior like smoking or exercise. While reinforcement will increase the frequency of a behavior, punishment will decrease the frequency of a behavior. However, both reinforcement and punishment can be either positive or negative. The terms *positive* and *negative* in this context do not mean good and bad; rather, *positive* means adding something (effects of the stimulus) to a situation, whereas *negative* means taking something away (removal or reduction of the effects of the stimulus) from the situation.

If individuals act in a certain way to produce a consequence that makes them feel good or that is enjoyable, it is labeled **positive reinforcement** (or *reward*). Examples of this would be an individual who is involved in an exercise program and "feels good" at the end of the workout, or one who participates in a weight loss program and receives verbal encouragement from the facilitator, again making that person "feel good." Stimulus response theorists would note that in both of these situations, the pleasant experiences (internal feelings and verbal encouragement, respectively) occur right after the behavior, which in turn increases the chances that the frequency of the behavior will increase.

While positive reinforcement helps individuals learn by shaping behavior, behavior that avoids punishment is also learned because it reduces the tension that precedes the punishment (Rosenstock et al., 1988). "When this happens, we are being conditioned by *negative reinforcement:* A response is strengthened by the *removal* of something from the situation. In such cases, the 'something' that is removed is referred to as a *negative reinforcer* or *aversive stimulus* (these two phrases are synonymous)" (Nye, 1979, p. 33). A good example of **negative reinforcement** is a weight loss program that requires weekly dues. When participants stop paying dues because they have met their goal weight, this removal of an obligation should increase frequency of the desired behavior (weight maintenance).

Some people think of negative reinforcement as a form of punishment, but it is not. While negative reinforcement increases the likelihood that a behavior will be repeated, punishment typically suppresses behavior. "Skinner suggests two ways in which a response can be punished: by *removing a positive reinforcer* or by *presenting a negative reinforcer* (aversive stimulus) as a consequence of the response" (Nye, 1979, p. 43). Punishment is usually linked to some uncomfortable (physical, mental, or otherwise) experience and decreases the frequency of a behavior. An aversive smoking cessation program that circulates cigarette smoke around those enrolled in the program as they smoke is an example of **positive punishment.** It decreases the frequency of smoking by presenting (adding) a negative reinforcer or **aversive stimulus** (smoke) as a consequence of the response. Examples of **negative punishment** (removing a positive reinforcer) would include not allowing employees to use the employees' lounge if they continue to smoke while using it, or reducing the health insurance benefits of employees who continue to participate in health-harming behavior such as not wearing a safety belt. Stimulus response theorists would note that taking away the privilege of using the employees' lounge or reducing health insurance benefits would cause a decrease in frequency of smoking among the employees and an increase in the wearing of safety belts, respectively. Figure 7.1 illustrates the relationship between reinforcement and punishment.

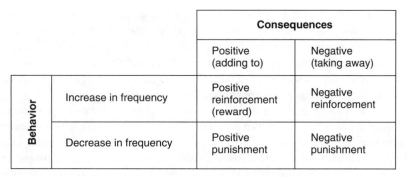

		Consequences	
		Positive (adding to)	Negative (taking away)
Behavior	Increase in frequency	Positive reinforcement (reward)	Negative reinforcement
	Decrease in frequency	Positive punishment	Negative punishment

Figure 7.1 2 X 2 table of the stimulus response theory

Finally, if reinforcement is withheld—or, stating it another way, if the behavior is ignored—the behavior will become less frequent and eventually will not be repeated. Skinner (1953) refers to this as extinction. Teachers frequently use this technique with disruptive children in the classroom. If a child is acting up in class, the teacher may choose to ignore the behavior in hopes that the nonreinforced behavior will go away.

Social Cognitive Theory (SCT)

The social learning theories (SLT) of Rotter (1954) and Bandura (1977b)—or, as Bandura (1986) relabeled them, the *social cognitive theory (SCT)*—combine SR theory and cognitive theories. Stimulus response theorists emphasize the role of reinforcement in shaping behavior and believe that no "thinking" or "reasoning" is needed to explain behavior. However, Bandura (2001) stated "If actions were performed only on behalf of anticipated external rewards and punishments, people would behave like weather vanes, constantly shifting directions to conform to whatever influence happened to impinge upon them at the moment" (p. 7). Cognitive theorists believe that reinforcement is an integral part of learning, but emphasize the role of subjective hypotheses or expectations held by the individual (Rosenstock et al., 1988). In other words, reinforcement contributes to learning, but reinforcement along with an individual's expectations of the consequences of behavior determine the behavior. "Behavior, in this perspective, is a function of the subjective value of an outcome and the subjective probability (or 'expectation') that a particular action will achieve that outcome. Such formulations are generally termed 'value-expectancy' theories" (Rosenstock et al., 1988, p. 176). In brief, SCT explains human functioning in terms of triadic reciprocal causation (Bandura, 1986). "In this model of reciprocal causality, internal personal factors in the form of cognitive, affective, and biological events, behavioral patterns, and environmental influences all operate as interacting determinants that influence one another bidirectionally" (Bandura, 2001, pp. 14–15). The constructs of the SCT that have been most often used in designing health promotion interventions will be presented here.

As already noted, reinforcement is an important component of SCT. According to SCT, reinforcement can be accomplished in one of three ways: directly, vicariously, or through self-reinforcement (Baranowski, Perry, & Parcel, 2002). An example of **direct reinforcement** is a group facilitator who provides verbal feedback to participants for a job well done. **Vicarious reinforcement** is having the participants observe some-one else being reinforced for behaving in an appropriate manner. This has been re-ferred to as *observational learning* (Baranowski et al., 2002) or *social modeling*. In a system of reinforcement by **self-reinforcement,** the participants would keep records of their own behavior, and when the behavior was performed in an appropriate man-ner, they would reinforce or reward themselves.

If individuals are to perform specific behaviors, they must know first what the be-haviors are and then how to perform them. This is referred to as **behavioral capa-bility.** For example, if people are to exercise aerobically, first they must know that aerobic exercise exists, and second they need to know how to do it properly. Many people begin exercise programs, only to quit within the first six months (Dishman, Sallis, & Orenstein, 1985), and some of those people quit because they do not know how to exercise properly. They know they should exercise, so they decide to run a few miles, have sore muscles the next day, and quit. Skill mastery is very important. The construct of **expectations** refers to the ability of human beings to think, and thus to anticipate certain things to happen in certain situations. For example, if people are en-rolled in a weight loss program and follow the directions of the group facilitator, they will expect to lose weight. **Expectancies,** not to be confused with expectations, are the values that individuals place on an expected outcome. "Expectancies influence behavior according to the hedonic principle: if all other things are equal, a person will choose to perform an activity that maximizes a positive outcome or minimizes a neg-ative outcome" (Baranowski et al., 2002, p. 173). Someone who enjoys the feeling of not smoking more than that of smoking is more likely to try to do the things necessary to stop. The construct of **self-control** or **self-regulation** states that individuals may gain control of their own behavior through monitoring and adjusting it (Clark et al., 1992). When helping individuals to change their behavior, it is a common practice to have them monitor their behavior over a period of time, through 24-hour diet or smoking records or exercise diaries, and then to have them reward (reinforce) them-selves based upon their monitored performance.

One construct of SCT that has received special attention in health promotion pro-grams is **self-efficacy** (Strecher et al., 1986), which refers to the internal state that individuals experience as "competence" to perform certain desired tasks or behavior, "including confidence in overcoming the barriers to performing that behavior" (Bara-nowski et al., 2002, p. 173). "Unless people believe they can produce desired results and forestall detrimental ones by their actions, they have little incentive to act or to persevere in the face of difficulties" (Bandura, 2001, p. 10). Self-efficacy is situation specific; that is, individuals may be self-efficacious when it comes to aerobic exercise but not so when faced with reducing the amount of fat in their diet. People's compe-tency feelings have been referred to as **efficacy expectations.** Thus, people who think they can exercise on a regular basis no matter what the circumstances have ef-ficacy expectations. Even though people have efficacy expectations, they still may not want to engage in a behavior because they may not think the outcomes of that be-havior would be beneficial to them. Stated another way, they may not feel that the reward (reinforcement) of performing the behavior is great enough for them. These beliefs are called **outcome expectations.** For example, in order for individuals to quit smoking for health reasons (behavior), they must believe both that they are ca-pable of quitting (efficacy expectation) and that cessation will benefit their health

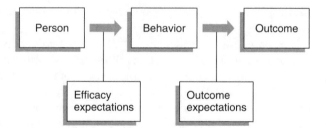

Figure 7.2 Diagrammatic representation of the difference between efficacy and outcome expectations
Source: Social Learning Theory by Bandura, Albert, © 1977. Reprinted by permission of Pearson Education, Inc., Upper Saddle River, NJ.

(outcome expectation) (I. M. Rosenstock, personal communication, April 1986). Figure 7.2 (Bandura, 1977b) illustrates efficacy and outcome expectations.

Individuals become self-efficacious in four main ways:

1. Through performance attainments (personal mastery of a task)
2. Through vicarious experience (observing the performance of others)
3. As a result of verbal persuasion (receiving suggestions from others)
4. Through emotional arousal (interpreting one's emotional state)

The construct of **emotional-coping responses** states that for people to learn, they must be able to deal with the sources of anxiety that may surround a behavior. For example, fear is an emotion that can be involved in learning; according to this construct, participants would have to deal with the fear before they could learn the behavior.

The construct of **reciprocal determinism** states, unlike SR theory, that there is an interaction among the person, the behavior, and the environment, and that the person can shape the environment as well as the environment shaping the person. All these relationships are dynamic. Glanz and Rimer (1995, p. 15) provide a good example of this construct:

> A man with high cholesterol might have a hard time following his prescribed low-fat diet because his company cafeteria doesn't offer low-fat food choices that he likes. He can try to change the environment by talking with the cafeteria manager or the company medical or health department staff, and asking that healthy food choices be added to the menu. Or, if employees start to dine elsewhere in order to eat low-fat lunches, the cafeteria may change its menu to maintain its lunch business.

Finally, there is one other construct that grew out of the social learning theory of Rotter (1954) that needs to be mentioned because of its association with health behavior. "Rotter posited that a person's history of positive or negative reinforcement across a variety of situations shapes a belief as to whether or not a person's own actions lead to those reinforcements" (Wallston, 1994, p. 187). Rotter referred to this construct as **locus of control.** Thus he felt that people with internal locus of control perceived that reinforcement was under their control, whereas those with external locus of control perceived reinforcement to be under the control of some external force. In the 1970s, Wallston and his colleagues at Vanderbilt University began testing the usefulness of this construct in predicting health behavior (Wallston, 1994). They explored the concept of whether individuals with internal locus of control were more likely to participate in health-enhancing behavior than those with external locus of control. They began their work by examining locus of control as a two-dimensional construct (internal vs. external), then moved to a multidimensional construct when they split the external dimension into "powerful others" and "chance" (Wallston, Wallston, & DeVellis, 1978). After a number of years of work by many different researchers, Wallston has come to the conclusion that locus of control accounts for only a small amount of the variability in health behavior (Wallston, 1992). The internal locus of control belief about one's own health status is a necessary but not sufficient determinate of health-enhancing behavior (Wallston, 1994). Since the rise of the construct of self-efficacy, Wallston (1994) feels that self-efficacy is a better predictor of health-promoting behavior than locus of control. This is not to say that locus of control is not a useful construct in developing health promotion programs. Knowing the locus of control orientation of those in the priority population can provide planners with valuable information when considering social support as part of a planned intervention. Table 7.2 provides a summary of the constructs of the SCT and an example of how each construct might be operationalized.

Theory of Reasoned Action (TRA)

Another theory that has received considerable attention in the literature of health behavior change is Fishbein's *theory of reasoned action (TRA)* (Fishbein 1967). Like the theories already discussed, this theory was developed to explain not just health behavior but all volitional behaviors. The theories discussed earlier in this chapter were directly concerned with behavior; however, this one provides a framework to study attitudes toward behaviors.

Fishbein and Ajzen (1975) distinguish among *attitude, belief, behavioral intention,* and *behavior,* and they present a conceptual framework for the study of the relationship among these four constructs. **Behavioral intention** is viewed as a special type of belief and is indicated by individuals' subjective perceptions and report of the probability that they will perform the behavior (Parcel, 1983). According to this theory, individuals' intention to perform given behaviors are functions of their *attitudes* toward the behavior and their *subjective norms* associated with the behaviors. **Attitude toward the behavior** "is determined by the individual's beliefs about outcomes or attributes of performing the behavior (*behavioral beliefs*) weighted by evaluations of those outcomes or attributes" (Montano & Kasprzyk, 2002, p. 70). Thus a person who has strong beliefs about positive attributes or outcomes from performing the behavior will have a positive attitude toward behavior (Montano & Kasprzyk, 2002). For example, if a person feels strongly about exercise being able to help control weight, then that person will have a positive attitude toward exercise. The converse is true as well. Weak beliefs about the outcomes or attributes of exercise will produce a negative attitude toward it.

Subjective norm is determined by *normative beliefs.* Normative beliefs are those beliefs held by the individual about whether important referent others approve or disapprove of the behavior, weighted by the individual's motivation to comply with

Table 7.2 Often-used constructs of the social cognitive theory and examples of their application

Construct	Definition	Example
Behavioral Capability	Knowledge and skills necessary to perform a behavior	If people are going to exercise aerobically, they need to know what it is and how to do it.
Expectations	Beliefs about the likely outcomes of certain behaviors	If people enroll in a weight-loss program, they expect to lose weight.
Expectancies	Values people place on expected outcomes	How important is it to people that they become physically fit?
Locus of Control	Perception of the center of control over reinforcement	Those who feel they have control over reinforcement are said to have internal locus of control. Those who perceive reinforcement under the control of some external force are said to have external locus of control.
Reciprocal Determinism	Behavior changes result from an interaction between the person and the environment; change is bidirectional (Glanz & Rimer, 1995)	Lack of use of vending machines could be a result of the choices within the machine. Notes about the selections from the nonusing consumers to the machine's owners could change the selections and change the behavior of the consumers to that of users.
Reinforcement (directly, vicariously, self)	Responses to behaviors that increase the chances of recurrence	Giving verbal encouragement to those who have acted in a healthy manner.
Self-Control or Self Regulation	Gaining control over own behavior through monitoring and adjusting it	If clients want to change their eating habits, have them monitor their current eating habits for seven days.
Self-Efficacy	People's confidence in their ability to perform a certain desired task or function	If people are going to engage in a regular exercise program, they must feel they can do it.
Emotional-Coping Response	For people to learn, they must be able to deal with the sources of anxiety that surround a behavior	Fear is an emotion that can be involved in learning, and people would have to deal with it before they could learn a behavior.

Source: Cottrell, Girvan, and McKenzie (2002), p.123. Reprinted by permission.

those referents (Montano & Kasprzyk, 2002). For many health behaviors, the referents may include a person's peers, parents, partner, close friends, teachers, role models, boss, and coworkers, as well as experts or professionals like physicians or lawyers. Thus individuals who believe that certain referents think they should perform a behavior and are motivated to meet the referents' expectations will hold a positive subjective norm (Montano & Kasprzyk, 2002). Similar to behavioral beliefs, the converse is also true. An example of a positive subjective norm are employees who see their coworkers as important referents and believe that these referents approve of them participating in a company exercise program.

Theory of Planned Behavior (TPB)

The theory of reasoned action has proved to be most successful when dealing with purely volitional behaviors, but complications are encountered when the theory is applied to behaviors that are not fully under volitional control. A good example of this is a smoker who intends to quit but fails to do so. Even though intent is high, nonmotivational factors—such as lack of requisite opportunities, skills, and resources—could prevent success (Ajzen, 1988).

The *theory of planned behavior (TPB)* (see Figure 7.3) is an extension of the theory of reasoned action that addresses the problem of incomplete volitional control. The major difference between TPB and TRA is the addition of a third, conceptually independent determinant of intention. Like TRA, TPB includes attitude toward the behavior and subjective norm, but it has added the concept of perceived behavioral control. Perceived behavioral control is similar to the SCT's concept of self-efficacy. **Perceived behavioral control** "is determined by *control beliefs* concerning the presence or absences of facilitators or barriers to behavioral performance, weighted by *perceived power* or impact of each factor to facilitate or inhibit the behavior" (Montano & Kasprzyk, 2002, p. 75). Stated differently, perceived behavioral control refers to the perceived ease or difficulty of performing the behavior and is assumed to reflect past experience as well as anticipated impediments and obstacles. As a general rule, the more favorable the attitude and subjective norm with respect to a behavior, and the greater the perceived behavioral control, the stronger

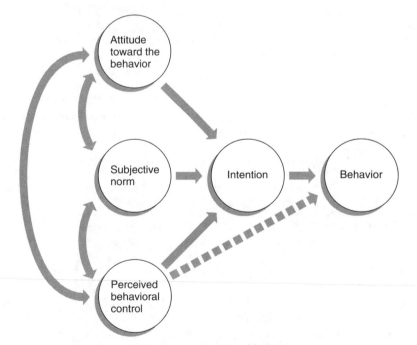

Figure 7.3 Diagram of the theory of planned behavior
Source: I. Ajzen, Diagram of Planned Behaviour, from *Attitudes, Personality, and Behaviour.* Copyright © 1988 Dorsey Press. The material is reproduced with the kind permission of the Open University/McGraw-Hill Publishing Company.

should be the individual's intentions to perform the behavior under consideration (Ajzen, 1988).

Figure 7.3 illustrates two important features of this theory. First, perceived behavioral control has motivational implications for intentions. That is, without perceived control, intentions could be minimal even if attitudes toward the behavior and subjective norm were strong. Second, there may be a direct link between perceived behavioral control and behavior. Behavior depends not only on motivation but also on adequate control. Thus it stands to reason that perceived behavioral control can help predict goal attainment independent of behavioral intention (Ajzen, 1988). To use the example of smoking once again as a behavior not fully under volitional control, TPB predicts that individuals will give up smoking if they:

1. Have a positive attitude toward quitting
2. Think others whom they value believe it would be good for them to quit
3. Perceives that they have control over whether they quit

Evidence to support the usefulness of the TPB to explain a variety of health behaviors seems to be mounting (Godin & Kok, 1996; Montano, Kasprzyk, von Haeften, & Fishbein, 2001; Montano, Phillips, & Kasprzyk, 2000; and Montano, Thompson, Taylor, & Mahloch, 1997). Godin and Kok (1996) presented a review of 58 studies where the theory was applied to health-related behaviors. They found that the efficiency of the theory seemed "to be quite good for explaining intention, perceived behavioral control being as important as attitude across behavioral categories. The efficiency of the theory, however, varied between health-related behavior categories" (Godin & Kok, 1996, p. 87).

Theory of Freeing (TF)

A theory that takes a much different approach from the other theories presented is the theory of freeing (TF) (Freire, 1973, 1974). Like the others, it is not specific to health promotion, but it does have application to health promotion. It is a theory aimed at empowering education. Wallerstein and Bernstein (1988, p. 380) define empowerment as "a social action process that promotes participation of people, organizations, and communities in gaining control over their lives in their community and larger society. With this perspective, empowerment is not characterized as achieving power to dominate others, but rather power to act with others to effect change."

The theory was first used in the late 1950s when the late Paulo Freire, a Brazilian educator, initiated a successful literacy and political consciousness program for shantytown dwellers and peasants in Brazil (Freire, 1973). Since that time, the theory has been applied to many other problems.

One of the first to apply this theory to health promotion was Greenberg. He stated (1978, p. 20) that the task of health education should be to "free people so they may make health-related decisions based upon their needs and interests as long as these needs and interests do not adversely affect others." In essence, Freire's concept of freeing contrasts "being free with being oppressed" (Walker & Bibeau, 1985/1986, p. 5). People become free by being critically conscious.

The underlying concept of this theory is that critical consciousness is determined by the interaction with culture. Consciousness is influenced by and influences the culture. Oppressed people are "of the world," and their consciousness is a product of the culture. Being "of the world" is defined by the lack of the person's ability to perceive, respond, and act with power to change concrete reality (Walker & Bibeau, 1985/1986). Free people are "in the world," and their consciousness is a producer of culture.

Education is the key to becoming critically conscious. However, the education that is meant here is not education in the traditional sense. Education occurs through dialogue, not through lecture. People who use dialogue are teachers, whereas those who just talk are lecturers. And in this type of education, participants replace pupils. All those involved in the educational process learn from one another.

A very useful summary of the applications of Freire's work to health promotion has been presented by Wallerstein and Bernstein (1988) and Wallerstein (1994). They state that Freire's theory includes three stages. Stage 1 is the listening stage, in which those in the priority population have the opportunity to share their thoughts, identify the problems, and set the priorities. Unlike in a more traditional planning process, the program planners do not collect data and determine the needs. Instead, the priority population is identifying the issues and prioritizing the needs.

Stage 2 is a dialogue process. The dialogue revolves around a *code*. "A 'code' is a concrete physical representation of an identified community issue in any form: role plays, stories, slides, photographs, songs, etc." (Wallerstein & Bernstein, 1988, p. 383). After experiencing a code, group facilitators lead the priority population through a discussion that helps the people move from a personal to a social analysis and action level. They do this by asking the priority population to respond to these five statements (Wallerstein & Bernstein, 1988):

1. Describe what you see and feel.
2. As a group, define the many levels of the problem.
3. Share similar experiences from your lives.
4. Question why this problem exists.
5. Develop action plans to address the problem.

Stage 3 of this theory is the action stage, in which those in the priority population try out the plans that came from the listening and dialogue stages. As the people put their plans into action, they reflect on their new experiences and create a thinking-acting cycle. "This recurrent spiral of action-reflection-action enables people to learn from their collective attempts at change and to become more deeply involved to surmount the cultural, social, or historic barriers" (Wallerstein & Bernstein, 1988, p. 383).

Health Belief Model (HBM)

The **health belief model (HBM),** which is the one most frequently used in health behavior applications, is also a value-expectancy theory. It was developed in the 1950s by a group of psychologists to help explain why people would or would not use health services (Rosenstock, 1966). The HBM is based on Lewin's decision-making model (Lewin, 1935, 1936; Lewin et al., 1944). Since its creation, the HBM has been used to help explain a variety of health behaviors (Becker, 1974; Janz & Becker, 1984).

The HBM hypothesizes that health-related action depends on the simultaneous occurrence of three classes of factors:

1. The existence of sufficient motivation (or health concern) to make health issues salient or relevant.

2. The belief that one is susceptible (vulnerable) to a serious health problem or to the sequelae of that illness or condition. This is often termed **perceived threat.**

3. The belief that following a particular health recommendation would be beneficial in reducing the perceived threat, and at a subjectively acceptable cost. Cost refers to the **perceived barriers** that must be overcome in order to follow the health recommendation; it includes, but is not restricted to, financial outlays (Rosenstock et al., 1988, p. 177). In fact, the lack of self-efficacy is also seen as a perceived barrier to taking a recommended health action (Strecher & Rosenstock, 1997).

Figure 7.4 provides a diagram of the HBM as presented by Becker, Drachman, and Kirscht (1974).

In recent years, self-efficacy has become a more meaningful concept in the perceived barriers construct of the HBM. When the HBM was first conceived, self-efficacy was not explicitly a part of it. "The original focus of the model was on

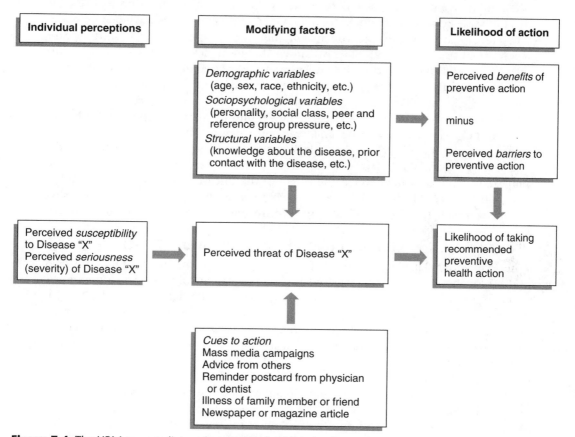

Figure 7.4 The HBM as a predictor of preventive health behavior
Source: M. H. Becker, R. H. Drachman, and J. P. Kirscht, "A New Approach to Explaining Sick-Role Behavior in Low Income Populations," *American Journal of Public Health, 64* (March 1974): 205–216. © 1974 American Public Health Association. Reprinted by permission.

circumscribed preventive actions, usually one-shot in nature, such as accepting a screening test or an immunization, actions that generally were simple behaviors to perform" (Janz, Champion, & Strecher, 2002, p. 50) and ones for which most people in the priority populations had adequate self-efficacy (Janz et al., 2002). However, when program planners want to use the HBM to plan health promotion interventions for priority populations in need of lifestyle behaviors requiring long-term changes, self-efficacy must be included in the model. "For behavior change to succeed, people must (as the original HBM theorizes) feel threatened by their current behavioral patterns (perceived susceptibility and severity) and believe that change of a specific kind will result in a valued outcome at acceptable cost. They must also feel themselves competent (self-efficacious) to overcome perceived barriers to taking action" (Janz et al., 2002, p. 51).

Here is an example of the HBM applied to exercise. Someone watching television sees an advertisement about exercise. This is a cue to action that starts her thinking about her own need to exercise. There may be some variables (demographic, sociopsychological, and structural) that cause her to think about it a bit more. She remembers her college health course that included information about heart disease and the importance of staying active. She knows she has a higher than normal risk for heart disease because of family history, poor diet, and slightly elevated blood pressure. Therefore, she comes to the conclusion that she is susceptible to heart disease **(perceived susceptibility).** She also knows that if she develops heart disease, it can be very serious **(perceived seriousness/severity**). Based on these factors, the individual thinks that there is reason to be concerned about heart disease (perceived threat). She knows that exercise can help delay the onset of heart disease and can increase the chances of surviving a heart attack if one should occur **(perceived benefits).** But exercise takes time from an already busy day, and it is not easy to exercise in the variety of settings in which she typically finds herself, especially during bad weather (perceived barriers). Her confidence in being able to exercise regularly will also be important. She must now weigh the threat of the disease against the difference between benefits and barriers. This decision will then result in a likelihood of exercising or not exercising **(likelihood of taking recommended preventive health action).**

The Elaboration Likelihood Model of Persuasion (ELM)

The Elaboration Likelihood Model of Persuasion, or Elaboration Likelihood Model (ELM) for short, was initially developed to help explain inconsistencies in the results from research dealing with study of attitudes (Petty, Barden, & Wheeler, 2002). Specifically, the model was designed to help explain how persuasion messages (communications), aimed at changing attitudes, were received and processed by people. "Although the model has a rich history in the field of psychology, its application to health promotion is newly emerging" (Crosby, Kegler, & DiClemente, 2002, p. 9). Since its development, the framework has been found useful for interpreting and predicting the impact that health messages (communications) have on subsequent attitudes and behavior (Petty et al., 2002).

Before we continue with our explanation of this model, it is necessary to define what is meant by the term elaboration. **Elaboration** refers to the amount of effortful processing people put into receiving messages. By effortful processing, we mean careful cognitive consideration of the message, or stated another way "careful thinking about" the message. With that definition out of the way, let's examine the three major elements of this model (see Figure 7.5).

First, the ELM organizes multiple persuasion processes into two routes of attitude change; *peripheral* and *central*. The peripheral processes are those that require little thought about issue-relevant information and instead rely on simple cues or mental shortcuts, called *heuristics*, as the primary means of attitude change (Petty et al., 2002). For example, a person may form an attitude after hearing a persuasive message simply because the person delivering the message is recognized as an expert in the field, such as when the Surgeon General makes a statement about a certain health behavior. Or, a person may form an attitude based solely on hearing the same message over and over. On the other hand, the central processes are those that require thoughtful consideration of issue-relevant information and its relationship to pertinent knowledge that one already has to form the primary bases for attitude change (Petty et al., 2002). "Two conditions are necessary for effortful processing to occur: the recipient of the message must be motivated and able to process it thoroughly" (Petty et al., 2002, p. 74). An example of central route processing would be a person's formation of an attitude about safety belt use based upon careful consideration of a message about the pros and cons of its use along with recalling the knowledge gained in drivers' education class and possibly the results of an automobile crash in which his/her cousin was involved.

It should be clear, that the distinction between the peripheral and central routes is the amount of consideration given to the issue-relevant information and how the information is processed, not the type of information itself (Petty, Wheeler, & Bizer, 1999). Yet not all messages fall neatly into either peripheral or central categories of processing. People really receive messages along an *elaboration likelihood continuum*. The continuum stretches from one end anchored with processes requiring no thinking, like classical conditioning (see discussion of the Stimulus Response Theory earlier in this chapter), to processes requiring some effortful thinking such as making inferences based on ones experiences, to processes requiring careful consideration (Petty et al., 2002).

Second, when comparing the consequences of the two routes, research has shown that even though both routes "can sometimes result in attitudes with similar valence, the two processes typically lead to attitudes with different consequences" (Petty et al., 2002, p. 93). According to this model, the more effortful processing (or the more elaboration) people put into receiving messages the more likely they are to form attitudes that are persistent over time, resistant to counterattack, and influential in guiding thought and behavior (Krosnick & Petty, 1995). Just the opposite is also true; the less elaboration, the less stable the attitude over time.

"Third, the model specifies how variables have an impact on persuasion" (Petty et al., 2002, p.82). The variables can influence a person's motivation to think or ability to think, as well the valence of one's thought or the confidence in the thoughts generated (Petty et al., 2002). Typical variables that have an influence on how persuasive messages are processed include the source of the message (i.e., Is the source credible? Is the source friendly? Is it coming from a friend, an authoritative figure, an expert?), the message itself (e.g., Is it understandable? Is it simple? Complex? Funny?), the context in which the message is presented (e.g., Is it delivered person-to-person? Where is the message received? Is the message coming by way of television or radio? Is the message being delivered to a group?), and the characteristics of the message recipient

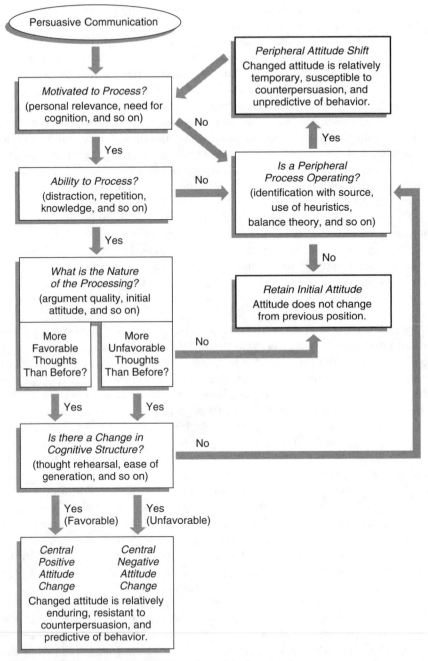

Figure 7.5 The elaboration likelihood model of persuasion
Source: "The Elaboration Likelihood Model of Persuasion," by Petty et al, *Emerging Theories In Health Promotion Practice & Research,* (DiChimente), p. 83. Copyright © 2002 by John Wiley & Sons, Inc. This material is used by permission of John Wiley & Sons, Inc.

(e.g., How intelligent is the recipient? How attentive? In what mood is the recipient? How relevant is the topic to the recipient?) (Petty et al., 2002).

The ELM has been used to develop a variety of interventions for health promotion programs. The one area where the ELM has been most useful in health promotion has been with message tailoring. Tailored messages are those that are "crafted for and delivered to each individual based on individual needs, interests, and circumstances" (NCI, 2002, p. 251). In other words, tailored messages are matched to the needs, interests, and circumstances of the intended recipient. It has been found that the more tailored the persuasive communication, the more relevant it is to the recipient, and the more likely the message will be processed through the central route. And, if a message is processed through the central route the more likely it will impact attitude and behavior change.

For those readers who want more information on tailoring messages, please refer to the work of Kreuter, Farrell, Olevitch, & Brennan (2000).

Stage Theories

All of the theories presented in this chapter so far fall into a subcategory of behavior change theories refereed to as **continuum theories.** The approach of such theories

> is to identify variables that influence action (such as perceptions of risk and precaution effectiveness) and to combine them in a prediction equation. When applied to a particular individual, the value generated by the equation indicates the probability that this person will act. Thus, each person is placed along a continuum of action of likelihood. Because each theory has only a single prediction equation, the way in which variables combine to influence action is expected to be the same for everyone (Weinstein, Rothman, & Sutton, 1998, p. 291).

The other subgroup of behavior change theories is referred to as **stage theories.** A stage theory is one that is comprised of an ordered set of categories into which people can be classified, and for which factors could be identified that could induce movement from one category to the next (Weinstein & Sandman, 2002b). More specifically, stage theories have four principal elements (Weinstein & Sandman, 2002a): 1) a category system to define the stages, 2) an ordering of stages, 3) common barriers to change that face people in the same stage, and 4) different barriers to change that face people in different stages. Several different stage models have been proposed, but the two most commonly reported in the literature are the Transtheoretical Model (TTM) (Prochaska, 1979; Prochaska & DiClemente 1983) and the Precaution Adoption Process Model (PAPM) (Weinstein, 1988; Weinstein et al., 1998). Each is presented below.

The Transtheoretical Model (TTM).   "The Transtheoretical Model is an integrative framework for understanding how individuals and populations progress toward adopting and maintaining health behavior change for optimal health. The Transtheoretical Model uses stages of change to integrate processes and principles of change from across major theories of intervention, hence the name 'Transtheoretical'" (Prochaska, Johnson, & Lee, 1998, p. 59). The model has its roots in psychotherapy and was developed by Prochaska (1979) after he completed a comparative analysis of 18 therapy systems and a critical review of three–hundred therapy outcome studies. From the analysis and review, Prochaska found that some common processes were involved in change.

As this model has evolved, researchers have applied it to many different types of health behavior change, including but not limited to "alcohol and substance abuse, anxiety and panic disorders, delinquency, eating disorders and obesity, high-fat diets, HIV/AIDS prevention, mammography screening, medication compliance, unplanned pregnancy prevention, pregnancy and smoking, sedentary lifestyles, sun exposure, and physicians practicing preventive medicine" (Prochaska, Redding, & Evers, 2002, p. 99–100.)

The core constructs of the transtheoretical model include the stages of change, the processes of change, the pros and cons of changing, and self-efficacy (see Table 7.3). In addition, this model is "based on critical assumptions about the nature of behavior change and interventions that can best facilitate change" (Prochaska et al., 1998, p. 60). These constructs and assumptions will be discussed next.

Behavioral change does not occur overnight. A person does not go to bed at night as a nonexerciser and wake up the next morning as an exerciser. Behavior change occurs over a period of time. Thus the **stage** construct is an important part of the trans-theoretical model because it represents the temporal dimension of change (Prochaska et al., 2002). The model suggests that "people move from *precontemplation*, not intend-ing to change, to *contemplation*, intending to change within 6 months, to *preparation*, actively planning change, to *action*, overtly making changes, and into *maintenance*, tak-ing steps to sustain change and resist temptation to relapse" (Prochaska, Redding, Harlow, Rossi & Velicer, 1994). The **precontemplation stage** is defined as a time when people are not seriously thinking about changing their behavior during the next six months. "Many individuals in this stage are unaware or underaware of their problems" (Prochaska, DiClemente, & Norcross, 1992, p. 1103). People in this stage "tend to avoid reading, talking, or thinking about their high-risk behaviors" (Prochaska et al., 1998). The second stage, **contemplation** occurs when people are aware that a problem exists and are seriously thinking about a behavior change but have not yet made a commitment to take action. They are more open to feedback and information about the problem behavior than those in the precontemplation stage (Redding et al., 1999). For example, most smokers know that smoking is bad for them and consider quitting, but are not quite ready to do so. The third stage is called **preparation** and combines intention and behavioral criteria. "Individuals in this stage are intending to take action in the next month and have unsuccessfully taken action in the past year" (Prochaska, DiClemente, & Norcross, 1992, p. 1104). In this stage, they may have taken some small steps toward action, such as buying the necessary clothes for exer-cising or cutting back on the fat grams they consume or the cigarettes they smoke, but they have not reached an effective criterion for effective action (Prochaska, Norcross, Fowler, Follick, & Abrams, 1992). "These are the people we should recruit for such action-oriented programs as smoking cessation, weight loss, or exercise" (Prochaska et al., 1998, p. 61).

People are in the fourth stage, the **action stage,** when they are overtly making changes in their behavior, experiences, or environment in order to overcome their problems. This stage of change reflects a consistent behavior pattern, is usually the most visible, and receives the greatest external recognition (Prochaska, DiClemente, & Nor-cross, 1992). Since the behavior change is very new in this stage and the chance of re-lapse is high, considerable attention still must be given to relapse prevention (Redding et al., 1999). Also, "not all modifications of behavior count as action in this model. Peo-

Table 7.3 Transtheoretical Model Constructs

Constructs	Description
Stages of Change	
Precontemplation	No intention to take action within the next 6 months
Contemplation	Intends to take action within the next 6 months
Preparation	Intends to take action within the next 30 days and has taken some behavioral steps in this direction
Action	Has changed overt behavior for less than 6 months
Maintenance	Has changed overt behavior for more than 6 months
Decisional Balance	
Pros	The benefits of changing
Cons	The costs of changing
Self-Efficacy	
Confidence	Confidence that one can engage in the healthy behavior across different challenging situations
Temptation	Temptation to engage in the unhealthy behavior across different challenging situations
Processes of Change	
Consciousness Raising	Finding and learning new facts, ideas, and tips that support the healthy behavior change.
Dramatic Relief	Experiencing the negative emotions (fear, anxiety, worry) that go with unhealthy behavioral risks
Self-Reevaluation	Realizing that the behavior change is an important part of one's identity as a person
Environmental Reevaluation	Realizing the negative impact of the unhealthy behavior, or the positive impact of the healthy behavior, on one's proximal social and/ or physical environment
Self-Liberation	Making a firm commitment to change
Helping Relationships	Seeking and using social support for the healthy behavior change
Counterconditioning	Substitution of healthier alternative behaviors and/or cognitions for the unhealthy behavior
Reinforcement Management	Increasing the rewards for the positive behavior change and/or decreasing the rewards of the unhealthy behavior
Stimulus Control	Removing reminders or cues to engage in the unhealthy behavior and/ or adding cues to reminders to engage in the healthy behavior
Social Liberation	Realizing that social norms are changing in the direction of supporting the healthy behavior change.

Source: Redding et al. (1999). Reprinted by permission.

ple must attain a criterion that scientists and professionals agree is sufficient to reduce risks of disease" (Prochaska et al., 1998, p. 61). For example, in smoking, reduction in the number of cigarettes smoked does not count, only total abstinence (Prochaska et al., 1998). If those making changes continue with their new pattern of behavior, they will move into the fifth stage, maintenance.

Working to prevent relapse is the focus of the **maintenance stage.** People in this stage have changed their problem behavior for at least six months and are increasingly more confident that they can continue their changes (Prochaska et al., 1998; Redding et al., 1999). The person's change has become more of a habit and the chance of relapse is lower, but it still requires some attention (Redding et al., 1999).

The final stage is **termination.** This stage is defined as the time when individuals who have changed have zero temptation to return to their old behavior and they have 100% self-efficacy—that is, a lifetime of maintenance. No matter what their mood, they will not return to their old behavior (Prochaska et al., 1998). This is a stage that few people reach with certain behaviors (i.e., alcoholics). Since this may not be a practical goal for the majority of people, it has been given less attention in the research (Prochaska et al., 1998). Figure 7.6 provides a summary of the stages of change.

The second major construct of the transtheoretical model is the **processes of change** (see Table 7.3 for an explanation of the 10 processes). "These are the covert and overt activities that people use to progress through the stages" (Prochaska et al., 1998, p. 62). Study over the years has indicated that some of the processes are more useful at specific stages of change. The experimental set of processes (consciousness raising, dramatic relief, self-reevaluation, environmental reevaluation, and social liberation) are most often emphasized in earlier stages (precontemplation, contempla-

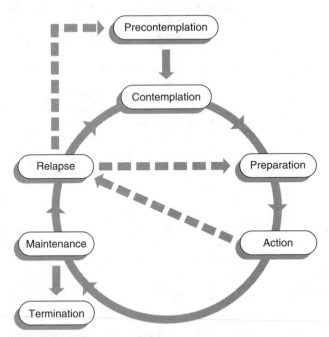

Figure 7.6 The stages of change
Source: "Models for Provider-Patient Interaction: Applications to Health Behavior Change," by M.G Goldstein, J. DePue, A. Kazura, and R. Niaura, in *The Handbook of Health Behavior Change,* 2nd edition, S.A. Shumaker, E.B. Schron, J.K. Ockene, and W.L. McBee (Eds.), © 1998 Springer Publishing Company, Inc., New York 10012. Used by permission of the publisher.

tion, and preparation) to increase intention and motivation, whereas the behavioral set of processes (helping relationships, counterconditioning, reinforcement management, stimulus control, and self-liberation) are most often utilized in the later stages (preparation, action, maintenance) as observable behavior change efforts get underway and need to be maintained (Redding et al., 1999) (see Table 7.4).

The construct of **decisional balance** refers to the pros and cons of the behavioral change. That is, individuals' decisions to move from one stage to the next is based on the relative importance (pro), or the lack thereof (con), of the behavior change for the individuals. "Characteristically, the pros of healthy behavior are low in the early stages and increase across the stages of change, and the cons of the healthy behavior are high in the early stages and decrease across the stages of change" (Redding et al., 1999, p. 90).

The final construct of the transtheoretical model is **self-efficacy.** The developers of this model see self-efficacy as it was defined by Bandura (1977b) earlier in this chapter. As used in the TTM, Prochaska and colleagues (2002) break self-efficacy into two components; confidence and temptation. *Confidence* refers to the feelings of being able to engage in healthy behaviors across different challenging situations. While *temptation* refers to the situational temptation of those making change to engage in the unhealthy behavior. "Typically, three factors reflect the most common types of tempting situations: negative affect or emotional distress, positive social situations, and craving" (Prochaska et al., 2002, p. 103). As one might guess, temptation decreases as one moves through the stages; however, even in the maintenance stage temptation is still present.

As noted at the beginning of this discussion, the transtheoretical model not only includes the four core constructs but it is also based on five critical assumptions. The assumptions (Prochaska et al., 2002) include:

1. No single theory can account for all the complexities of behavior change. Therefore a more comprehensive model will most likely emerge from an integration across major theories.

2. Behavior change is a process that unfolds over time through a sequence of stages.

Table 7.4 Stages of change in which processes are most emphasized

	Stages of Changes				
Processes	Precontemplation	Contemplation	Preparation	Action	Maintenance
	Consciousness raising				
	Dramatic relief				
	Environmental reevaluation				
		Self-reevaluation	Self-liberation		
				Contingency management	
				Helping relationship	
				Counterconditioning	
				Stimulus control	

Source: "The Transtheoretical Model of Behavior Change," by O.J. Prochaska, S. Johnson, and P. Lee, in *The Handbook of Health Behavior Change,* 2nd edition, S.A. Shumaker, E.B. Schron, J.K. Ockene, and W.L. McBee (Eds.), © 1998 Springer Publishing Company, Inc., New York 10012. Used by permission of the publisher.

3. Stages are both stable and open to change just as chronic behavioral risk factors are stable and open to change.

4. The majority of at-risk populations are not prepared for action and will not be served by traditional action-oriented prevention programs.

5. Specific processes and principles of change should be applied at specific stages if progress through the stages is to occur (p. 104).

Since its development, the transtheoretical model has been useful in several different ways. The first is that it makes program planners aware that not everyone is ready for change "right now," even though there is a program that can help them modify their behavior. People proceed through behavior change at different paces. Second, if individuals are not ready for action right now, then other programs can be developed to help them become ready for action. This second aspect fits in nicely with the effort to market a program and is discussed further in Chapter 11.

Precaution Adoption Process Model (PAPM). The Precaution Adoption Process Model has been more recently developed than the transtheoretical model (TTM) (Weinstein, 1988; Weinstein & Sandman, 1992), and has been referred to as an *emerging theory* by DiClemente and colleagues (2002). Its goal "is to explain how a person comes to the decision to take action, and how he or she translates that decision into action" (Weinstein & Sandman, 2002a, p. 124). Though the TTM and PAPM are both stage models and appear similar, "it is mainly the names that have been given to the stages that are similar. The number of stages is not the same in the two theories, and those with similar names are defined quite differently" (Weinstein & Sandman, 2002a, p. 125). The PAPM is most applicable for use with the adoption of a new precaution, or the abandonment of a risky behavior that requires a deliberate action. It can also be used to explain why and how people make deliberate changes in habitual patterns. It is not applicable for actions that require the gradual development of habitual patterns of behavior such as exercise and diet (Weinstein & Sandman, 2002b). Weinstein and Sandman (2002a) report that PAPM has been successfully applied to osteoporosis prevention, mammography, hepatitis B vaccination, and home testing to detect radon gas.

The PAPM includes seven stages along the full path from ignorance to action (see Figure 7.7).

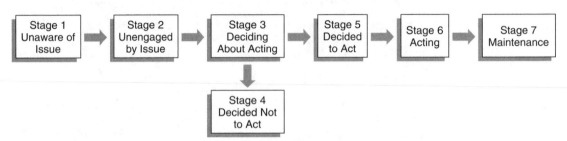

Figure 7.7 Stages of the precaution adoption process model
Source: "Stages of the Precaution Adoption Process Model," by Weinstein & Sandman, *Health Behavior & Health Education*, K. Glanz, B.K. Rimer, & F.M. Lewis (Eds.), 3rd edition, p. 125. Copyright © 2002 by John Wiley & Sons, Inc. This material is used by permission of John Wiley & Sons, Inc.

At some initial point in time, people are unaware of the health issue (Stage 1) [Unaware]. When they first learn something about the issue, they are no longer unaware, but they are not necessarily engaged by it either (Stage 2) [Unengaged]. People who reach the decision-making stage (Stage 3) [Deciding about acting] have become engaged by the issue and are considering their response. This decision-making process can result in one of two outcomes. If the decision is to take no action, the precaution adoption process ends (Stage 4) [Decide not to act], at least for the time being. But if people decide to adopt the precaution (Stage 5) [Decide to act], the next step is to initiate the behavior (Stage 6) [Acting]. A seventh stage, if appropriate, indicates that the behavior has been maintained over time (Stage 7) [Maintenance] (Weinstein & Sandman, 2002b, p. 21. Note: name of the stages have been inserted by McKenzie, Neiger, & Smeltzer).

Like with the TTM, the usefulness of this model is its ability to identify various stages of the behavior change process. Once it is known what stage the program participants are in, then the program planners can develop a stage-specific intervention to move the participants toward action. Table 7.5 presents the important issues that need to be addressed to move participants from one stage to the next.

Cognitive-Behavioral Model of the Relapse Process

For most people, relapse is a part of change. **Relapse** "refers to the breakdown or failure in a person's attempt to change or modify a particular habit pattern, such as stopping 'bad habits' or developing new, optimal health behaviors" (Marlatt & George, 1998, p. 33). Marlatt and George (1998) differentiate between relapse (an indication of total failure) and a **lapse** (a single slip or mistake). The first drink or cigarette following a period of abstinence would be considered a lapse. It has been said that getting

Table 7.5 Issues likely to determine progress between stages of the PAPM

Stage Transition	Important Issues
Stage 1 to stage 2	• Media messages about the hazard and precaution
Stage 2 to stage 3	• Communication from significant other • Personal experience with hazard
Stage 3 to stage 4 or stage 5	• Beliefs about hazard likelihood and severity • Beliefs about personal susceptibility • Beliefs about precaution effectiveness and difficulty • Behaviors and recommendations of others • Perceived social norms • Fear and worry
Stage 5 to stage 6	• Time, effort, and resources needed to act • Detailed "how-to" information • Reminders and other cues to action • Assistance in carrying out action

Source: "Precaution Adoption Model," by Weinstein & Sandman, *Health Behavior & Health Education*, K. Glanz, B.K. Rimer, & F.M. Lewis (Eds.), 3rd edition, p. 130. Copyright © 2002 by John Wiley & Sons, Inc. This material is used by permission of John Wiley & Sons, Inc.

people to change behavior is hard, but having them maintain the behavior is much harder. This is nicely illustrated by the old saying "Giving up smoking is easy; I've done it a hundred times." At one time, it was enough for program planners just to get people to change their behavior; now they need to do more. Because of the difficulty of maintaining a new behavior, program planners need to give special attention to helping those in the priority population avoid slipping back to their previous behaviors.

Although much of the early research dealing with this concept of slipping back was conducted using addictive behaviors, such as substance abuse and gambling, the concept applies to all behavior change, including preventive health behaviors. Marlatt (1982) indicates that a high percentage of individuals who enter programs for health behavior change relapse to their former behaviors within one year. More specifically, researchers have warned program planners of **recidivism** problems with participants in exercise (Dishman, Sallis, & Orenstein, 1985; Horne, 1975; Simkin & Gross, 1994), oral health care treatment (McCaul et al., 1990), weight loss (Stunkard & Braunwell, 1980), and smoking cessation (Leventhal & Cleary, 1980) programs. Therefore, planners need to make sure that program interventions include the skills necessary for dealing with those difficult times during behavior change.

Marlatt (1982) refers to the process of trying to prevent slipping back as relapse prevention. Relapse prevention which is based on the social cognitive theory, combines behavioral skill-training procedures, cognitive therapy, and lifestyle rebalancing (Marlatt & George, 1998). **Relapse prevention (RP)** is "a self-control program designed to help individuals to anticipate and cope with the problem of relapse in the habit-changing process" (Marlatt & George, 1998, p. 33). Relapse is triggered by *high-risk situations.* "A high-risk situation is defined broadly as any situation (including emotional reactions to the situation) that poses a threat to the individual's sense of control and increases the risk of potential relapse" (Marlatt & George, 1998, p. 38). Cummings, Gordon, and Marlatt (1980), in a study of clients with a variety of problem behaviors (drinking, smoking, heroin addiction, gambling, and overeating), found high-risk situations to fall into two major categories: intrapersonal and interpersonal determinants. They found that 56% of the relapse situations were caused by intrapersonal determinants, such as negative emotional states (35%), negative physical states (3%), positive emotional states (4%), testing personal control (5%), and urges and temptations (9%). The 44% of the situations represented by interpersonal determinants included interpersonal conflicts (16%), social pressure (20%), and positive emotional states (8%). These determinants can be referred to as the *covert antecedents* of relapse. That is to say, these high-risk situations do not just happen; instead, they are created by what Marlatt (1982) calls *lifestyle imbalances.*

People who have the coping skills to deal with a high-risk situation have a much greater chance of preventing relapse than those who do not. Figure 7.8 illustrates the possible paths one may take in a high-risk situation (Marlatt, 1982).

Marlatt has developed both global (Figure 7.9) and specific (Figure 7.10) self-control strategies for relapse intervention. Specific intervention procedures are designed to help participants anticipate and cope with the relapse episode itself, whereas the global intervention procedures are designed to modify the early antecedents of relapse, including restructuring of the participant's general style of life. A complete application of the relapse prevention model would include both specific and global interventions (Marlatt, 1982).

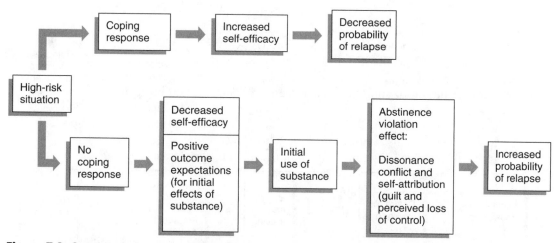

Figure 7.8 Cognitive-behavioral model of the relapse process
Source: "Relapse Prevention: Theoretical Rationale and Overview of the Model," by G. A. Marlatt, in G. A. Marlatt and J. R. Gordon (Eds.), *Relapse Prevention* (p. 38), 1985, New York: Guilford Press. Reprinted by permission of Guilford Press.

Applying Theory to Practice

Learning and understanding the theories presented in this chapter are manageable tasks. However, learning "how to apply given theories to 'real life' projects where theories usually have to be bent and twisted and adapted to uncontrollable conditions" (Hochbaum et al., 1992, p. 311) is a much more difficult task. Several authors (Burdine & McLeroy, 1992; Crosby et al., 2002; D'Onofrio, 1992; Glanz et al., 2002b; Hochbaum et al., 1992; McLeroy, 1993; van Ryn and Heaney, 1992) have reported the difficulties practitioners have had in applying theory. In the sections below, we will discuss the reported barriers to applying theory in the field and provide suggestions for choosing and applying theory.

Barriers to Applying Theory

Burdine and McLeroy (1992) have reported on semistructured interviews with health professionals on the use of theory in practice. Though the group was not randomly selected—it was part of a workgroup in eastern Pennsylvania—it was thought to be broadly representative of "practicing health educators." From these interviews came three primary reasons why practitioners were not using theory learned in their professional preparation courses in college. They included "(1) the failure of theory to adequately guide practice in specific settings or contexts; (2) the lack of appropriate theories to guide community-oriented interventions; and (3) difficulties in transferring theories from the academic training context to the practice environment" (Burdine & McLeroy, 1992, p. 336).

The concern about the failure of theory to adequately guide practice in specific settings or contexts stems from the fact that the theory on which the health promotion profession was built is borrowed from the social and behavioral sciences. It primarily revolves around individual behavior change. Even though behavior change

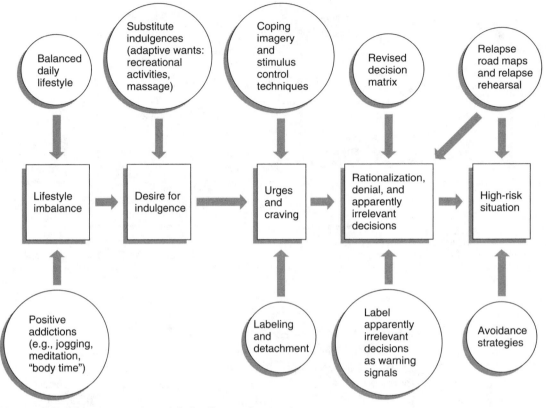

Figure 7.9 Relapse prevention: global self-control strategies
Source: "Relapse Prevention: Theoretical Rationale and Overview of the Model," by G. A. Marlatt, in G. A. Marlatt and J. R. Gordon (Eds.), *Relapse Prevention* (p. 61), 1985, New York: Guilford Press. Reprinted by permission of Guilford Press.

is an important part of the work of health educators, the theories do not match well with the expanded role of health educators when they address problems such as controlling environmental health hazards, increasing access to and utilization of health care facilities, limiting the commercial promotion of alcohol and tobacco (D'Onofrio, 1992), and organizing committees to deal with these problems (Burdine & McLeroy, 1992).

The issue of the lack of appropriate theory to guide community-oriented interventions speaks to the fact that the profession lacks process or practical guide theory. The profession needs a theory to take one from the social science theory to creating appropriate interventions for a specific priority population (Burdine & McLeroy, 1992).

The third reason shared by Burdine and McLeroy (1992) for practitioners not using theory in practice is the means by which theory is taught by academicians. Instead of presenting the theories and asking how they apply to a problem, it is suggested (Burdine & McLeroy, 1992; D'Onofrio, 1992) that academicians should be teaching theory by starting with a specific health problem and asking how each of the theories helps one understand the problem.

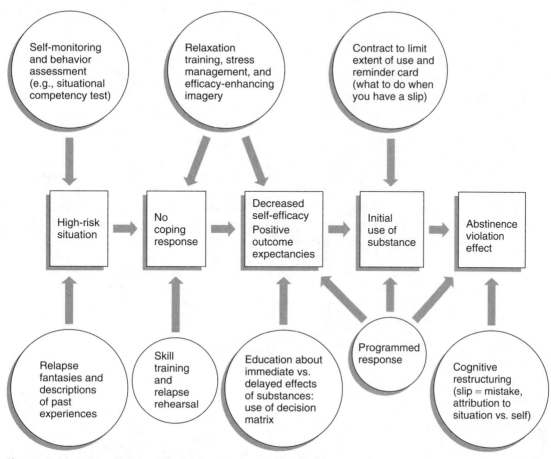

Figure 7.10 Relapse prevention: specific intervention strategies
Source: "Relapse Prevention: Theoretical Rationale and Overview of the Model," by G. A. Marlatt, in G. A. Marlatt and J. R. Gordon (Eds.), *Relapse Prevention* (p. 54), 1985, New York: Guilford Press. Reprinted by permission of Guilford Press.

Now that you know a bit about what appears to be some of the reasons for not using theory in practice, let's look at how it can be implemented.

Suggestions for Applying Theory to Practice

"Behavioral and social science theory provides a platform for understanding why people engage in health-risk or health-compromising behavior and why (as well as how) they adopt health-protective behavior" (Crosby et al., 2002, p. 1). Using the most appropriate theory and practice strategies for a given situation greatly enhances the chances for effective health promotion practice (Glanz et al., 2002b).

Several authors (D'Onofrio, 1992; Hochbaum et al., 1992; McGuire, 1983; van Ryn & Heaney, 1992) have suggested ideas for applying theory to practice. Following is a summary compilation of their ideas.

The first step is to have a basic grasp of the theories—old and new (D'Onofrio, 1992). Practitioners should take the time to review the theories and not depend on memory. Theories, like most other knowledge, are forgotten over time if they are not used. Also, the very nature of theory suggests that it can change and be updated. The theory of reasoned action and the theory of planned behavior are good examples. Practitioners also need to become familiar with new theories and models.

Once practitioners feel comfortable with the theories and models, they should examine their applicability to the problem they are addressing (D'Onofrio, 1992; van Ryn & Heaney, 1992). This can be done by taking the goals of a proposed program and matching them with the most applicable theories. For example, some theories were developed to help explain behavior change of individuals, whereas others were developed to help explain change at the community level. Thus some theories work better in some situations than others, depending on which level of influence the program is being planned. The concept of the level of influence is included in the ecological perspective (McLeroy et al., 1988). The **ecological perspective** "recognizes that health behaviors are part of the larger social system (or ecology) of behaviors and social influences, much like a river, forest or desert is part of a larger biological system (or ecosystem), and that lasting changes in health behaviors require supportive changes in the whole system, just as the addition of a power plant, the flooding of a reservoir, or the growth of a city in a desert produce changes in the whole ecosystem" (O'Donnell, 1996, p. 244). The ecological perspective includes five levels of influence on health-related behaviors and conditions:

1. Intrapersonal (or individual) factors
2. Interpersonal factors
3. Institutional (or organizational) factors
4. Community factors
5. Public policy factors

Here is how the levels of influence might be applied to assisting individuals in starting an exercise program. At the *intrapersonal (or individual) level*, a health promotion program could be planned for the priority population to present the knowledge and skills necessary to begin regular exercise. Going beyond the individual level, program planners could consider setting up social support networks of family and friends to help encourage those in the priority population. Such an approach would be at the *interpersonal level*. If planners worked with and through the institutions in which the members of the priority population were associated (e.g., churches and worksites) to get the priority population exercising, they would be working at the *institutional (or organizational) level* of influence. Creating a *community culture* that favors active community members would be a strategy for influencing at the next level. And finally, planners can work to influence *public policy* that encourages physically active community members. This may take the form of getting the city council to pass an ordinance that would establish bike lanes in the roads. Some good examples of the application of the ecological perspective to worksite health promotion are provided by Watts, Donahue, Eddy and Wallace (2001) and Eddy, Donahue, Webster, and Bjornstad (2002).

To assist program planners with matching theories with the appropriate level of influence, Glanz and Rimer (1995) modified the five levels of influence into three.

Table 7.6 Theories categorized by level of influence

Level of Influence	Theory	Where Discussed in This Book
Intrapersonal	Stimulus Response Theory	Chapter 7
	Theory of Planned Behavior	Chapter 7
	Health Belief Model	Chapter 7
	Elaboration Likelihood Model of Persuasion	Chapter 7
	Transtheoretical Model	Chapter 7
	Precaution Adoption Process Model	Chapter 7
Interpersonal	Social Cognitive Theory	Chapter 7
	Social Support/Networks	Chapter 8
Community	Community Organization	Chapter 9
	Diffusion Theory	Chapter 11
	Theory of Freeing	Chapter 7

They have done this by using the first two levels, intrapersonal and interpersonal, and combining institutional, community, and public policy into one level called *community*. Table 7.6 categorizes, by level of influence, the theories presented in this book.

Knowing that several theories are applicable to the problem they are addressing, planners should look for evidence that the theories or models will work in their particular situation. Have others used theories with success with the same or a similar problem or priority population (McGuire, 1983; van Ryn & Heaney, 1992)? Some theories may have to be adjusted or modified to be applicable to certain priority populations. For example, can the same theory apply to people from different cultural backgrounds within the United States? Or, what is the applicability of behavioral theories based on Western thought to people from non-Western cultures (D'Onofrio, 1992)?

It is also important to remember that seldom does a single theory address all the complexities of a problem. Planners will more than likely have to use more than one theory to adequately address all the components of the problem. To do so, planners will need to synthesize and integrate the theories to fit their particular situation (D'Onofrio, 1992). In bringing theories together, planners are warned against using only selected parts of a theory. Theories are based on the interaction of several variables. When some of those variables are removed, the theory is not the same. For example, if cues to action or motivation are removed from the health belief model, planners will not know the true effectiveness of the model. Thus the most effective use of a theory is to use it in total (Hochbaum et al., 1992).

In the final step in choosing a theory, planners need to select "a theory that makes sense to them, given their experience and what they know and believe about the world" (van Ryn & Heaney, 1992, p. 320). This is not to say that planners should not consider theories that may be different from their own views, but it "does not make sense to base a program on theoretical ideas that are at odds with one's own philosophy or belief system" (van Ryn & Heaney, 1992, p. 320).

Table 7.7 Major components of the theories that underlie health promotion interventions

Stimulus Response Theory	Social Cognitive Theory	Theory of Reasoned Action	Theory of Planned Behavior	Theory of Freeing
Operant behavior	Reinforcement 1. Direct 2. Vicarious 3. Self-management	Attitude toward behavior	Attitude toward behavior	Free
Consequences	Behavioral capability	Subjective norm	Subjective norm	Oppressed
Positive reinforcement	Expectations	Intentions	Perceived behavioral control	Critical consciousness
Negative reinforcement	Expectancies	Behavior	Intentions	Education
Positive punishment	Self-control		Behavior	
Negative punishment	Self-efficacy			
	Emotional coping response			
	Reciprocal determinism			

(Table 7.7 continues)

(Table 7.7 continued)

Health Belief Model	Transtheoretical Model	Cognitive-Behavior Model of the Relapse Process	Elaboration Likelihood Model of Persuasion	Precaution Adoption Process Model
Perceived susceptibility	Stages of change	High-risk situation	Central route	Stages
Perceived seriousness	Decisional balance	Global self-control strategies	Peripheral route	Issues
Perceived benefits	Processes of change	Specific intervention strategies	Elaboration likelihood continuum	
Perceived barriers	Self-efficacy		Variables	
Motivation (cues to action)				
Self-efficacy				

SUMMARY

This chapter presents an overview of several theories that underlie the interventions used in many of today's health promotion programs. These theories are important components for planning and evaluating health promotion programs because they provide planners with ideas that have been tried and tested. They provide the framework on which to build. The theories reviewed include stimulus response theory, the social cognitive theory, the theory of reasoned action, the theory of planned behavior, the theory of freeing, the health belief model, elaboration likelihood model of persuasion, the transtheoretical model, precaution adoption process model, and the cognitive-behavioral model of the relapse process (see Table 7.7 for a summary of the major components).

Finally, the chapter provides a discussion of some of the roadblocks to using theory and suggestions for applying theory to practice.

REVIEW QUESTIONS

1. Define *theory*, using your own words.
2. How is a theory different from a model?
3. How do concepts, constructs, and variables relate to theories?
4. Why is it important to use theories when planning and evaluating health promotion programs?
5. What is the underlying concept for each of the following theories?
   a. Stimulus response theory
   b. Social cognitive theory
   c. Theory of reasoned action
   d. Theory of planned behavior
   e. Theory of freeing
   f. Elaboration Likelihood model of persuasion
6. What are the major components of the Health Belief Model? Explain each.
7. What makes stage theories different from continuum theories?
8. What is the major difference between the transtheoretical model and the precaution adoption process model?
9. What are the constructs of the transtheoretical model? Why is it important to understand this model?
10. How can program planners help to prepare those in the priority population for relapse prevention?
11. What are the major barriers to using theories in practice?
12. How can the ecological perspective be used in applying theories?

ACTIVITIES

1. Assume that you have identified a need (health problem) for a given priority population. In a two-page paper:
   a. State who the priority population is and what the need is.
   b. Select a theory to use as a guide in developing an intervention to address the problem.
   c. Explain why you chose the theory that you did.

    d. Defend why you think this is the best theory to use.

    e. Show how the problem "fits into" the theory.

2. In a two-page paper, identify a theory that you plan to use in developing the intervention for the program you are planning. Explain why you chose the theory, and why you think it is a good fit for the problem you are addressing.

3. Write a paragraph on each of the following:

    a. Using the stimulus response theory, explain why a person might smoke.

    b. Using the social cognitive theory, explain how you could help people change their diets.

    c. Explain how the SCT construct of behavioral capability applies to managing stress.

    d. Explain the differences between and the relationship of the SCT constructs of expectations and expectancies.

    e. Explain what would have to take place for individuals to be self-efficacious with regard to taking their insulin.

    f. According to the theory of reasoned action, what would increase intent to exercise?

    g. Use the theory of planned behavior to explain how a smoker stops smoking.

    h. Using the theory of freeing, describe an ideal teacher.

    i. Apply the health belief model to getting a person to take a "flu shot."

    j. Apply the transtheoretical model to get a person to change any health behavior.

    k. Using the precaution adoption process model, explain how a person decides to get screened for blood cholesterol.

WEBLINKS

1. **http://www.uri.edu/research/cprc/**
   Cancer Prevention Resource Center (CPRC), University of Rhode Island

   This is the website for the CPRC which is the home of the Transtheoretical Model. Information about the model as well as measures that can be used to "stage" a person can be found at this site.

2. **http://www.cdc.gov/std/program/community/9-PGcommunity.htm**
   National Center for HIV, STD, and TB Prevention, Division of Sexually Transmitted Diseases

   This website provides an overview of the following behavior change theories: Health Belief Model, Theory of Reasoned Action, Social (Cognitive) Learning Theory, Transtheoretical Model (stages of change), Diffusion of Innovations, and Empowerment Theory/Popular Education.

3. **http://oc.nci.nih.gov/services/Theory_at_glance/HOME.html**
   National Cancer Institute (NCI)

   The web page is part of the NCI website. This site presents the primer Theory at a Glance: A Guide for Health Promotion Practice. This volume explains why theories and models are important, how to use theory, provides explanations of several behavior change theories, as well as a couple of program planning models.

CHAPTER 8

Interventions

Chapter Objectives

After reading this chapter and answering the questions at the end, you should be able to:

- Define the word *intervention* and apply it to a health promotion setting.
- Provide a rationale for selecting an intervention strategy.
- Explain the advantages of using a combination of several intervention strategies rather than a single intervention strategy.
- List and explain the different categories of intervention strategies.
- List some of the documents that provide guidelines or criteria for developing health promotion interventions.
- Discuss the ethical concerns related to intervention development.
- Create an intervention for a health promotion program.

Key Terms

codes of practice	disincentive	risk appraisal
communication channel	ethics	risk reduction
community advocacy	incentives	segmenting
community building	intervention	tailored
community organization	penetration rate	treatment

Once the goals and objectives have been developed, planners need to decide on the most appropriate means of reaching or attaining the goals and objectives. The planners must design an activity or set of activities that would permit the most *effective* (leads to desired outcome) and *efficient* (uses resources in a responsible manner) achievement of the outcomes stated in the goals and objectives. These planned activities make up the **intervention,** or what some refer to as **treatment.** The intervention is the theory-based strategy or experience to which those in the priority population will be exposed or in which they will take part. In the strictest sense, *intervention* means "to occur, fall, or come between points of time or events" (Woolf, 1979, p. 600). When applied to the planning of health promotion programs, it is usually thought of as something that occurs between the beginning and the end of a program or between pre- and postprogram measurements. For example, let's say that you want the employees of Company S to increase their use of safety belts while riding in company-owned vehicles. You can measure their safety belt use before doing anything else, by observing them driving out of the motor pool. This would be a preprogram measure. Then you can intervene in a variety of ways. For example, you could provide an incentive by stating that all employees seen wearing their safety belts would receive a $10 bonus in their next paycheck. Or you could put in each employee's pay envelope a pamphlet on the importance of wearing safety belts. You could institute a company policy requiring all employees to wear safety belts while driving company-owned vehicles. Each of these activities for getting employees to increase their use of safety belts would be considered part of an intervention. After the intervention, you would complete a postprogram measurement of safety belt use to determine the success of the program.

The term *intervention* is used to describe all the activities that occur between the two measurement points. Thus an intervention may use a single strategy, or it may be a combination of two or more strategies. In the case of the example just given, you could use an incentive by itself and call it an intervention, or you could use an incentive, pamphlets, and a company policy all at the same time to increase safety belt use and refer to the combination as an intervention.

With regard to the number of activities that should be included in an intervention, research (Erfurt et al., 1990; Kline & Huff, 1999; Shea & Basch, 1990) shows that interventions that include several activities are more likely to have an effect on the priority population than are those that consist of a single activity. In other words, the size of the "dose" is important in health promotion. Few people change their behavior based on a single exposure (or dose); instead, multiple exposures (doses) are generally needed to change most behaviors. It stands to reason that "hitting" the priority population from several angles or through multiple channels should increase the chances of making an impact. Although research has shown that using several strategies is better than one, it has not identified an exact number of strategies or a specific combination of strategies that will ensure the most effective results (Kline & Huff, 1999). It is still a best guess situation.

Types of Intervention Strategies

As mentioned earlier, there are many different types of strategies that planners can use as part of an intervention. Here, we present several categories of intervention strategies based on a modification of the Centers for Disease Control and Prevention's (2003) terminology for intervention strategies. These categories cover the more common strategies used by planners, but in actuality the variety of strategies is limited only by the planner's imagination. Note that the categories presented here are not always independent of each other—that is, some of the examples that we use to help explain the strategies could be used in more than one category. Even with this limitation, the strategies have been categorized into the following groups:

1. Health communication strategies
2. Health education strategies

3. Health policy/enforcement strategies

4. Health engineering strategies

5. Health-related community service strategies

6. Community mobilization strategies

7. Other strategies

Health Communication Strategies

We present health communication strategies first for several reasons. First, almost all interventions include some form of communication, whether it be as simple as speaking, reading, or writing, or more complex, such as the production of small media (i.e., handouts, brochures, etc.), or very complex in the development of mass media (i.e., radio, TV, or newspaper) campaigns. Second, communication strategies are very useful in reaching so many of the goals and objectives of health promotion programs, such as the following:

1. Increasing awareness.

2. Increasing knowledge.

3. Increasing attitudes (for example, about blood pressure, cancer screenings, and the ills of smoking).

4. Reinforcing attitudes (for example, about smoking in public places).

5. Maintaining interest (for example, for those contemplating a behavior change).

6. Providing cues and motivation for action.

7. Demonstrate simple skills (as in self-screening) (Bellicha & McGrath, 1990; Erickson, McKenna, & Romano, 1990).

8. Increasing demand and support for health services (NCI, 2002).

9. Increasing perceptions of one's ability to perform a behavior (NCI, 2002).

10. Reinforcing behaviors (NCI, 2002).

11. Building social norms (NCI, 2002).

Third, communication strategies probably have the highest **penetration rate** (number in the priority population exposed or reached) of any of the intervention strategies. And fourth, they are also much more cost effective and less threatening than many other types of strategies.

The literally hundreds of communication activities can be sub-divided by communication channels. A **communication channel** is the route through which a message is disseminated to the priority population. The four primary communication channels include intrapersonal (one-on-one communication), interpersonal (small group communication), organization and community, and mass media. These channels are hierarchical in nature with regards to the number of people they reach. The intrapersonal channel typically reaches the fewest number of people, while the mass media channel reaches the largest number of people.

Over the years, the *intrapersonal channel* has most often been used, but by no means exclusively, in health care settings when the health care provider and patient interact. This is a familiar channel for most people and one they trust. It is typically an effective communication channel, but it is also typically the most time and resource intensive channel for the number of people reached. In more recent years, this channel of communication has been greatly enhanced by the use of technology. For example, computers have been used to deliver tailored electronic mail messages. Also, though most do not think of the telephone as "technology" it too is being used for health promotion interventions via the intrapersonal channel. Planners have used it for "gathering information, disseminating information, providing health education and counseling, promoting health education programs, offering cues to action and social support" (Soet & Basch, 1997, p. 760). Health education delivered by telephone "can be classified into two broad categories: *individual initiated,* where the individual must actively seek contact and assistance from a health information hotline; and *outreach,* where the individual is called by a health educator or counselor" (Soet & Basch, 1997, p. 760). Individual-initiated health information hot lines usually provide information, and sometimes education and counseling, whereas outreach activities range from brief, one-time preappointment reminders to long-term interactive professional health counseling (Soet & Basch, 1997). Telephone-delivered intervention activities have been created for a variety of topics, including but not limited to cancer screening (Davis et al., 1997; Ludman et al., 1999; McDowell, Newell, & Rosser, 1989b), medical appointments (Linkins et al., 1994), hypertension screening (McDowell, Newell, & Rosser, 1989a), smoking cessation (Koffman et al., 1998; Simmons, 1998), and weight loss (Hellerstedt & Jeffery, 1997). Soet and Basch (1997) present a generic process for developing a telephone intervention activity that includes three areas: "designing the intervention protocol, selection and training of the health educator/counselor(s), and developing the documentation and data collection protocol" (p. 763).

Examples of the *interpersonal channel* are support groups and small classes. This channel has many of the same characteristics of the intrapersonal channel, but reaches larger numbers of people with fewer resources.

Many people receive a lot of information through *organization* and *community channels.* Often health promotion programs have priority populations that are part of or entirely comprise already existing groups (i.e., workers of a particular company, social groups, or members of a religious organization), or who may participate in a community activity. As such, organizational and community channels provide excellent ways of reaching priority populations. Thus church bulletins, company or agency newsletters, organizations or community bulletin boards, and community activities are often used as a part of communication activities (i.e., an AIDS walk, the American Cancer Society's Great American Smokeout, and health fairs).

Probably the most visible communication channel to most people is the *mass media channel.* This channel includes both print and electronic media formats such as: billboards; direct mail; daily papers with national or local circulation; local weekly newspapers; local, public, and network television, including cable television; public and commercial radio stations; and magazines with either a broad readership or a narrow focus. There are many ways to convey a message using the mass media. These include news coverage (see Appendix A for an example of a news release and copy for a newspaper column), public affairs coverage, talk shows, public service roundtables, entertainment, public service announcements (PSAs) (see Appendix B for an example of a radio PSA and a TV PSA), paid advertisements, editorials, letters to the editor, comic strips, and columnists' commentaries (Arkin, 1990).

Box 8.1 Producing Materials for Special Populations

Although planners should create/select materials that are applicable to each priority population , extra attention needs to be given to materials that are prepared for special populations. Consider the following:

A. For culturally diverse populations, remember:

1. Interaction with the priority population and "intermediaries" familiar with the culture is especially important.

2. Use of language may vary for different cultural groups (e.g., a word may have different meanings to different groups).

3. Differences in priority populations extend beyond language to include diverse values and customs.

4. Different channels of communication may be credible and more capable of reaching certain cultural groups.

5. Don't assume that "conventional wisdom," published research studies or "common knowledge" will hold true for different cultural groups. The degree of assimilation and mainstreaming is ever changing, so current information will be needed to choose the best channels and message strategies.

6. Message appeals should be developed separately for each cultural group, since the perceived needs, values, and beliefs of one culture may differ from others.

7. Print materials should be simply written, reinforced with graphics, and pretested. People perceive graphics and illustrations in different ways, just as their language skills differ.

8. Bilingual materials assure that intermediaries and family members who are most comfortable with English can help the reader understand the content.

9. Print materials should never be simply translated from English; concepts and appeals may differ by culture, just as the words do.

10. Audiovisual materials or interpersonal communication may be more successful for some messages and audiences.

B. For patient populations, remember:

1. Patients and their families facing a disorder or a disease may require different information in different formats at various points in the disease continuum.

2. All patients are not alike, and may have nothing in common except their illness. Therefore, their interests in information and ability to understand the illness may vary.

3. Few patients and family members can handle everything they need to know at once, and may find it particularly difficult to absorb information at the time of diagnosis.

4. Patients' information needs may change as they emotionally adjust to their illness.

Source: Adapted from U.S. Department of Health and Human Services (1989).

The cost of communication activities can range from almost nothing (e.g., elementary school children making posters for a health awareness campaign) to moderately priced (e.g., production of a brochure) to expensive (e.g., personal counseling) to very expensive (e.g., a prime-time television commercial). However, no matter what form the communication activities take or their cost, to be effective, they need to be carefully planned. See Chapter 2 for more information about health communication and the models commonly used to plan interventions using communication activities. Also, we recommend that health educators obtain a copy of the book *Making Health Communication Programs Work* (NCI, 2002), also fondly referred to as the "Pink Book" by visiting NCI's website at www.cancer.gov or by calling NCI's Cancer Information Service at 1-800-4-CANCER.

Before leaving our discussion on communication strategies, we would like to share some guidelines that we have found useful in preparing communication materials for priority populations with special needs. Box 8.1 presents a list of items to consider when preparing materials for culturally diverse and patient populations. Planners also need to be concerned with creating written communication materials that are appropriate for the reading abilities of the priority population. Many health promotion materials are written at a reading level too difficult for many people in the general public to understand. That holds for both printed materials (Buxton, 1999; Davis et al., 1994; Dollahite, Thomson, & McNew, 1996) and those on the World Wide Web (Graber, Roller, & Kaeble, 1999). Meyer and Rainey (1994) created a set of guidelines for health educators to follow when creating health promotion materials for low-literacy populations. We found their guidelines to be useful regardless of the priority population. Their eight guidelines have been modified and are summarized in Table 8.1. The only addition we would make to their list would be to check the reading level of the written materials. "For the general public, writing at the 6th grade reading level is usually safe. You can check if you're on target by using a readability test such as the SMOG, the Fog-Gunning Index, or the Fry Readability Formula" (USDHHS, 1991, p. 3). You can find such formulas in most reading methods books and on selected computer word-processing programs. Box 8.2 presents the steps in the process of testing readability using the SMOG.

Health Education Strategies

Some authors include health education strategies as part of communication strategies, but because of the variety of health education activities available to planners we have separated them as a category of their own. Thus we see health education strategies as those usually associated with formal education in courses, seminars, and workshops. This includes educational methods—such as lecture, discussion, and group work—as well as audiovisual materials, computerized instruction, laboratory exercises, and written materials (books and periodicals). Box 8.3 provides a more complete listing of educational activities, and Gilbert and Sawyer (2000) have provided a detailed discussion of these methods.

Health Policy/Enforcement Strategies

Health policy/enforcement strategies include executive orders, laws, ordinances, policies, position statements, regulations, and formal and informal rules. These could be classified as mandated activities or regulated activities because they are activities that

Table 8.1 Guidelines for preparing written materials

Guideline	Explanation
1. Needs and priority population identification	Identify the topic and the priority population (e.g., middle-aged women and mammography).
2. Plan the project	Develop a work plan and budget for your material.
3. Audience research	Segment your priority population using such factors as experience, attitude, culture, etc.
4. Material development	
a. Style	Use an active voice with familar terms that highlight key points. If possible, develop a behaviorally oriented interactive message.
b. Organization	Sequence or prioritize the message.
c. Content	Write using words and terms that are understandable to lay people. Use short sentences and paragraphs.
d. Format	Make it appealing to the eye, making sure the reader can identify the main points.
5. Graphics and illustrations	Graphics and illustrations should be positive and easy to understand, and should summarize the message.
6. Pretesting	Make sure the materials work before you use them with the priority population . Also, make sure the reading level is appropriate.
7. Printing	Consider paper color, size, and cost.
8. Distribution and training	Develop a distribution system and instructions for use.

Source: Adapted from Meyer and Rainey (1994), pp. 372–374.

Box 8.2 The SMOG Readability Formula

To calculate the SMOG reading grade level, begin with the entire written work that is being assessed, and follow these four steps:

1. Count off ten consecutive sentences near the beginning, in the middle, and near the end of the text.
2. From this sample of thirty sentences, circle all of the words containing three or more syllables (polysyllabic), including repetitions of the same word, and total the number of words circled.
3. Estimate the square root of the total number of polysyllabic words counted. This is done by finding the nearest perfect square, and taking its square root.
4. Finally, add a constant of three to the square root. This number gives the SMOG grade, or the reading grade level that a person must have reached if he or she is to fully understand the text being assessed.

A few additional guidelines will help to clarify these directions:

- A sentence is defined as a string of words punctuated with a period (.), an exclamation point (!), or a question mark (?).
- Hyphenated words are considered as one word.

(Box 8.2 *continues*)

(Box 8.2 *continued*)
- Numbers that are written out should also be considered, and if in numeric form in the text, they should be pronouned to determine if they are polysyllabic.
- Proper nouns, if polysyllabic, should be counted, too.
- Abbreviations should be read as unabbreviated to determine if they are polysyllabic.

Not all pamphlets, fact sheets, or other printed materials contain thirty sentences. To test a text that has fewer than thirty sentences:

1. Count all of the polysyllabic words in the text.
2. Count the number of sentences.
3. Find the average number of polysyllabic words per sentence as follows:

$$\text{Average 5} \frac{\text{Total \# of polysyllabic words}}{\text{Total \# of sentences}}$$

4. Multiply that average by the number of sentences *short of thirty.*
5. Add that figure to the total number of polysyllabic words.
6. Find the square root and add the constant of three.

Perhaps the quickest way to administer the SMOG grading test is by using the SMOG conversion table. Simply count the number of polysyllabic words in your chain of thirty sentences and look up the appropriate grade level on the chart.

SMOG Conversion Table*

Total Polysyllabic Word Counts	Aproximately Grade Level (±1.5 Grades)
0–2	4
3–6	5
7–12	6
13–20	7
21–30	8
31–42	9
43–56	10
57–72	11
73–90	12
91–110	13
111–132	14
133–156	15
157–182	16
183–210	17
211–240	18

*Developed by Harold C. McGraw, Office of Educational Research, Baltimore County Schools, Towson, Maryland.

Source: U.S. Department of Health and Human Services (1989).

Box 8.3 Commonly Used Educational Strategies

A. Audiovisual materials and equipment
1. Audiotapes, records, and CDs
2. Bulletin, chalk, cloth, flannel, magnetic, and peg boards
3. Charts, pictures, and posters
4. Films and filmstrips
5. Instructional television
6. Opaque projector
7. Slides and slide projectors
8. Transparencies and overhead projector
9. Video (DVDs and tapes)
B. Computer based
1. World Wide Web
2. Desktop Publishing
3. Presentation programs
4. Individualized learning programs
5. Video conferencing
C. Printed educational materials
1. Instructor-made handouts and worksheets
2. Pamphlets
3. Study guides (commercial and instructor made)
4. Text and reference books
5. Workbooks
D. Teaching strategies and techniques for the classroom
1. Brainstorming
2. Case studies
3. Cooperative learning
4. Debates
5. Demonstrations and experiments
6. Discovery or guided discovery
7. Discussion
8. Group discussion
9. Guest speakers
10. Lecture
11. Lecture/discussion
12. Newspaper and magazine articles
13. Panel discussions
14. Peer group teaching/coaching
15. Poems, songs, and stories
16. Problem solving

(Box 8.3 *continues*)

(Box 8.3 *continued*)

17. Puppets
18. Questioning
19. Role playing and plays
20. Simulation, games, and puzzles
21. Tutoring
22. Values clarification activities

E. Teaching strategies and techniques for outside of the classroom
   1. Community resources
   2. Field trips
   3. Health fairs
   4. Health museums
   5. Health education centers

are required by an administrator, board, or legislative body to guide individual or collective behavior (Schmid, Pratt, & Howze, 1995). Examples include state laws requiring the use of safety belts and motorcycle helmets or raising the taxes on cigarettes, company policy stating that there will be no smoking in corporate offices and company-owned vehicles, and a board of education adopting a position statement that it will provide only well-balanced meals in its cafeterias. "An example of an executive order is a ban on tobacco advertising on city-owned buses" (Brownson et al., 1995, p. 479).

This type of intervention strategy may be controversial. It has been criticized by some because it mandates a particular response from an individual. It takes away individual freedoms and sometimes plays on a person's pride, "pocketbook," and psyche. This type of strategy must be sold on the basis of "common good." That is, the justification for this type of societal action is to protect the public's health. Health policy/enforcement strategies exist for the protection of the community and of individual rights.

> Officials are willing to intercede into the private activities and lives of people in order to protect the larger population. When such intervention occurs it is usually very narrow and very specifically defined. There also tend to be sanctions attached if people do not comply. For example, in the case of inoculations, if a mother and father did not have their child inoculated that child cannot attend school. If parents do not send their child to school they are in violation of the law, and there are criminal and civil penalties that are involved. (Rich & Sugrue, 1989, p. 33)

Some would say that health policy/enforcement strategies do not allow for the "voluntary actions conducive to health" that are suggested by Green and Kreuter (1999, p. 27) in their definition of health education. But, at the same time, this kind of activity can get people to change their behavior when other strategies have failed. For example, before the passage of safety belt laws, most states were reporting about a 14% use rate by drivers of automobiles and were trying to attack the problem through communication strategies using the mass media. Now that safety belt laws are in effect in many states, usage rates in those states are closer to 75%; in some states where there is strict enforcement, usage rates approach 90%. Another example is the work of Sorensen and colleagues (1991), which showed a 21% reduction in the number of employees who smoked in a company that put a nonsmoking policy in effect. Both of these examples show that health policy/enforcement strategies are necessary to reinforce and support prevention messages.

Since health policy/enforcement strategies are often mandatory, it is particularly important to use good judgment and show respect for others when implementing them. In some instances, planners will be faced with ethical decisions. Also, if a program uses health policy/enforcement strategies, the planner should remember that, as in any political process, there is likely to be both pro and con feelings toward the "mandatory" action. Thus when developing and implementing any mandatory action, planners should bear in mind the following points:

1. Have top-level support for the mandated action (Emont & Cummings, 1989; Mikanowicz & Altman, 1995).

2. Have a representative group (committee) from the priority population help formulate the "mandatory" action.

3. Consider surveying those in the priority population to gain additional information regarding policy change (Mikanowicz & Altman, 1995).

4. Make sure expert advice on the subject of the mandated action is available to the group developing it.

5. Seek a legal opinion if necessary.

6. Examine the work of others and review the issues they faced when implementing "mandatory" actions.

7. Be sure that health policy/enforcement strategies are based on sound principles and, if possible, good research.

8. Seek input and debate/discussion concerning the mandated action from the priority population while it is being formulated.

9. Develop health policy/enforcement strategies that are written simply and include a rationale, a general policy statement, specific areas affected, and clearly defined complaint, grievance, and enforcement procedures (Mikanowicz & Altman, 1995).

10. Consider phasing in the new regulation a little bit at a time. For example, if a no-smoking policy is going to be implemented, the planner may want to begin by restricting smoking in certain areas before banning it altogether. This not only helps people change gradually but it also expresses concern for them.

11. Provide education and behavior change programs to assist those in the priority population with the implementation of the "mandatory" actions (Mikanowicz & Altman, 1995).

12. Ensure that, once formulated, the "mandatory" actions

    a. are actively communicated to those in the priority population.

    b. are reviewed on a regular basis for the purposes of evaluating and revising if necessary.

    c. apply to all in the priority population and not just to select groups.

d. are consistently enforced. Be prepared to deal with the complaint and grievance processes (Mikanowicz & Altman, 1995).
e. are enforced as a shared responsibility of all in the institution.

To help gain a sense of the difficulty of dealing with health policy/enforcement strategies, let's examine the options available to a group of department heads who are trying to decide whether they should continue to allow the public to smoke in the lobby of the building and employees to smoke in their individual, self-contained offices. Several options are available to this administrative group:

1. Decide to have no explicit policy.
2. Make no changes and continue with the status quo.
3. Eliminate only public smoking in the building.
4. Designate a different area within and/or outside the building for public smoking.
5. Allow smoking only in individual offices.
6. Designate the entire building as a "smoke-free building."
7. Request that all employees hired in the future be nonsmokers.
8. A combination of items 1–7.

Each of these options poses special concerns for administrative groups. Policies are seldom easy to develop, but looking at others that have already been developed helps in the creation of a new policy. Appendix C presents two example nonsmoking policies created by the Coalition for a Smoke-Free Valley in Allentown, PA. (*Note:* Planners interested in developing policies regulating smoking should also review these works CDC (1999b), Mikanowicz & Altman [1995] and USDHHS [1985].)

Health Engineering Strategies

Another group of strategies that have proved useful in reaching desired outcomes is the category of health engineering strategies. Health engineering strategies are those designed to change the structure or types of services, or systems of care to improve the delivery of health promotion services (CDC, 2003). Examples of such strategies include equipping automobiles with safety belts, air bags, and child safety seats, placing speed bumps in parking lots by playgrounds to slow traffic where children are present, or installing fire and safety doors in apartments buildings to make them safer for the residents. These strategies are characterized by changes in those things "around" individuals that may influence their awareness, knowledge, attitudes, skills, or behavior. Often health engineering strategies do not necessarily require action on the part of the priority population (CDC, 2003) as noted in the examples above. Yet, some of these strategies provide a "forced choice" situation, as when the selection of foods and beverages in vending machines or cafeterias are changed to include only "healthy" foods. If people want to eat foods from these sources, they are forced to eat certain types of foods. French and colleagues (1997) used a similar idea to the forced choice idea when they lowered the price by 50% on low-fat snacks in vending machines to try to influence food choices.

Other activities in this category may provide those in the priority population with health messages and environmental cues for certain types of behavior. Examples would be posting of no-smoking signs, eliminating ashtrays, providing lockers and showers, using role modeling by others, playing soft music in a work area, organizing a shuttle service or some other type of transportation system to get seniors to congregate for meals or to a health care provider, and providing point-of-purchase education, such as a sign on a vending machine or food labeling on the food lines in the cafeteria.

Finally, like so many of the other intervention strategies health engineering strategies often are more effective when combined (i.e., an increased "dose") with intervention strategies from the other categories. For example, the inclusion of safety belts in automobiles is important but when combined with strict enforcement of safety belt laws (a health policy/enforcement strategy) it makes for a much more effective intervention.

Health-Related Community Service Strategies

Health-related community service strategies include things such as services, tests, or treatments to improve the health of those in the priority population (CDC, 2003). Examples of this type of intervention strategy include, but are not limited to, completing a health risk appraisal (HRA) form (see Chapter 4 for a discussion of HRAs), offering low-cost flu shots or child immunizations, providing clinical screenings (sometimes called biometric screenings) for cancer, diabetes, blood pressure, or cholesterol, and providing professional health check-ups and examinations. Because a health-related community service strategy requires action on the part of those in the priority population, an important component of this type of strategy is to reduce the barriers to obtaining the service. Thus planners must be mindful of the affordability and accessibility of such services. Also, planners must weigh the consequences of including this type of strategy in an intervention. For example, if abnormal readings are found during a screening, those conducting the screening have an ethical obligation to follow up and make sure appropriate referrals for care are made. Chapman (2003a) has provided a nice review of many of the concerns associated with biometric screening.

Health-related community service strategies are often offered in settings such as grocery stores, shopping malls, health fairs, worksites, personal residencies, in mobile units (e.g., vans equipped with mammography units), and easily accessible health care facilities. Such strategies usually have high credibility with priority populations because of their link with health care providers.

Community Mobilization Strategies

"Community mobilization strategies involve helping communities identify and take action on shared concerns using participatory decision making, and include such methods as empowerment" (Barnes, Neiger, & Thackeray, 2003, p. 60). In this book we present two subcategories of community mobilization strategies; 1) community organization and community building, and 2) community advocacy.

Community Organization and Community Building   Other than defining the terms community organization and community building little will be presented here about these terms because all of Chapter 9 is dedicated to the discussion of these processes. **Community organization** has been defined "as the process by which community groups are helped to identify common problems or goals, mobilize resources, and in other ways develop and implement strategies for reaching the goals they have collectively set" (Minkler & Wallerstein, 2002, p. 279). **Community building** is not so much a process but rather "an orientation to community that is strength based rather than need based and stresses the identification, nurturing, and celebration of community assets" (Minkler, 1997b, p. 5–6).

Community Advocacy **Community advocacy** is a process in which the people of the community become involved in the institutions and decisions that will have an impact on their lives. It has the potential for creating more support, keeping people informed, influencing decisions, activating nonparticipants, improving service, and making people, plans, and programs more responsive (Checkoway, 1989). But community advocacy is not without costs; in most situations it requires time and effort, as well as persistence. Yet it can have a big impact on social change issues involving health. Techniques often used in advocacy activities include: (1) personal visits to educate or lobby the key people; (2) a community rally; (3) telephone call campaigns to the offices of the decision makers; (4) TV or radio appearances to express views; (5) letter-writing campaigns (see Figure 8.1) to the key people who educate/influence decision makers; (6) letter-writing campaigns to newspaper editors, expressing concern (congratulations or "shame-on-you") about the results of a vote by decision makers on a particular issue; and (7) letter-writing campaigns to decision makers, thanking them for support on a key issue.

Auld (1997) offered a set of practical tips for influencing public policy. They are adapted here to apply to influencing public policy at the local as well as the state and federal levels.

1. *Opening doors.* Establish relationships that build trust and rapport with staff, legislative assistants, and, if possible, the elected officials themselves so that you can approach them for their support on an issue of concern. Know what committees your elected officials sit on and how they have voted on the issues.

2. *Identifying the players.* Identify who the stakeholders are on a particular issue and find out why they are.

3. *Making the link.* Find out how the issues you are interested in are linked to the health problems of the population/constituency of the elected officials. For example, if you are interested in chronic diseases, show how they are linked to the elderly in the population/constituency.

4. *Crafting your position.* Make sure your position on the issue(s) is (are) developed on the best available science and data.

5. *Organizing the troops.* Organize others who may be interested in your issue to show broad representation from the population/constituency (see Chapter 9 for organizing techniques).

6. *Visiting policymakers.* Schedule appointments with the elected official or staff to express your views on the issues. Take others with you who can help explain your views. Be on time, be brief, yet be prepared to educate by using practical examples.

7. *Demonstrating the power of press.* Demonstrate your link to the media and how you and your organization can get positive press for the elected official by activating (i.e., letters to the editor, etc.) your link.

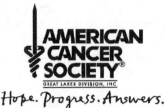

AMERICAN CANCER SOCIETY
GREAT LAKES DIVISION, INC.

Hope. Progress. Answers.

Senators and Representatives pay attention to their constituents. It is good politics. Responding to constituents is the "bread and butter" of a legislative office. A member knows your approval can be won or lost by his or her response to your concerns.

The most effective means of communication with your legislator, aside from a personal visit, is a personal letter (not a form letter). It should be concise, informed and polite.

Date

Your address

Legislator's address

Dear Senator/Representative:

- Try to stick to one typewritten page. Don't type or write on the back of a page. If writing longhand, take care to write legibly.
- In a short first paragraph, *state your purpose.* Stick with *one* subject or issue. Support your position with the rest of the letter.
- If a bill is the subject, cite it by name and number.
- Be factual and support your position with information about how legislation is likely to affect you and others. Avoid emotional, philosophical arguments.
- Explain how you intend to help the cause. *Ask what else you can do to help change things.*
- *State one more time what you would like your legislator to do.*
- Be sure you include your name and address
- Follow up your letter with a phone call.

Sincerely,

Jane Doe

U.S. CONGRESS ADDRESSES	INDIANA LEGISLATURE	MICHIGAN STATE LEGISLATURE
The Honorable ... U.S. Senate Washington, DC 20510 The Honorable... U.S. House of Representatives Washington, DC 20515	The Honorable... Indiana State House 200 W. Washington St. Indianapolis, IN 46204	The Honorable... Michigan State Senate P.O. Box 30036 Lansing, MI 48909 The Honorable... Michigan House of Representatives P.O. Box 30014 Lansing, MI 48909

Figure 8.1 Tips for writing effective letters

Source: American Cancer Society, Great Lakes Division, Inc. Used with permission.

8. *Reinforcing your message.* End your visit or follow up the visit with a packet that summarizes your position on the issues. Supporting scientific data should be included. Also, send a thank you letter. As the issue moves through the legislative process, let your elected official know your views on its direction.

9. *Serving as a resource.* Stay in contact with the staff and elected official and offer to be a resource person to help them as needed on the issue.

10. *Responding quickly.* Be prepared to respond quickly when asked to be a resource person or testify to a legislative group. Requests often come at the last minute.

11. *Reaching the finish line.* Follow up on a piece of legislation after it has been passed to help those who have to implement it and to advocate for funding to help the implementation.

To further assist planners with community advocacy activities the Coalition of National Health Education Organizations (CNHEO) maintains a website for advocacy information. The website features advocacy alerts, federal legislation, testimony, fact sheets, and other policy tools for health education and health promotion (SOPHE, 2003) (see the *Weblinks* at the end of this chapter for more information about the site).

Other Strategies

The "Other Strategies" category includes a variety of intervention activities that do not fit neatly into one of the six categories noted above.

Behavior Modification Activities   Behavior modification activities, often used in intrapersonal-level interventions, includes techniques intended to help those in the priority population experience a change in behavior. *Behavior modification* is usually thought of as a systematic procedure for changing a specific behavior. The process is based on the stimulus response and social cognitive theories. As applied to health behavior, emphasis is placed on a specific behavior that one might want either to increase (such as exercise or stress management techniques) or to decrease (such as smoking or consumption of fats). Particular attention is then given to changing the events that are antecedent or subsequent to the behavior that is to be modified.

In changing a health behavior, the behavior modification activity often begins by having those in the priority population keep records (diaries, logs, or journals) for a specific period of time (24 to 48 hours, one week, or one month) concerning the behavior (such as eating, smoking, or exercise) they want to alter. Using the information recorded, one can plan an activity to modify that behavior. For example, facilitators of smoking cessation programs often will ask participants to keep a record of all the cigarettes they smoke from one class session to the next (see Figure 8.2 for an example of such a record). After keeping the record, participants are asked to analyze it to see what kind of smoking habit they have. They may be asked questions such as these: "What three cigarettes seem to be the most important of the day to you?" "In what three places or activities do you find yourself smoking the most?" "With whom do you find yourself smoking most often?" "Is there a primary reason or mood for your smoking?" "When during the day do you find yourself smoking the most and the least?" Once the participant has answered these questions, appropriate interventions can be designed to deal with the problem behavior. For example, if participants say they only smoke when they are by themselves, then activities would be planned so that they do not spend a lot of time alone. If other participants seem to do most of their smoking while drinking coffee, an activity would be developed to provide some type of substitute. If participants seem to smoke the most while sitting at the table after meals, activities could be planned to get them away from the dinner table and doing something that would occupy their hands.

Another way of leading into a behavior modification activity is through a health status evaluation, or what is often referred to as a *health screening*. Such screenings

Name _____

Date _____

Number of Cigarettes during the Day	Time of Day	Need Rating*	Place of Activity	With Whom	Mood or Reason
1.	_____	1 2 3	_____	_____	_____
2.	_____	1 2 3	_____	_____	_____
3.	_____	1 2 3	_____	_____	_____
4.	_____	1 2 3	_____	_____	_____
5.	_____	1 2 3	_____	_____	_____
6.	_____	1 2 3	_____	_____	_____
7.	_____	1 2 3	_____	_____	_____
8.	_____	1 2 3	_____	_____	_____
9.	_____	1 2 3	_____	_____	_____
10.	_____	1 2 3	_____	_____	_____
11.	_____	1 2 3	_____	_____	_____
12.	_____	1 2 3	_____	_____	_____
13.	_____	1 2 3	_____	_____	_____
14.	_____	1 2 3	_____	_____	_____
15.	_____	1 2 3	_____	_____	_____
16.	_____	1 2 3	_____	_____	_____
17.	_____	1 2 3	_____	_____	_____
18.	_____	1 2 3	_____	_____	_____
19.	_____	1 2 3	_____	_____	_____
20.	_____	1 2 3	_____	_____	_____
21.	_____	1 2 3	_____	_____	_____
22.	_____	1 2 3	_____	_____	_____
23.	_____	1 2 3	_____	_____	_____
24.	_____	1 2 3	_____	_____	_____
25.	_____	1 2 3	_____	_____	_____
26.	_____	1 2 3	_____	_____	_____
27.	_____	1 2 3	_____	_____	_____
28.	_____	1 2 3	_____	_____	_____
29.	_____	1 2 3	_____	_____	_____
30.	_____	1 2 3	_____	_____	_____

*Need rating: How important is the cigarette to you at this time?
        1 = Most important; I would miss it very much.
        2 = Average
        3 = Least important; I would not miss it.

Figure 8.2 Twenty-four-hour cigarette count

could happen at home (e.g., BSE, TSE, hemocult, etc.), at a community health fair (e.g., blood pressure, cholesterol), or in the office of a health care professional (e.g., breast examination). Like record keeping via diaries, logs, or journals, health screenings can "grab the attention" (develop awareness) of those in the priority population to begin the behavior modification process.

Organizational Culture Activities   Closely aligned with health engineering strategies are activities that affect organizational culture. Culture is usually associated with norms and traditions that are generated by and linked to a "community" of people. Organizations, which are made up of people, also can have their own culture. The culture of an organization can be thought of as its personality. The culture expresses what is and what is not considered important to the organization. The nature of the culture depends on the type of organization—corporation, school, or nonprofit group.

Many people think that it takes a long time to establish norms and traditions, and it often does. Still, change can occur very quickly if the decision makers in an organization support it. For example, if organizational decision makers believe exercise is important, they may provide employees with an extra 20 minutes at lunchtime for exercise. Similarly, it is surprising to see how many young executives will use a corporation's exercise facility because the chief executive officer does. Other examples of organizational culture activities might include changing the types of foods found in vending machines, closing the "junk food" machines during lunch periods at school, offering discounts on the health foods found in the company cafeteria, and getting retailers to change the way they have done things in the past, such as moving their tobacco products from in front of a counter to behind a counter, so that an employee has to get them for the customer. Because these activities affect groups of people, they are usually used at the organizational or institutional level.

Incentives and Disincentives   The use of incentives and disincentives to influence health outcomes is a common type of activity. This type of intervention activity is based on many health behavior theories that suggest that it is the anticipation of rewards—and tangible ones at that—that increases the probability of an individual engaging in desired behavior (Lefebvre, 1992). An **incentive** can increase the perceived value of an activity (Patton et al., 1986), motivate people to get involved, and remind program participants of their commitment to and goals for behavior change (Wilbur, 1983). The key to motivating someone with an incentive is to know what will incite an individual to action. Thus for this type of activity to work, the planners need to match the incentives with the needs, wants, or desires of the priority population. However, this is not easy, for what is an incentive for one person may be a deterrent for another, and vice versa. It has been suggested that incentives should even be tailored to the socioeconomic characteristics of the participants (Chenoweth, 1987) and, for that matter, the individual characteristics of each person.

For the planners, the task becomes one of matching the needs of the program participant or potential program participant with available incentives. Two approaches have been used to accomplish this. The first is to include questions about incentives as part of any needs assessment conducted in program planning. For example, a workforce needs survey might include a question on incentives, such as "What incentives would entice you to participate in the exercise program?" or "What would it take to get you to participate in this program?" or "What would it take to keep you involved in a health promotion program?" or "Would you continue to participate in an exercise program if you knew you were going to be given a nice tee shirt after logging 100 miles running or walking, or participating for 50 days in an aerobic dance or swimming program?" The responses to these questions should provide some indication of the type of incentives that would be most useful for this priority population. The second is the shotgun approach, based on previous experience or the experience reported by others. The shotgun approach offers a variety of incentives to meet the needs of a large percentage of the program's priority population. However, the former approach is recommended as being more likely to meet the targeted needs and wants.

Based on the idea that incentives should meet the individual needs of the priority population, the number of different types of incentives is almost endless. Feldman (1983) suggests two major categories of incentives or reinforcers. The first group includes incentives that would be considered social reinforcers; the second group includes incentives that are considered material reinforcers, or what may be referred to as economic incentives (see Figure 8.3).

The following advice is offered to planners who choose to use incentives:

1. Make sure everyone can receive one, whatever the incentive may be (Kendall, 1984).

2. Make the incentives useful and meaningful (Kendall, 1984).

3. Ensure that the ground rules are fair, understandable, and followed by everyone (Kendall, 1984).

4. Make a big deal of awarding the incentive.

5. Use incentives that are consistent with health promotion philosophies. For example, avoid incentives of alcoholic beverages, high fat or high sugar foods, or other mixed-message prizes.

As a final comment on incentives, several authors (French, Jeffery, & Oliphant, 1994; Jeffery et al., 1993; Matson, Lee, & Hopp, 1993; Price et al., 1992) have reported on the effectiveness of using incentives for program participation and behavior change. From these works, it appears that incentives are useful in getting people to participate and change their behavior for a short period of time. Also, more recent studies (Pescatello et al., 2001; Poole, Kumpfer, & Pett, 2001) have shown that incentives have also been useful in changing and maintaining health behavior change over time.

Just as incentives can be used to get people involved in behavior change, **disincentives** can be used to discourage a certain behavior. For example, Penner (1989) reports on the use of a surcharge for health insurance to influence the behavior of those who continue to use tobacco products. Another example would be not allowing the use of something because of a certain behavior, such as not allowing employees who smoke to use the employee lounge or company vehicles.

Up to this point, our discussion of incentives and disincentives has been mostly aimed at the intrapersonal, interpersonal, and institutional/organizational levels of influence. However, incentives and disincentives have also been effective when incorporated into the community and public policy levels of influence. "Sustained increases in excise taxes, constraining advertising and marketing, constricting use in public places, and penalizing the sale and distribution to minors have all worked to help drive down the use of tobacco" (McGinnis et al., 2002, pp. 88–89). The campaign

I. Social Reinforcers
   A. Special attention or recognition from instructors, peers, classmates, coworkers, or chief executive officers (Feldman, 1983; Shepard, 1985)
   B. Praise/verbal reinforcement (Feldman, 1983; Shepard, 1985)
   C. Public and other recognition (i.e., name in newsletter, name on bulletin board) (Koffman et al., 1998)
   D. Encouragement (Feldman, 1983; Shepard, 1985)
   E. Friendship (Feldman, 1983; Shepard, 1985)
   F. Inclusion of family members in the program (Feldman, 1983; Shepard, 1985)
   G. Personal letter to those reaching goals (Bensley, 1991)
II. Material Reinforcers
   A. Inexpensive "token" incentives
      1. T-shirts, hats, caps, visors, warm-up jackets, calendars, key chains, flashlights, pens, windshield scraper, wallets, tape measures, vacuum bottles, mugs, home fire extinguishers, smoke detectors, and auto safety kits (Cinelli, Rose-Colley, & Hayes, 1988; Kendall, 1984)
      2. Certificates
      3. Pins, buttons, patches, and decals that can be worn and plaques or markers that can be displayed in the work area
      4. Towels, lockers
      5. Preferred or free parking
   B. Program cost sharing between employer and employee
      1. Cost of registering for a program (Pollock et al., 1982)
      2. Membership at a fitness center/club
      3. Sliding-scale fee based on the ability to pay
      4. Refund of part or all of program fee based on participant's completion of a strategy
      5. Money to be used as an incentive (Koffman et al., 1998)
   C. Health Insurance
      1. Sharing between employer and employee of money saved on health insurance from one year to the next (Toufexis, 1985)
      2. Alteration of fringe benefit package to reward good health practices
      3. Employer picking up more of the insurance costs to reward good health practices (Toufexis, 1985)
      4. Provision of a fund for each employee to pay for the person's health care costs during the year, with any unused money from this account given to the employee at the end of the year (Hosokawa, 1984; Toufexis, 1985)
      5. Lower premiums for employees with fewer health risks (i.e., nonsmoker or exerciser) (Hosokawa, 1984)
   D. Monetary
      1. Tokens, Monopoly-style dollars, stamps, coupons, or points that are redeemable at a company store or a retail store, or for catalog shopping for prizes or merchandise (Kendall, 1984; Piniat, 1984; Toufexis, 1985)
      2. Drawings, lotteries, and raffles open to those who have participated or met a goal (Cinelli et al., 1988; Emont & Cummings, 1992; Health Insurance Association of America, 1983; Toufexis, 1985)
      3. Bonus, extra pay, rebates, or just plain pay for completion of contract, participation, not smoking on the job, or quitting (DiBlase, 1985; Pescatello et al., 2001; Poole, Kumpfer, & Pett, 2001; Toufexis, 1985)
      4. Financial rewards for both individuals and groups who have fewer and/or no work accidents during the year (DiBlase, 1985) or better smoking cessation rate (Koffman et al., 1998)

(continues)

Figure 8.3 Incentives: Social and material reinforcers

5. "Well pay" for unused sick days (DiBlase, 1985)
6. Gift certificates, from a small value, such as for a free ice cream cone, to something of greater value, such as a U.S. savings bond (Kendall, 1984)
7. Registration fee refund for completing a program (Pescatello et al., 2001)
8. Retail store gift card for completing a health risk appraisal (B. Neilson Hahn, personal communication, October 17, 2003)

E. Work Hours
1. Flex-time (flexible work hours) in order to participate
2. Released time to participate
3. Time off (Cinelli et al., 1988)

F. Contracts
1. Contract (competition) with a buddy
2. Contract with instructor to reach a specific goal, with a material incentive provided by instructor

3. Forfeiture of money or time to charity for not fulfilling a contract (Bloomquist, 1981)
4. Contract is entered into with the instructor in which money is withheld (via payroll deduction) while the person is enrolled in the program, so that if goal is met, the money is refunded; if not, it is forfeited (Bensley, 1991; Forster et al., 1985)

III. Miscellaneous
A. Special medical examinations and screenings for those who participate.
B. Special events, such as contests or luncheons (Kendall, 1984; Patton et al., 1986)
C. Providing special "space," such as a table in the lunchroom for those on a special diet (Bensley, 1991)

Figure 8.3

to raise the tobacco tax in Massachusetts is a good example of this (Heiser & Begay, 1997). Other forms of using incentives and disincentives at the community and public policy levels could include advertising the identity of restaurants in violation of food safety protocols, grants-in-aid to encourage communities to develop bike paths, and economic incentives to encourage health care providers to take a broader perspective for keeping people healthy such as reimbursement for brief interventions to assist smokers to quit or nonexercisers to exercise (McGinnis et al., 2002).

Social Activities   The importance of social support for behavior change and its relationship to health have been noted by several researchers (Becker & Green, 1975; Berkman & Syme, 1979; Cohen & Lichtenstein, 1990; Colletti & Brownell, 1982; Horman, 1989; Kviz et al., 1994; Kaplan & Cassel, 1977; Cummings, Becker, & Maile, 1980). Many people find it much easier to change a behavior if those around them provide support or are willing to be partners in the behavior change process. One of the major reasons why worksite health promotion programs have been so well received is because of the built-in social support from coworkers (Behrens, 1983).

Reference has already been made to how social support could work as an incentive. That would be one form of a social activity. Other social interventions could include support groups or buddy support, social gatherings, and social networks.

Support Groups and Buddy System.   The importance of support groups as part of comprehensive interventions has been well established. One need only look to the 12-step programs (such as Alcoholics Anonymous, Overeaters Anonymous, and Gamblers

Anonymous) and commercial programs (such as Weight Watchers) to realize the importance of people coming together to share their experiences and support one another's efforts. A support group need not be large; it might be as small as just two people. A buddy system is an example of a two-person group. A buddy system can take one of two different forms. In the first, both individuals are trying to change a behavior. In such a relationship, the two individuals support each other, whether this means helping each other stay on a special diet or meeting each other at 6 A.M. for exercise. In the other form, only one of the two is trying to change a behavior. The one not changing the behavior may have already changed (e.g., has already quit smoking or is exercising regularly) and is acting as a mentor to the one trying to change, or may not be trying to change but provides support at regular intervals or as problems arise.

Special elements that can be added to the support group or buddy system are the use of competition or a contract. Competition can take place among individual group members over such things as who can lose the most weight, who can walk/run the most miles, or who can go the longest without a cigarette. Competition could also be based on teams within the priority population (such as two different companies, two schools, or departments within an organization), using similar criteria but now based on group total figures (pounds, miles, or cigarettes). See Chapter 11 for more on competitions.

Contracts could be used by having one member of the priority population enter into an agreement with another member or with another person (such as the program facilitator, a friend, or spouse) over a change in some health behavior. The major component of a contract is the contingency. The *contingency* is a statement of what will happen if a contract is met or not met. For example, if a person meets the terms of his contract by losing 10 pounds in five weeks, he can then expect to receive something specified (an intangible, such as praise, or a material object) from the person who agreed to the contract. If the terms are not met, then the person for whom the contract was written must forfeit something specified (perhaps time volunteered to a community service or a material object of his own). See Chapter 11 for more on contracts.

Social Gatherings.   Social gatherings can be an important type of social intervention. Bringing together people who may be confronting similar problems for the purpose of purely social interaction not related to the problem can indirectly help them deal with the problem. Examples of such activities might be single parents having a cookout or a group of senior citizens attending a play. Although these gatherings do not deal directly with these people's common problems, they do help fill voids in their lives and thus indirectly help with the problem.

Social Networks.   Social networks are another type of social intervention. *Networks* are matrices linked by relationships or "ties." The nature of a tie can be quite varied, consisting of almost anything that creates a special feeling: need, concern, loyalty, frustration, power, affection, or obligation to name just a few. When people are "networking," they are said to be looking for relationships that would be useful in helping them with their concerns, such as problem solving, program development, resource identification, and others. As part of a health promotion intervention, social networking may take the form of having program participants trade telephone numbers for the purpose of calling each other when they are trying to resist smoking a cigarette or trying to locate a needed resource to solve a problem.

It should also be noted that although most social support and buddy systems take place between individuals, they can also be established at the institutional level. Like individuals, institutions can be paired up to help one another. For example, if two companies are interested in establishing health promotion programs, they could work together on their programs and share information and resources where appropriate. Or, if one company has a well-established program in place, then that company could "mentor" another company in setting up a program.

Creating Health Promotion Interventions

Once program planners have completed a needs assessment, written program goals and objectives, and considered different types of intervention strategies, they are in a position to begin designing an appropriate intervention.

Criteria and Guidelines for Developing Health Promotion Interventions

There is no one best way of intervening to accomplish a specific program goal that can be generalized to all priority populations. Each priority population has its own needs and wants that must be addressed. Nevertheless, successful and responsible health promotion programs generally adhere to some common set of guidelines, standards, or criteria around which their interventions are planned (Ad Hoc Work Group, 1987). Such guidelines help standardize and ensure the quality of the program, give credibility to a program, help with program accountability, provide a legal defense if a liability situation might arise, and identify ethical concerns that need to be addressed as a part of planning, implementing, and evaluating programs.

In 1987, the American Public Health Association (APHA), in collaboration with the Center for Health Promotion and Education of the Centers for Disease Control (CDC), developed a set of criteria to serve as guidelines for establishing the feasibility and/or the appropriateness of health promotion programs in a variety of settings (industrial, hospital, worksite, voluntary and official agencies) before making a decision to implement them. The criteria were not developed to assure successful programs, but rather to suggest issues that need to be considered in the decision-making process leading to the allocation of resources or the setting of program priorities (Ad Hoc Work Group, 1987, pp. 89–92). The five criteria suggested by the Work Group are:

1. A health promotion program should address one or more risk factors that are carefully defined, measurable, modifiable, and prevalent among the members of a chosen target group, and these factors that constitute a threat to the health status and the quality of life of target group members.
2. A health promotion program should reflect a consideration of the special characteristics, needs, and preferences of its target group(s).
3. Health promotion programs should include interventions that will clearly and effectively reduce a target risk factor and are appropriate for a particular setting.
4. A health promotion program should identify and implement interventions that make optimum use of the available resources.

5. From the outset, a health promotion program should be organized, planned, and implemented in such a way that its operation and effects can be evaluated.

In addition to the criteria set forth by APHA and CDC, other agencies and organizations have suggested criteria and guidelines. The Society of Prospective Medicine has developed the Ethics Guidelines for the Development and Use of Health Assessments (SPMBoD, 1999). Some organizations and professionals have set guidelines, criteria, or **codes of practice** for specific types of health promotion programs. Examples are the criteria set forth by the American College of Sports Medicine (Franklin, 2000) for exercise programs, the guidelines established by the American College of Obstetricians and Gynecologists for exercise during pregnancy, and the clinical practice guidelines for smoking cessation available from the Agency for Health Care Policy and Research (AHCPR, 1996) as well as those by Bartlett and colleagues (1986). Obviously, these guidelines and criteria are not all that are available. Prudent planners should seek out, through inquiry and networking, other criteria and guidelines that apply to programs they are planning.

Designing Appropriate Interventions

Selection of interventions for a health promotion program should be based on a sound rationale as opposed to chance; a strategy should not be selected just because the planners think it "sounds good" or because they have a "feeling" that it will work. As mentioned earlier, planners should choose an intervention that will be both effective and efficient. Although no prescription for an appropriate intervention has been developed, experience has indicated that the results of some interventions are more predictable than others. In this section, we present eight major questions that planners need to consider when creating health promotion interventions. Figure 8.4 summarizes these major considerations.

1. **Do the intervention strategies fit the goals and objectives of the program?** It is important that there be a good fit between the goals and objectives of a program and the intervention strategies used to reach the desired outcomes. If the single purpose of a program were to increase the awareness of the priority population, the intervention would be very different from what it would be if the purpose were to change behavior. Matching goals and objectives sounds easy enough, but creating such a match is a bit more difficult because of the "gray areas" created by the lack of empirical data to support such claims. Anderson and O'Donnell (1994) created such an intervention-outcome matrix based upon work presented in the *American Journal of Health Promotion*. Figure 8.5 presents a similar matrix using the terminology presented in this textbook.

2. **At what level of prevention will the program be aimed?** Because the needs and wants of those in the priority population, planners need to consider at which level or levels of prevention the program will be aimed. For example, a program aimed at increasing the level of exercise is likely to be received differently by asymtomatic nonexercisers than by a patient recovering from a heart attack.

3. **At what level(s) of influence will the intervention be focused?** Program planners must recognize that those in the priority population "live in social, political, and economic systems that shape behaviors and access to the resources they

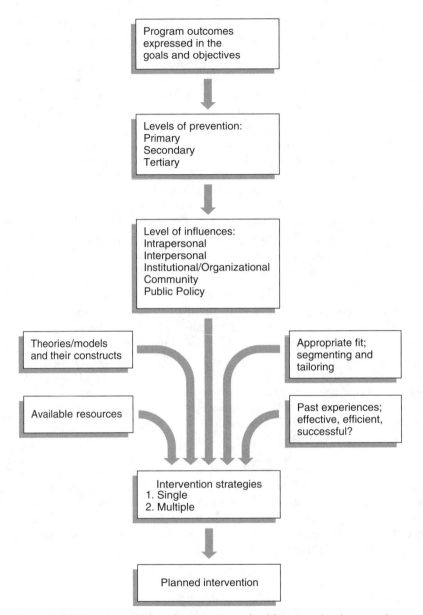

Figure 8.4 Items to consider when creating a health promotion intervention

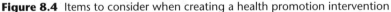

need to maintain good health" (Pellmar, Brandt, & Baird, 2002, p. 210). As such, planners need to decide at what level or levels of influence they can best obtain the goals and objectives of the program. For example, if the goal of the program is to increase safety belt use, can that best be accomplished by trying to intervene at an intrapersonal level with an individual education program, at the institutional level with a company policy, or at the public policy level with a enhanced state safety belt law?

Intervention Strategies

Type of Objective	Program Outcome	Communication	Educational	Health Policy/Enforcement	Health Engineering	Health-Related Community Service	Community Mobilization	Other
PROCESS/ADMINISTRATION	1. Activities presented	X	X	X	X	X	X	X
	2. Tasks completed							
LEARNING	1. Awareness	X	X	X	X	X	X	X
	2. Knowledge	X	X	X	?	X	X	X
	3. Attitudes	X	X	?	?	X	X	X
	4. Skills	X	X	X	X	X	?	X
ACTON/BEHAVIORAL	1. Behavioral change	X	?	X	X	X	?	X
ENVIROMENTAL	1. Environmental change	X	?	X	X	X	X	X
OUTCOME/PROGRAM	1. Quality of life	X	?	?	?	X	X	X
	2. Health status	X	?	X	X	?	X	X
	3. Health risks	X	?	X	X	X	X	X
	4. Social benefits	X	?	X	?	?	X	X

Figure 8.5 Matrix of intervention strategies, objectives, and program outcomes

4. **Are the strategies based on an appropriate theory?** Interventions have a much greater chance of reaching the desired outcome if they are planned using sound learning and educational theories that have proved their worth through experience and social science research. Interventions should not be without a solid basis in theory. Refer to Chapter 7 to review (1) the relationship between the levels of influence and the theories and (2) Table 7.7 for a listing of the constructs of the various theories.

5. **Is the intervention an appropriate fit for the priority population?** Intervention strategies need to be designed to "fit" the priority population. Each priority population has certain characteristics that impact how it will receive an intervention. It is important for planners to try to identify these characteristics in order to segment a priority population. **Segmenting** is the process of dividing a broader population into smaller groups with similar characteristics that are likely to exhibit similar behavior/reaction to an intervention (Wright, 1997) (see Box 11.3 for ways by which planners can segment the priority population). Segmentation allows planners to create an intervention to fit the needs and characteristics of a priority audience (Pasick, D'Onofrio, & Otero-Sabogal, 1996). Following are a few examples of how priority population segmentation can be applied. If program planners are developing written materials as part of their intervention, they need to make sure that the materials are written at an acceptable reading level for the priority population. From a developmental stage perspective, it is not reasonable to expect kindergartners to sit still for a one-hour lesson. Interventions also need to "fit" culturally within the priority population (Huff & Kline, 1999; LeMaster & Connell, 1994; Luquis & Perez, 2003; Pahnos, 1992) and be culturally sensitive. Cultural-sensitive interventions are those "that are relevant and acceptable within the cultural framework of the population to be reached" (Frankish, Lovato, & Shannon, 1998).

   If an intervention activity is created specifically for an individual's needs, interests, and circumstances it is referred to as a **tailored** activity. The rationale for tailoring an intervention activity is based on research that shows people pay more attention to information that is personally relevant to them (NCI, 2002). Tailored intervention activities have been used in a variety of programs including, but not limited to, AIDS (Bakker, 1999), cancer screening (Skinner, Strecher, & Hospers, 1994), exercise (Marcus et al., 1998), immunizations (Kreuter, Vehige, & McGuire, 1996), nutrition (Campbell et al., 1994), smoking cessation (Strecher et al., 1994), and weight loss (Kreuter, Bull, Clark, & Oswald, 1999). See Kreuter and colleagues (2000) for a review of tailoring.

   One final item to consider when thinking about the appropriateness of an intervention strategy for the priority population is to ask if there is any chance that the strategy could cause any unintended effects in the priority population. For example, could the strategy threaten the physical safety or raise undue anxiety in the priority population (CDC, 2003)?

6. **Are the necessary resources available to implement the intervention selected?** Obviously some intervention strategies require more money, time, personnel, or space to implement than others. For example, it may be prudent to provide each person in the priority population with $100 for participating in the health promotion program, but it may not be possible because of budget limitations.

7. **What types of intervention strategies are known to be effective (i.e., have been successfully used in previous programs) in dealing with the program focus?** By networking with others and by reviewing the literature, planners can find out what interventions have been effective with certain priority populations or in dealing with specific health problems.

8. **Would it be better to use an intervention that consists of a single strategy or one that is made up of multiple strategies?** A single-strategy intervention would most likely be easier and less expensive to implement and easier to evaluate. There are, however, some real advantages to using several strategies. These advantages include: (1) "hitting" the priority population with a message in a variety of ways; (2) appealing to the variety of learning styles within any priority population; (3) keeping the health message constantly before the priority population; (4) hoping that at least one strategy appeals enough to the priority population to help bring about the expected outcome; (5) appealing to the various senses (such as sight, hearing, or touch) of each individual in the priority population; and 6) increasing the chances that the combined strategies would help reach the goals and objectives of the program (e.g., communication used to publicize a policy change) (CDC, 2003). Probably the biggest drawback to using multiple strategies is the difficulty of separating the effects of one strategy from the effects of others in evaluating the impact of the total program and of individual components (Ad Hoc Work Group, 1987). However, Glasgow, Vogt, and Boles (1999) have developed an evaluation model titled RE-AIM (acronym for reach, efficacy, adoption, implementation, and maintenance) for use with multistrategy interventions.

SUMMARY

Interventions are strategies used by planners to bring about the outcomes identified in the program objectives. Interventions are also sometimes referred to as *treatments*. Although many times an intervention is made up of a single strategy, it is more common for planners to use a variety of strategies to make up an intervention for a program. In this chapter, intervention strategies were categorized into the following groups:

1. Health communication strategies
2. Health education strategies
3. Health policy/enforcement strategies
4. Health engineering strategies
5. Health-related community service strategies
6. Community mobilization strategies
7. Other strategies

Additionally, this chapter identified the need for program planners to be aware of recommended standards/criteria/guidelines when planning program interventions. Some examples of general, as well as program-specific, guidelines that have been set forth by both professional organizations and individual professionals, were reviewed. Finally, this chapter presented questions that planners need to consider when creating health promotion interventions.

REVIEW QUESTIONS

1. What is an intervention?

2. What are the advantages of using a multistrategy intervention over one that includes a single strategy? Are there any disadvantages? If so, what are they?

3. What are the major categories of interventions? Explain each.

4. Why should program planners be concerned with program guidelines that have been developed by professional organizations?

5. What are some of the documents and sponsoring groups that have suggested standards, criteria, or guidelines for program development?

6. Briefly discuss the questions set forth in this chapter that should be considered before creating an intervention.

ACTIVITIES

1. Create a multistrategy intervention for a program you are planning.

2. Create a multistrategy intervention for a program that has as its goal "to get third-grade students to wear helmets while riding their bicycles."

3. Create a multistrategy intervention for a program that has as its goal "to eliminate smoking of all employees of Company X."

4. Create a multistrategy intervention for a program that has as its goal "the rehydration of young children in the small village of Y in the Third World country of Q."

5. Design and present on a 8-1/2" x 11" piece of paper a bulletin board that could be used as part of the multiactivity intervention you are planning. Divide the piece of paper that represents the bulletin board into six equal sections and indicate what you will include in each section.

6. Interview a classmate to find out information about his or her health risks. Then, assuming you are a patient educator in a health clinic, create a one-page *tailored* letter to the person, urging him or her to seek an appropriate screening for the health risk(s).

7. Develop a three-fold pamphlet that can be used as an informational piece for a program you are planning.

8. With other students in your class, write a PSA script for a program you are planning. Then rehearse the script and have it videotaped.

9. Write a two-page, double-spaced news release that describes a program you are planning.

10. Write a letter to your state or federal senators or representatives and request their support of a piece of health-related legislation that is currently being considered.

WEBLINKS

1. **http://www.healtheducationadvocate.org**
   Health Education Advocate

   The Health Education Advocate website is sponsored by the Coalition of National Health Education Organizations (CNHEO). It was designed to provide a timely source of advocacy information related to the field of health education and promotion. This site includes a number of items to help health planners with advocacy activities. The site includes, but is not limited to, information about how to identify and contact their senators and congresspersons, the status of specific bills, health resolutions and policy statements of sponsoring agencies, and advocacy resources.

2. **http://www.cdc.gov/communication/cdcynergy.htm**
   CDCynergy

   This is a page at the Centers for Disease Control and Prevention website that presents background information about the CDCynergy health communication planning model. Also, the site provides the latest information on the various editions (i.e., cardiovascular, diabetes) of the CD-Rom program.

3. **http://www.americanheart.org/presenter.jhtml?identifier=2945**
   American Heart Association (AHA)

   This is the advocacy page of the AHA's website. Like most other voluntary health organizations, the American Heart Association has an active advocacy program to support its mission. This site provides an overview of the advocacy work in which the AHA is involved.

4. **http://www.welcoa.org/store/sidenav/incentivecampaigns.html**
   The Wellness Councils of America (WELCOA)

   This is a page at the WELCOA website that presents information on the incentive campaigns offered by the Council.

5. **http://www.nhlbi.nih.gov**
   National Heart, Lung, and Blood Institute (NHLBI)

   This is the homepage for the NHLBI. This site provides a wealth of information for both the lay public and health professionals. Of particular interest is the portion of the site that deals with health communications. By clicking on the communication link, one can find all the press releases distributed by the NHLBI over the past few years.

6. **http://www.sophe.org**
   Society for Public Health Education, Inc. (SOPHE)—Advocacy Matters

   This is the home page for SOPHE. SOPHE is a professional health education organization founded in 1950 and has a mission to provide leadership to the profession of health education and health promotion to contribute to the health of all people through advances in health education theory and research, excellence in health education practice, and the promotion of public policies conducive to health. At this site, health planners can click on the *Advocacy Matters* button to find out more about the Society's advocacy efforts.

Part II

Implementing a Health Promotion Program

The chapters in this section of the book present information used in implementing a health promotion program. The chapters identify important components related to implementation and address the challenges one may face during the implementation process. The chapters and topics presented in this section are:

CHAPTER 9

Community Organizing and Community Building

Chapter Objectives

After reading this chapter and answering the questions at the end, you should be able to:

- Define *community, community organizing, community building,* and *coalitions.*
- Outline the processes for organizing and building a community.
- Explain the term *mapping community capacity.*
- Provide an overview of PATCH.

Key Terms

active participants
bottom-up
citizen initiated
coalitions
community
community building
community organizing
executive participants

gatekeepers
grass-roots
locality development
mapping community
  capacity
occasional participants
ownership
PATCH

potential building blocks
primary building blocks
secondary building blocks
social action
social planning
stakeholders
supporting participants

A significant portion of the work of health educators involves implementing health promotion programs with small communities of people. **Community** means

a locale or domain that is characterized by the following elements: (1) membership—a sense of identity and belonging; (2) common symbol systems—similar language, rituals, and ceremonies; (3) shared values and norms; (4) mutual influence—community members have influence and are influenced by each other; (5) shared needs and commitment to meeting them; and (6) shared emotional connection—members share common history, experiences, and mutual support. Communality may be geographically bounded (e.g., a neighborhood) but is not necessary (e.g., an ethnic group) (Israel et al., 1994).

Thus it is not uncommon for planners to implement a smoking cessation program in a corporate setting, organize a support group for families affected by a chronic disease, or present a drug education program for school-age children. However, planners sometimes work with large communities, a task that involves organizing the people in a community to work together to implement a solution to a communitywide problem, concern, or issue. This chapter addresses the fundamental elements of organizing large communities for action.

Community Organizing and Its Assumptions

In recent years, there has been a shift in the focus of the work of planners and others in the helping professions. Where once the work of planners focused almost solely on the individual, today the focus is on broadening to the community. *Citizen participation, grass-roots participation, community participation, macro practice, community based, community empowerment,* and *community partnerships* are among the many terms that are being used more frequently by health agencies, outside funders, and policymakers (Minkler, 1997b). There are good reasons for the use of these terms and most revolve around the need for communities to organize.

In the early history of the United States, a sense of community was inherent in everyday life (Green, 1989). It was natural for communities to pool their resources to deal with shared problems. More recently, the need to organize communities has seemed to increase. Advances in electronics, communications, and increased opportunities for travel have resulted in a loss of the sense of community. Individuals are much more independent than ever before. The days when people knew everyone on their block are past (McKenzie et al., 2002).

Because of these changes in community social structure and the resources necessary to meet the needs of communities, it now takes a conserted effort to organize a community to act for the collective good.

"The term *community organization* was coined by American social workers in the late 1880s to describe their efforts to coordinate services for newly arrived immigrants and the poor" (Minkler & Wallerstein, 1997, p. 31). More recently, *community organization* has been used by a variety of professionals, including health educators, and refers to various methods of intervention to deal with social problems. "Community organization is important in health education in part because it reflects one of the field's most fundamental principles, that of starting where the people are" (Minkler & Wallerstein, 1997, p. 31). "The health education professional who begins with the community's felt needs, rather than with a personal or agency-dictated agenda, will be far more likely to experience success in the change process and to foster real community ownership of programs and actions than if he or she were to impose an agenda from outside" (Minkler & Wallerstein, 2002, p. 280).

Community organizing has been defined as "a process through which communities are helped to identify common problems or goals, mobilize resources, and in other ways develop and implement strategies for reaching their goals they have collectively set" (Minkler, 1997b, p. 5). It is not a science but rather an art of building consensus within the democratic process (Ross, 1967). (See Box 9.1 for definitions of related terms.) Although community organization may not be as "natural" as it once was, communities can still organize to analyze and solve problems through collective action. In working toward this end, those who assist communities with organizing must make several assumptions. Ross (1967, pp. 86–92) has stated these as follows:

Box 9.1 Terms Associated with Community Organizing

Citizen Participation	The bottom-up, grass-roots mobilization of citizens for the purpose of undertaking activities to improve the condition of something in the community.
Community Capacity	"Community characteristics affecting its ability to identify, mobilize, and address problems" (Minkler & Wallerstein, 2002, p. 288).
Community Development	"A process designed to create conditions of economic and social progress for the whole community with its active participation and the fullest possible reliance on the community's initiative" (United Nations, 1955, p. 6).
Community Participation	"A process of involving people in the institutions or decisions that affect their lives" (Checkoway, 1989, p. 18).
Empowered Community	"One in which individuals and organizations apply their skills and resources in collective efforts to meet their respective needs" (Israel et al., 1994).
Grass-Roots Participation	"Bottom-up efforts of people taking collective actions on their own behalf, and they involve the use of a sophisticated blend of confrontation and cooperation in order to achieve their ends" (Perlman, 1978, p. 65).
Macro Practice	The methods of professional change that deal with issues beyond the individual, family, and small group level.

1. Communities of people can develop capacity to deal with their own problems.

2. People want to change and can change.

3. People should participate in making, adjusting, or controlling the major changes taking place in their communities.

4. Changes in community living that are self-imposed or self-developed have a meaning and permanence that imposed changes do not have.

5. A "holistic approach" can deal successfully with problems with which a "fragmented approach" cannot cope.

6. Democracy requires cooperative participation and action in the affairs of the community, and that the people must learn the skills which make this possible.

7. Frequently communities of people need help in organizing to deal with their needs, just as many individuals require help in coping with their individual problems.

The Processes of Community Organizing and Community Building

There is no one specific method for organizing a community (Clapp, Packard, & Stanger, 1993). In fact, Rothman and Tropman (1987, pp. 4–5) have stated, "We should speak of community organization methods rather than the community organization method." Over the years, several different community organization methods have been used, including revolutionary techniques (Alinsky, 1971). However, the best known categories of community organization were the three put forth by Rothman and Tropman (1987) and include locality development, social planning, and social action. **Locality development** is most like community development and seeks community change through broad self-help participation from the local community. "It is heavily process oriented, stressing consensus, and cooperation and aimed at building group identity and a sense of community" (Minkler & Wallerstein, 1997, p. 34). **Social planning** "is heavily task oriented, stressing rational-empirical problem-solving" (Minkler & Wallerstein, 1997, p. 34) and includes various levels of participation, ranging from a little to a lot, and involves outside planners. **Social action** "is both task and process oriented" (Minkler & Wallerstein, 1997, p. 34) and deals with organizing a disadvantaged segment of the population. It aims at making changes in institutions and communities and often seeks a redistribution of resources and power. Although this model is no longer used as often as it once was, it was most useful during the civil rights and gay rights movements.

Though the concepts found in community organizing methods proposed by Rothman and Tropman (1987) have been the primary means by which communities have organized over the years, they do have their limitations. One of the greatest limitations is that they are primarily "problem-based and organizer-centered, rather than strength-based and community-centered" (Minkler & Wallerstein, 2002, pp. 284–285). Thus some of the newer models are based more upon collaborative empowerment and community building. Regardless of whether one talks about the "old models" or the "new models," they all revolve around a common theme: The work and resources of many have a much better chance of solving a problem or meeting a goal than the work and resources of a few.

Minkler and Wallerstein (2002) have done a nice job of summarizing the newer perspectives of community organizing with the older models by presenting a typology that incorporates both needs- and strength-based approaches. That typology is presented in Figure 9.1. This figure is divided into four quadrants with strength-based and needs-based on the vertical axis and consensus and conflict on the horizontal axis. Though this typology separates and categorizes the various methods of community organizing and building, Minkler and Wallerstein (2002, pp. 286–287) point out that

> "Community organizing and community building are fluid endeavors. Although some organizing efforts primarily have focused in one quadrant, the majority incorporate multiple tendencies, possibly starting as a result of a specific need or crisis and moving to a strength-based community capacity approach. Different organizing models, such as coalitions, lay health worker programs, political action groups, or grassroots organizing may incorporate needs- or strength-based approaches at different times as well, depending on the starting place and the ever changing social dynamic. It is important, however, that organizing efforts clarify their assumptions and make decisions on primary strategies based on skills of group members, history of the group, willingness to take risks, or comfort level with different approaches."

Since the purpose of this chapter is to provide an overview of the community organizing and community building processes, and at the risk of oversimplifying the processes, we would like to present a very general or generic approach to community organizing and community building (see Figure 9.2). It does not include everything

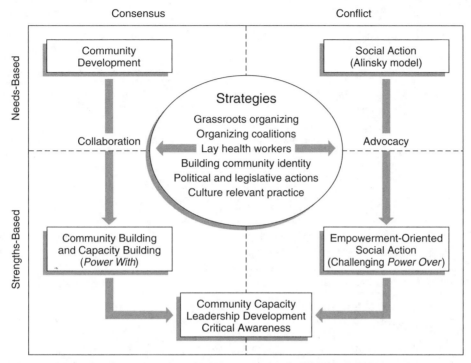

Figure 9.1 Community organization and community building typology

Source: "Improving Health Through Community Organization and Community Building," by Minkler, M., & Wallerstein, N.B., in *Health Behavior and Health Education: Theory, Research, and Practice*, K. Glanz, B.K. Rimer, & F.M. Lewis (Eds.), 3rd edition, p. 287. Copyright © 2002 by John Wiley & Sons, Inc. This material is used by permission of John Wiley & Sons, Inc.

planners need to know about community organizing and community building, but it does present the basic elements.

For further information about community organizing, refer to any of several references (Archer, Kelly, & Bisch, 1984; Brager, Specht, & Torczyner, 1987; Checkoway, 1989; Kretzmann & McKnight, 1993a; Minkler, 1997a; Minkler & Wallerstein, 2002; Langton, 1978; Rifkin, 1986; Ross, 1967; Rothman & Tropman, 1987; Rubin & Rubin, 1992) that are devoted entirely to the subject. Also, there are several works that deal specifically with the application of community organization to health promotion activities (Blackburn, 1983; Kumpfer, Turner, & Alvarado, 1991; Maccoby & Solomon, 1981; McAlister et al., 1982; Minkler, 1997c; Pentz et al., 1989; Wallenstein, Sanchez-Merki, & Dow, 1997).

Before presenting the generic process for community organizing and community building, we would like to comment on the role of the planner in this process. For many years, the planner was seen as a "leader" of the community organizing effort. However, more often than not, the planner is an "outsider" to the community being organized and, as such, has trouble gaining the credibility to serve as a leader. Yes, he/she may work in the "community" (remember that a community is often defined by something other than geographical boundaries) but often lives outside the "community" where the problem resides. Thus, the role that the planner should take is that

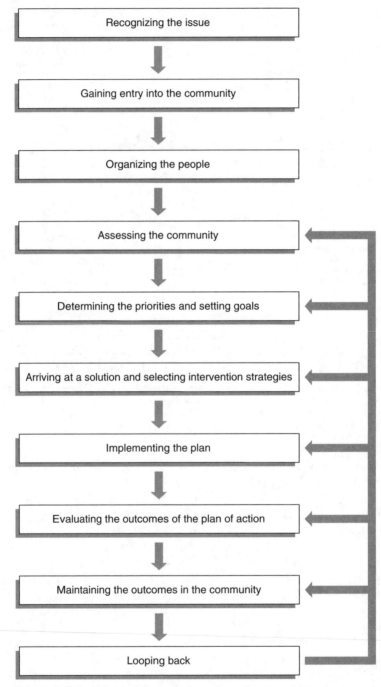

Figure 9.2 Summary of the steps in community organizing
and building

of a facilitator or assistant rather than the leader. Experience has shown that it is best if the leaders come from "within" the community. Keep this thought in mind as you read through the general model.

Recognizing the Issue

The processes of community organizing and building begin when someone recognizes that an issue exists in the community and that something needs to be done about it. For the purposes of this discussion, assume that the concern is a health problem, but remember that the community organization process may be used with any type of problem found in a community. Concerns can be as specific as trying to get a certain piece of legislation passed or as general as advocating for a drug-free community.

The recognition of an issue can occur from inside or outside the community. A citizen or a church leader from within the community may identify the issue, or it may first be identified by someone outside the community, such as an employee of a local or state health department, a state legislator, or someone from a local voluntary health agency. However, the community organizing efforts that have been most successful have been those that are recognized from the inside. "All historic evidence indicates that significant community development takes place only when local community people are committed to investing themselves and their resources in the effort" (Kretzmann & McKnight, 1993b, p. 11). The primary reason for this is that those within the community are much more likely to take ownership of the effort. It is difficult for someone from the outside coming in and telling community members that they have problems or issues that need to be dealt with and they need to organize to take care of them. When there is internal recognition of the issue or concern, it is referred to as **grass-roots, citizen-initiated,** or **bottom-up** organizing.

⤷ Starts w/ people directly impacted

Gaining Entry into the Community

The second step of this generic process of community organizing and community building may or may not be needed. If the issue identified in the previous step is recognized by someone from within the community, then this step of the process will, more than likely, not be needed. We say "more than likely" because those within a community do not need to gain entry into it. But there may be some cases when someone from within a community may identify the issue but has not lived in the community long enough or know enough about the interactions of the community to proceed with the process. In these later cases, the person may be treated or feel like an "outsider" and may have to proceed as an outsider would.

If the issue is identified by someone from outside the community this becomes a most critical step in the process. Recognition of a concern does not mean that people should immediately set about correcting it. Instead, they should follow a set of steps to deal with it, gaining proper "entry" into the community is the first step. Braithwaite and colleagues (1989) have stressed the importance of tactfully negotiating entry into a community with the individuals who control, both formally and informally, the "political climate" of the community. These individuals are referred to as **gatekeepers.** The term infers that one must pass through the "gate" in order to get at the people in the community (Wright, 1994). These "power brokers" know their community, how it functions, and how to accomplish tasks within it. Longtime residents are usually able to identify the gatekeepers of their community. They may include people such as business leaders, education leaders, heads of law enforcement agencies, leaders of community activist groups, parent and teacher groups, clergy, politicians, and others. Their support is absolutely essential to the success of any attempt to organize a community.

Organizers must approach the gatekeepers on the gatekeepers' terms and "play" the gatekeepers' "game." However, before making this contact, organizers must first be familiar with the community with which they are working. They must (1) know with whom the power lies, (2) know what type of political interactions take place within the community, (3) understand the culture or cultures that exist in the community, and (4) know whether the concern has been recognized before, and, if so, how it was addressed. In other words, community organizers must have a thorough knowledge of the community and the people living there before they try to enter the informal boundaries of the community (Braithwaite et al., 1989). Having a thorough understanding of the community and tactfully approaching its gatekeepers will help community organizers develop credibility and trust with those in the community, and, as noted earlier, it is not easy to bring a concern to the attention of those in the community. Few people are glad to know they have a problem, and fewer still like others to tell them they have a problem. Move with caution, and do not be too aggressive!

When people from outside the community are working to facilitate the organizing efforts, they will find it advantageous to enter the community through an already established, well-respected organization or institution in the community, such as a church, a service group, or another successful local group. Green (1990) has suggested that the academic health center might be the ideal convener to address health services, health protection, or health promotion issues. "It has the deep roots in the community, it is not typically beholden to an out-of-state master, it can cut deals with local organizations, and it can draw upon resources to leverage commitments and resources from other organizations" (p. 175). If those who make up an existing organization/ institution in the community can see that a problem exists and that solving the problem will improve the community, it can help smooth the way to gaining entry and achieving the remaining steps in the process.

Organizing the People

Obtaining the support of the community members to deal with the concern is the next step in the process. It is best to begin with those individuals who are already interested in addressing the concern. This is not the time to try to convert people to the cause or to make sure that all the key players of the community are involved. The initial group must be made up of those people most affected by the problem and who want to see change occur. For example, if the identified problem is teenage drug use, then teens needed to be included in the group. If the issue is housing for low income individuals, then those low income individuals need to be included. More often than not, this core group will be small and will consist of people who are committed to the resolution of the concern, regardless of the time frame. Brager and colleagues (1987) have referred to this core group as **executive participants.** From among the core group, a leader or coordinator must be identified. If at all possible, the leader should be someone with leadership skills, good knowledge of the concern and the community, and most of all, someone from within the community. One of the early tasks of the leader will be to help build group cohesion.

Not everyone is cut out to be an organizer or a leader. Researchers have found that good organizers are successful because of a combination of skills and attributes. These skills and attributes fall into three main areas: change vision attributes, technical skills, and interactional or experience skills. *Change vision attributes* are closely aligned with the organizer's view of the world political terms. These people see a need for change and are personally dedicated and committed to seeing the change occur—so much so that they are willing to put other priorities aside to see the project through (Mondros & Wilson, 1994).

Technical skills include two areas: those related to efficacy on issues and those related to organizational health and effectiveness. The former includes being able to analyze issues, opponents, and power structure; develop and implement change strategies; achieve goals; and have outstanding communication and public relation skills. Organizational health and effectiveness skills include building structures for the recruitment and involvement of others, forming and maintaining task groups, and implementing skills of fund-raising and organizational management (Mondros & Wilson, 1994).

The third characteristic of a good organizer is possessing *interactional or experience skills*. These include an ability to respond with empathy, to assess and intervene with individuals and groups, and to be able to identify, develop, educate, and maintain organizational members and leaders (Mondros & Wilson, 1994).

With the core group and leader in place, the next step is to expand the group to build support for dealing with the concern—that is, to broaden the constituency. Brager and colleagues (1987) have noted that other group participants will include active, occasional, and supporting participants. The **active participants** (who may also be executive participants) take part in most group activities and are not afraid to do the work that needs to be done. The **occasional participants** become involved on an irregular basis and usually only when major decisions are made. The **supporting participants** are seldom involved but help swell the ranks and may contribute in nonactive ways or through financial contributions. When expanding the group, look for others who may be interested in helping, and ask current group members for names of people who might be interested. Look for people who may already be dealing with the concern, affected by the problem through their present work, or who have resources to contribute. This search should include existing social groups, such as voluntary health agencies, agricultural extension services, church groups, hospitals, health care providers, political officeholders, policymakers, police, educators, lay citizens, or special interest groups. (See Box 9.2 on tips for understanding the diversity in a working group.)

Over the last few decades, in many communities the number of people interested in volunteering their time has decreased. Today, if you ask someone to volunteer, you may hear the reply, "I'm already too busy." There are two primary reasons for this response. First, there are many families in which both husband and wife work outside the home. Between 1970 and 2001, the proportion of married women with preschool-aged children who were in the labor force more than doubled, from 30.3% to 62.5%. Also during this same period of time, the proportion of married women with children

> ### *Box 9.2 Understanding Diversity*
>
> Members of a group come from many different backgrounds. Some members may be much older or much younger than other members; some may represent different cultural, racial, or ethnic groups; some may represent different educational levels and abilities. Extra awareness and flexibility are required for the facilitator and other group members to remain sensitive to different backgrounds. Below we suggest a few ways to improve your awareness of differences. In general, new information is acquired so that different perspectives can be understood and appreciated.
>
> - Become aware of differences in the group by asking questions and getting involved in small-group discussions.
> - Seek involvement and input and listen to persons of different backgrounds without bias, and avoid being defensive.
> - Learn the beliefs and feelings of specific groups about particular issues.
> - Read about current and emerging issues that concern different groups, and read literature that is popular among different groups.
> - Learn about the language, humor, gestures, norms, expectations, and values of different groups.
> - Attend events that appeal to members of specific groups.
> - Become attuned to cultural cliches, stereotypes, and distortions you may encounter in the media.
> - Use examples to which persons of different cultures and backgrounds can relate.
> - Learn the facts before you make statements or form opinions about different groups.
>
> *Source:* Centers for Disease Control and Prevention (no date), p. A2–15.

of school age who were in the labor force jumped from 49.2% to 77.7%. In 2001, 69% of married couples with children reported that both husband and wife were employed outside the home. Second, there are more single-parent households. Today, they constitute a little over one-fifth (27%) of all family households with children, and most (22% vs. 5%) are headed by women (USBC, 2002). (See Box 9.3 for tips on working with volunteers.)

These expanded community groups are sometimes referred to as *coalitions*. A **coalition** can be defined as a "formal, long-term alliance among a group of individuals representing diverse organizations, factors, or constituencies within the community who agree to work together to achieve a common goal" (Butterfoss & Whitt, 2003, p. 354) often, to compensate for deficits in power, resources and expertise. The underlying concept behind coalitions is collaboration, for several individuals, groups, or organizations where their collective resources have a better chance of solving the problem than any single entity (See Box 9.4 for characteristics of successful coalitions). "Building and maintaining effective coalitions have increasingly been recognized as vital components of much effective community organizing and community building" (Minkler, 1997b, p. 15). For those wanting more information about coalition development, Butterfoss and Whitt (2003) have provided a nice overview on the processes of building and sustaining coalitions.

Box 9.3 Tips on Working with Volunteers

Volunteers work for self-satisfaction, personal growth, fun, and other intangible rewards. Each volunteer should be treated as a colleague and recognized as an official part of the team. However, offer volunteers more flexibility than you can to employees, and adjust your expectations accordingly. For example, because volunteers cannot contribute as much time as paid, full-time workers do, they cannot complete tasks as quickly. When scheduling activities, be realistic about how long a busy PATCH participant will need to complete it.

Get to know each volunteer personally so that you can learn about special abilities and limitations and match responsibilities to skills. Vary responsibilities as desired by volunteers.

Be sure to assign specific and clearly defined tasks and to explain procedures and expectations. Develop a work plan or job description for the volunteer to help ensure that roles and responsibilities are understood. Provide training and give credit for work done. Give lots of feedback, encouragement, and signs of appreciation. Be willing to change the placement of volunteers, if that seems appropriate, or even dismiss a volunteer if necessary.

Keep in mind the following key points of working with volunteers. They want to be

- appreciated for the work that they do.
- busy with worthwhile and varied tasks.
- provided with clear communication about tasks and expectations.
- developed through training.

Source: Centers for Disease Control and Prevention (no date), p. A2–17.

Assessing the Community

Earlier in this chapter reference was made to the Rothman and Tropman's (1987) typology of community organization: locality development, social planning, and social action. Each of these community organizing strategies operates "from the assumption that problems in society can be addressed by the community becoming better or differently 'organized,' with each strategy perceiving the problems and how or whom to organize in order to address them somewhat differently" (Walter, 1997, p. 69). In contrast to these strategies is community building. **Community building** "is an orientation to community that is strength based rather than need based and stresses the identification, nurturing, and celebration of community assets" (Minkler, 1997b, pp. 5–6). Asset-based community building is intended to affirm the strong community-rooted traditions, and to build upon the good work already going on in communities (Kretzmann & McKnight, 1993b). One of the major differences between community organization and community building is the type of assessment that is used to determine where to focus the community's efforts. In the community organization approach, the assessment is focused on needs of the community, whereas in community building, the assessment focuses on assets and capabilities of the community. A clearer picture of the community will be revealed and a stronger base will be developed for change if the assessment includes the identification of both needs and assets, and involves those who live in the community. Hancock and Minkler (1997, p. 140) provide this illustration:

Box 9.4 Characteristics of Successful Coalitions

- Continuity of coalition staff, in particular the coordinator position.
- Ownership of the problem by coalition members and the community.
- Community leaders support the coalition and its efforts.
- Active involvement of community volunteer agencies.
- High level of trust and reciprocity among members.
- Frequent and ongoing training for coalition members and staff.
- Benefits of membership outweigh the costs.
- Active involvement of members in developing coalition goals, objectives, and strategies.
- Development of a strategic action plan rather than a project-by-project approach.
- Consensus is reached on issues instead of voting.
- Productive coalition meetings.
- Large problems are broken down into smaller, solvable pieces.
- Steering committee of elected leaders and staff guides coalition.
- Task or work groups of members design and implement strategies.
- Rules and procedures are formalized.
- Local media are actively involved.
- Coalition and its activities are evaluated continuously.

Source: Butterfoss, F.D., & Whitt, M.D., "Building and Sustaining Coalitions," in R.J. Bensley & J. Brookins-Fisher (Eds.), *Community Health Education Methods,* 2nd edition, p. 329. © 2003 Jones and Bartlett Publishers, Sudbury, MA. www.jbpub.com. Reprinted with permission.

For example, a narrowly defined needs assessment designed and conducted by out-side experts as a means of justifying and providing raw data for organizing around a predetermined community health need may be effective in achieving its objectives. But by failing to meaningfully involve community members in determining the goals of the assessment process, by focusing solely on needs rather identifying and building on community strengths, and by failing to make empowerment of people a central goal of the assessment process, such an approach would fail to meet several critical criteria of community organizing and community building practice.

Thus a community assessment conducted by the community and for the com-munity will produce needs data that will identify the deficiencies (Hancock & Min-kler, 1997) (see Figure 9.3). But the assessment will also uncover the capacities and assets of a community. It is from these capacities and assets that communities are built (McKnight & Kretzmann, 1997).

The steps to complete the needs identification of an assessment have already been discussed in this book (see Chapter 4). But what has not yet been discussed is the process of assessing the capacities and assets. McKnight and Kretzmann (1997) provide a technique for completing this portion of assessment called **mapping community capacity** (see Figure 9.4). They have categorized assets into three different groups based on their availability to the community and refer to them as *building blocks*. **Primary building blocks** are the most accessible assets. They are located in the neighborhood and are largely under the control of those who live in the neighborhood.

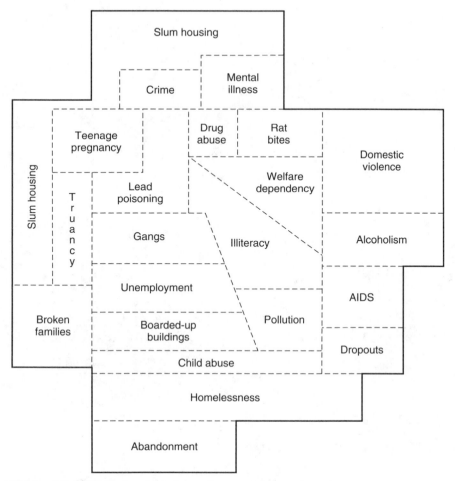

Figure 9.3 Neighborhood needs map

Source: McKnight, J.L., & Kretzmann, J.P., "Mapping Community Capacity," in M. Minkler (Ed.), *Community Organizing and Community Building For Health,* Rutgers University Press, 1997, p. 168. Reprinted by permission of the authors.

Primary building blocks can be organized into the assets of individuals and those of organizations or associations (see Box 9.5 for examples of each). The next most accessible building blocks are **secondary building blocks,** which are assets located in the neighborhood but largely controlled by people outside (see Box 9.5). The least accessible assets are referred to as **potential building blocks.** They are located resources originating outside the neighborhood and controlled by people outside (see Box 9.5). Knowing both the needs and the assets of the community, organizers can work to identify the true concerns of the community and the capacity to deal with them.

Determining Priorities and Setting Goals

Once the community has been assessed, the community group is ready to develop its goals. The goal-setting process includes two phases. The first phase consists of identifying the priorities of the group—what the group wants to accomplish. The priorities

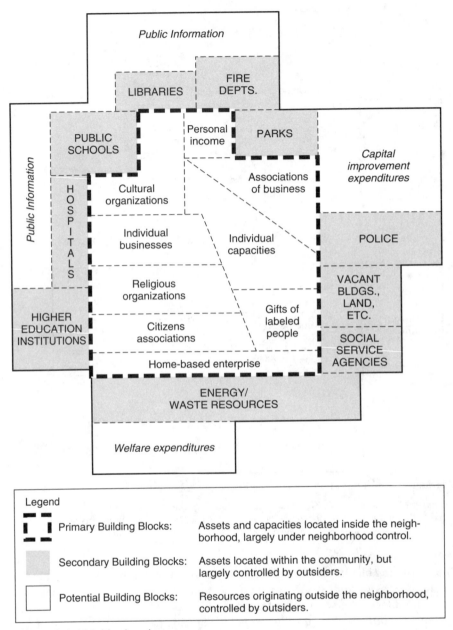

Figure 9.4 Neighborhood assets map

Source: McKnight, J.L., & Kretzmann, J.P., "Mapping Community Capacity," in M. Minkler (Ed.), *Community Organizing and Community Building For Health*, Rutgers University Press, 1997, p. 169. Reprinted by permission of the authors.

should be determined through consensus rather than through formal voting (see Box 9.6 for tips on how to reach consensus). The second phase consists of using the priority list to write the goals. To help ensure that the ideals of community organization take hold, the **stakeholders** (those in the community who have something to

---

Box 9.5 Building Blocks (Assets) of Communities

Primary Building Blocks

Individual assets

- Skills, talents, and experience of residents
- Individual businesses
- Home-based enterprises
- Personal income
- Gifts of labeled (disabled) people

Organizational assets

- Associations of businesses (i.e., Chamber of Commerce)
- Citizens' associations (i.e., neighborhood watch)
- Cultural organization (i.e., Old West End Festival, British Club)
- Communications organizations (i.e., newspapers, TV, radio)
- Religious organizations

Secondary Building Blocks

Private and nonprofit institutions

- Higher education institutions
- Hospitals and clinics
- Social service groups (i.e., United Way)

Public institutions and services

- Public schools
- Police, sheriff, and fire departments
- Libraries
- Parks and other recreational facilities

Physical resources

- Vacant land
- Commercial and industrial structures
- Housing
- Energy and waste resources

Potential Building Blocks

Welfare expenditures

Public capital information expenditures

Public information

Source: Adapted from McKnight, J.L., & Kretzmann, J.P., "Building Blocks of Communities," in M. Minkler (Ed.), *Community Organizing and Community Building For Health*, Rutgers University Press, 1997, pp. 157–172. Reprinted by permission of the authors.

---

gain or lose from the community organizing and building efforts) must be the ones to establish priorities and set goals. This may sound simple, but in fact it may be the most difficult part of the process. Getting the stakeholders to agree on priorities takes a skilled group facilitator, because there is sure to be more than one point of view.

> ### Box 9.6 Reaching Consensus
>
> Groups sometimes find it hard to reach a consensus, or general agreement. Remind participants of the following guidelines to group decision making.
> - Avoid the "one best way" attitude; the best way is that which reflects the best collective judgment of the group.
> - Avoid "either, or" thinking; often the best solution combines several approaches.
> - A majority vote is not always the best solution. When participants give and take, several viewpoints can be combined.
> - Healthy conflict, which can help participants reach a consensus, should not be smoothed over or ended prematurely.
> - Problems are best solved when participants try both to communicate and to listen.
>
> If a group has trouble reaching consensus, consider using some special techniques such as brainstorming, the nominal group process, and conflict resolution.
>
> *Source:* Centers for Disease Control and Prevention (no date), p. A2–12.

When working with coalitions and task forces, one is likely to find that determining priorities and setting goals causes *turf struggles* (disagreements over the control of resources and responsibilities). Even though individuals or representatives of their organizations have come together to solve a problem, many people will still be concerned with finding specific solutions to the problems faced by their organization. For example, in the case of drug abuse in the community, consensus may indicate that the majority of people believe the concerns lie in the educational system, but people who work in the treatment centers may believe that they lie in the treatment of drug abuse. The facilitator will need special skills to keep these treatment center people involved after the priority-setting process does not identify their concern as a problem the group will attack. One means of dealing with this is to have subgoals that can be worked on by special interest subcommittees. Such an arrangement will allow the subcommittee to have a feeling of **ownership** in the process.

Arriving at a Solution and Selecting Intervention Strategies

To achieve the goals that it has set, the group will need to identify alternative solutions and—again, through consensus—choose a course of action. Most concerns can be dealt with in any of several ways, however, each alternative has advantages and disadvantages. The group should examine the alternatives in terms of probable outcomes, acceptability to the community, probable long- and short-term effects on the community, and the cost of resources to solve the problem (Archer & Fleshman, 1985). Most of the intervention strategies discussed in Chapter 8 are means by which the group deal with the concerns.

Much of the work to identify the appropriate solution(s) can be accomplished through subcommittees. Subcommittees can complete specific tasks that will contribute to the larger plan of action. Their work should yield specific strategies that are culturally sensitive and appropriate for the community. The plan of action is usually written in a proposal format and will be given final approval at a meeting of the full committee or coalition. It is important to take care in putting together this proposal; as many as possible of the ideas of the various subcommittees should be included. This will help to ensure approval of the entire plan. In the end, the real test of the course of action selected is whether it can provide whatever it is the people are seeking (Brager et al., 1987).

Final Steps in the Community Organizing and Building Processes

The final four steps in a community organizing and building processes include implementing the plan, evaluating the outcomes of the plan of action, maintaining the outcomes in the community, and, if necessary, "looping" back to the appropriate point in the process to modify the steps and restructure the work plan. Once the work of the group has been completed (that is, either the issue has been solved or community empowerment achieved), the group can either disband or reorganize to deal with other issues.

Planned Approach to Community Health (PATCH)

So far, this chapter has presented a general description of the processes of organizing and building a community. However, there are some models for the community organization process that have been developed to guide community organizers. A couple of these models (Mobilizing for Action Through Planning and Partnerships [MAPP] and Healthy Communities) were presented as planning models in Chapter 2 of this book (see Chapter 2). However, one other that has received considerable use and attention in the area of health promotion is the Planned Approach to Community Health, better known by its acronym, **PATCH** (Kreuter et al., 1985) (see Figure 9.5).

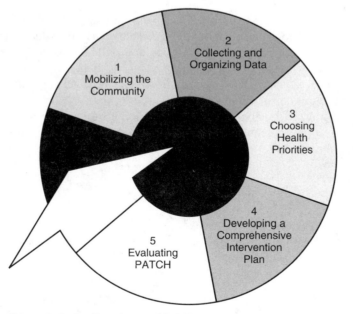

Figure 9.5 The five phases of PATCH

Source: Centers for Disease Control and Prevention (no date). *Planned Approach to Community Health.* Retrieved November 6, 2003 from http://www.cdc.gov/nccdphp/patch/index.htm

The concept of PATCH emerged in 1983 as the response of the Centers for Disease Control and Prevention (CDC) to the shift in the federal policy regarding the distribution of money to states via categorical (block) grants (Kreuter, 1992). PATCH was designed using the PRECEDE model and was created "to strengthen state and local health departments' capacities to plan, implement, and evaluate community-based health promotion activities targeted toward priority health problems" (Kreuter, 1992, p. 135). Since its development, PATCH has proved to be a useful process with a good "track record for facilitating collaborative, community-based programs" (Speers, 1992, p. 132). The use of PATCH also led to the inspiration for PROCEED (Green & Kreuter, 1992). (See the *Journal of Health Education*, April 1992, for accounts of some of the success stories.) The essential elements of PATCH include community organization with local support, participation, and leadership; community members using local health data to determine the health problems, prioritize the health problems, and set goals and objectives; carrying out interventions; and evaluating the results (Speers, 1992). PATCH is a team approach in which the people of the community make the decisions (via a consensus process) and do the work, with technical assistance from the state and local health departments and the Centers for Disease Control and Prevention. These team members not only facilitate the necessary work but also provide financial support for the project.

Boxes 9.2, 9.3, and 9.6 presented in this chapter have come from the "PATCH Guide for the Local Coordinator" (USDHHS, CDC, no date). For more information on PATCH, contact your local health department, state health department, or the Centers for Disease Control and Prevention.

Summary

Community organization refers to various methods of intervention whereby individuals, groups, and organizations engage in planned collective action to deal with social concerns. The literature on community organizing and building is not distinct; it is often intertwined with such terms as *citizen participation, community empowerment, community participation, grass-roots participation, macro practice,* and *community development*. The process of community organization has been used for many years in the area of social work, but its history in the area of health promotion is much more recent. Within this chapter generic processes for community organizing and building were presented, which should be an adequate introduction to the process. Finally, a brief overview of the PATCH model was presented.

Review Questions

1. What is meant by the term *community?*
2. How does community organization relate to community empowerment?
3. Community organization originated out of what discipline?
4. What is the underlying concept of community organization?
5. What are some of the assumptions under which planners work when organizing a community?
6. What are the basic steps in the community organizing and building processes?
7. What is meant by the term *gatekeepers?*

8. What is the difference between the assessments for community organizing and community building?

9. What is meant by *mapping community capacity?*

10. What are the differences among primary, secondary, and potential building blocks (assets)?

11. What does the acronym PATCH stand for? What are the major components of this process?

ACTIVITIES

1. Assume that a core group of individuals have come together to deal with the concern of a high rate of teenage pregnancy in the community. Identify (by job title/function) others who you think should be invited to be part of the larger group. In addition, provide a one-sentence rationale for inviting each. Assume that this community is large enough to have most social service organizations.

2. Provide a list of at least 10 different community agencies that should be invited to make up an antismoking coalition in your home town. Provide a one-sentence rationale for including each.

3. Assume that you want to make entry into a community, with which you are not familiar, in order to help to organize and build the community. Describe such a community, and then write a two-page paper to tell what steps you would take to gain entrance into the community.

4. If you wanted to find out more about your community's resources regarding exercise programs, with whom would you network? Provide a list of at least five contacts, and provide a one-sentence rationale for why you selected each.

5. Ask your professor if he or she is aware of any community organizing or building efforts in a local community. If such exists, make an appointment along with some of your classmates to interview the organizers. Ask the organizers to respond to the following questions:
   a. What is the concern being tackled?
   b. Who identified the initial concern?
   c. Who makes up the core group? How large is it?
   d. Did the group complete an assessment?
   e. What type of intervention is being used?
   f. What type of community organizing or building model was used?

WEBLINKS

1. **http://www.northwestern.edu/ipr/abcd.html**
   Asset-Based Community Development (ABCD) Institute, Northwestern University

   This is the web page of the Asset-Based Community Development Institute (ABCD) established in 1995 at Northwestern University's Institute for Policy Research. The ABCD was built on the community development research of John Kretzmann and John L. McKnight. The website provides background information on many of the projects sponsored by the ABCD Institute.

2. **http://ctb.ku.edu/about**
   The Community Tool Box (CTB), University of Kansas

The CTB provides practical information to support work in promoting community health and development. This website is created and maintained by the Work Group on Health Promotion and Community Development at the University of Kansas in Lawrence, Kansas (U.S.A) in collaboration with AHEC/Community Partners in Amherst, MA. The core of the CTB is the "topic sections" that include practical guidance for the different tasks necessary to promote community health and development. Each section includes a description of the task, advantages of doing it, step-by-step guidelines, examples, checklists of points to review, and training materials.

3. **http://www.nhlbi.nih.gov/health/prof/heart/obesity/hrt_n_pk/hnp_resg.htm**
   National Heart, Lung, and Blood Institute (NHLBI)

   This is a web page of the NHLBI where the Community Mobilization Guide, developed by the NHLBI and the National Recreation and Park Association, can be found. The guide was created to assist planners at the community level with implementing a Hearts N' Parks program which is aimed at promoting heart-healthy lifestyle and changes such as increased physical activity and heart-healthy eating among children and adults. The guide provides all the necessary tools for implementing this program including background information and materials, techniques for creating and delivering heart-healthy activities to participants, tools and strategies for reaching targeted groups, forming partnerships, and working with the media, as well as assessment tools to measure program performance.

4. **http://www.cdc.gov/nccdphp/patch/index.htm**
   Planned Approach to Community Health (PATCH)

   This is the web page for PATCH. Visitors to this site can download the PATCH guide and supporting visual materials. The PATCH Guide is designed to be used by the local coordinator and contains "how to" information on the process, things to consider when adapting the process to your community, and sample overheads and handout materials.

5. **http://www.hospitalconnect.com:80/DesktopServlet**
   Association for Community Health Improvement (ACHI)

   This is the home page for the ACHI. The ACHI was conceived in mid–2002 as a successor to three national community health initiatives that were approaching the end of their grant cycles or were otherwise ripe for renewal and growth: the Community Care Network Demonstration Program, ACT National Outcomes Network, and Coalition for Healthier Cities and Communities. The mission of ACHI is to strengthen community health through education, peer networking and practical tools. This site provides a variety of information pertaining to work of community health including: news and updates, resources, as well as, networking, education, and professional conference opportunities.

CHAPTER 10

Identification and Allocation of Resources

Chapter Objectives

After reading this chapter and answering the questions at the end, you should be able to:

- Define *resources*.
- List the common resources used in most health promotion programs.
- Identify the tasks to be carried out by program personnel.
- Explain the difference between *internal* and *external* resources.
- Define *culturally sensitive* and *culturally competent*.
- Explain what is meant by the term *canned health promotion programs*.
- Identify questions to ask vendors when they are selling their programs, products, and services.
- List and explain common means of financing health promotion programs.
- Define *budget*.
- Identify and explain the major components of a grant proposal.

Key Terms

canned program	hard money	request for proposals (RFP)
culturally competent	in-house materials	resources
culturally sensitive	in-kind support	seed dollars
curriculum	internal resources	sliding-scale fee
external resources	ownership	soft money
flex time	peer education	speaker's bureau
grant money	profit margin	vendors
grantsmanship	proposal	

For a program to reach the identified goals and objectives, it must be supported with the appropriate resources. **Resources** include all the people and things needed to carry out the desired program. The quantity or amount of resources needed to plan, implement, and evaluate a program depends on the scope and nature of the program. Most resources carry a "price tag," which planners must take into account.

Thus planners face the task of securing the financial resources necessary to carry out a program. However, several different resources are provided by organizations, mostly voluntary or governmental health organizations, that are free or inexpensive. This chapter identifies, describes, and suggests sources for obtaining the resources commonly needed in planning, implementing, and evaluating health promotion programs.

Personnel

The key resource of any program is the individuals needed to carry out the program. Instead of trying to identify all the individuals necessary to ensure the program's success (because many times the same person is responsible for several different program components), planners should focus on the tasks that need to be completed by the program personnel. These tasks include planning; identifying resources; advertising; marketing; conducting the program, including having the necessary interpreters for those who speak a different language than the one in which the program is offered and accommodating those with disabilities; evaluating the program; making arrangements for space and program materials; handling clerical work; and keeping records (for program sign-up, collection of fees, attendance, and budgeting).

In some cases, the program participants themselves constitute a program resource. For example, in the case of a worksite health promotion program, planners will need to find out whether the employees will participate on company time, on their own time before or after work hours, on a combination of company time and employee time, or on their own anytime during the work day as long as they put in their regular number of work hours. (This last option is known as **flex time.**) The current trend in worksite health promotion programs is to ask the employees to participate at least partially on their own time. The reasoning behind this trend is that this investment by the participant helps to promote a sense of program **ownership** ("I have put something into this program, and therefore I am going to support it") and thus build loyalty among participants.

Internal Resources

When identifying the personnel needed to conduct a program, planners have three basic options. One, referred to as **internal resources,** uses individuals from within the planning agency/organization or people from within the priority population to supply the needed labor. For example, if a local health department was planning a health promotion program in a community, the employees of the health department might handle the planning, implementation, and evaluation of the program. If that same health department was planning a health promotion program for the faculty and staff of a school district, there would likely be many school employees (i.e., school nurse, health educator, physical education instructor, family and consumer science teacher) who have the expertise (knowledge and skills) to carry out much of the program. If the department was planning a worksite program, there would probably be some employees who would be qualified to conduct at least a portion of the program (for example, an employee who is certified to teach first aid or cardiopulmonary resuscitation).

Another internal resource that health promotion planners are using successfully in a variety of settings, especially in schools (from kindergarten to college), is **peer education.** The process is simple: Individuals who have specific knowledge, skills, or understanding of a concept help to educate their peers. For example, college students may work with other college students to help educate them about the dangers of drinking and driving. The major advantages of peer education are its low cost and the credibility of the instructor. Children, for example, are greatly influenced by slightly older peers.

External Resources

A second source of personnel for a program is to bring in individuals from outside the planning agency/organization or the priority population to conduct part or all of the program. Such individuals are considered **external resources.** Typically, these individuals are brought in when it is found that there is a gap between what can be provided internally and what ultimately must be provided to accomplish the program goals and objectives (Harris, 2001). There are now many companies that offer or sell programs, services, or consulting to groups wanting health promotion programs. These companies are referred to as **vendors.** Some vendors are for-profit groups—such as hospitals, consulting agencies, health promotion companies, or related businesses—whereas others are nonprofit organizations—such as voluntary health agencies, YMCAs, YWCAs, governmental health agencies, universities/colleges, extension services, or professional organizations.

Planners must be careful when using vendors because the quality of vendors can vary greatly. Figure 10.1 provides a checklist (Harris, 2001) that can be used to assist planners in screening vendors. It should be noted that the checklist has not been standardized and there is no set score that will assure that a vendor will be a good supplier of health promotion services. However, vendors who receive "yes checks" in a vast majority of the questions are likely to be highly qualified. Those who have a large number of "no checks" should be viewed skeptically (Harris, McKenzie, & Zuti, 1986).

An often untapped inexpensive source of personnel for health promotion programs is experts available through **speaker's bureaus.** Most local offices of voluntary health agencies, hospitals, and other health-related organizations maintain speaker's bureaus. The services of these experts are usually available at little or no cost to groups. With some inquiry and a little networking, it is not difficult for planners to identify organizations that have individuals available to speak on a variety of health-related topics, or health care organizations willing to send their medical experts into the community to share their knowledge. The speaker's bureau is a win-win concept for both the group offering the service and the one receiving it. Groups that take advantage of a speaker's bureau gain access to expert information, but those delivering the information gain in terms of public relations and recognition.

There are advantages and disadvantages connected with using either internal or external personnel to conduct health promotion programs. Table 10.1 lists the pros and cons of each.

Combined Resources

The third option for obtaining personnel to carry out a program is a combination of internal and external resources. This option is the one most commonly used because it allows the program planners to make use of the advantages of the first two options and avoid many of the disadvantages. In fact, in worksite health promotion there is evidence (Elliott, 1998) to support the use of both internal and external resources by those in best-practice (i.e., the most successful) organizations.

Code:	Yes = Yes, the vendor does/did this. No = No, the vendor does not/did not do this.			NA = Not applicable NS = Not sure	
1. Initial experience with the vendor		**Yes**	**No**	**NA/NS**	**Comments**
A.	Did the vendor present a good professional image?				
B.	Did the vendor do his/her homework on your company prior to the initial meeting?				
C.	Is the vendor's philosophy of health promotion consistent with your company's philosophy?				
D.	Can the vendor explain why his/her product can meet the needs of your company?				
E.	Did the vendor appear responsive to your company's needs?				
F.	Did the vendor explain how his/her product can meet the needs of your company?				
G.	Was the vendor willing to listen to you or was he/she too busy trying to sell his/her product?				
H.	Is the vendor willing to make a presentation to your company's management?				
I.	Did the vendor demonstrate his/her organization's expertise with regard to the product?				
J.	Did the vendor provide you with a reference list of other customers?				
K.	Did the vendor leave written materials that summarize his/her product?				
2. Product quality					
A.	Did the vendor provide an overview of the product content?				
B.	Can the vendor provide careful documentation of the product effectiveness?				
C.	Does the vendor have evaluative data to back up the product?				
D.	Does the vendor have data to compare success rates of the product to those of his/her competitors?				
E.	Can the vendor provide data which show the adequacy of his/her product with a population similar to yours?				
F.	Can the vendor provide several different products (health promotion activities), or does he/she just specialize in one area?				
G.	Did the vendor explain the types of interventions (behavior modification, aversive techniques, etc.) that are used with the product?				
H.	Will the vendor "customize" the product to meet the needs of your company?				

Figure 10.1 Checklist for selecting health promotion vendors

2. **Product quality** *(continued)*		Yes	No	NA/NS	Comments
I.	Can the vendor offer a variety of interventions (i.e., different approaches to smoking cessation) from which you can choose to best meet the needs of your employees?				
J.	Can the vendor offer a product which can meet special needs of your employees (e.g., reading levels, various levels of health status, etc.)?				
K.	When appropriate, does the vendor provide written instructional materials to accompany the product?				
L.	If written informational materials are provided, are they written clearly and presented in an attractive way?				
3. Individuals who provide the service					
A.	What type of education and training do the staff and/or instructors have?				
B.	Are the instructors certified by a professional and/or health organization?				
C.	Are the instructors required to update their training periodically?				
D.	Are the instructor-to-participate ratios reasonable?				
4. Product delivery and service					
A.	Can the vendor put in writing the actual services that will be provided?				
B.	If a written presentation of services is made, does it spell out the responsibilities of both parties?				
C.	Is the vendor willing to market the product inside your company?				
D.	Does purchase of the product include an evaluation?				
E.	Can the vendor appropriately serve the size of your company's population?				
F.	Can the vendor provide the product at all sites desired?				
G.	Can the vendor provide the product at the time desired?				
H.	Are the length of the product sessions appropriate for your work day?				
I.	Does the vendor provide you with the name of one of his/her employees who can act as a troubleshooter?				
J.	Does the vendor provide you with other products/services to other departments (units) (i.e., the safety division, health policy, etc.) in your company?				
K.	Has the vendor been in business for at least five years?				

Figure 10.1 *(continued)*

4. Product delivery and service *(continued)*	Yes	No	NA/NS	Comments
L. Is the vendor's company well managed and financially sound?				
M. Does the vendor enjoy a good reputation in the community?				
5. Product cost				
A. Is the cost of the product competitive with the cost of other vendors?				
B. Does the vendor provide written bids for the product?				
C. Does the cost per unit go down when the number of participants increases?				
D. Does the cost per unit go down if additional products are purchased from the same vendor?				
E. Does the vendor offer corporate discounts?				
6. General concerns				
A. Does the vendor carry adequate liability insurance?				
B. Does the vendor put in writing a "statement of reasonable expectations" for the product?				
C. Is the vendor willing to sign a contract?				
D. If you buy the product of this vendor, will it improve the image of your company in the community?				
E. If you buy the product of this vendor, will it improve the image of your company with the employees?				

Figure 10.1 *(continued)*

Source: This checklist appeared in *Absolute Advantage*, [Harris, J. H. (2001). Selecting the right vendor for your health promotion program. *Absolute Advantage*, 1(4), 4–5.] a publication of the Wellness Councils of America (www.welcoa.org). This checklist is a revised version of the one created earlier by Harris, McKenzie, & Zuti (1986).

One special concern for personnel, regardless of whether they are internal, external, or a combination of the two, is that they are both culturally sensitive and culturally competent. **Culturally sensitive** means having a basic understanding and appreciation of the importance of sociocultural factors (Kim, McLeod, & Shantzis, 1992). Cultural competence goes beyond just being culturally sensitive. **Culturally competent** is defined as the "process for effectively working within the cultural context of an individual or community from a diverse cultural or ethnic background" (Campinha-Bacote, 1994, pp. 1–2). Luquis and Pe'rez (2003) have provided a discussion of some of the issues surrounding cultural competence and some strategies by which planners can become more culturally competent. One strategy is becoming familiar with Standards for Culturally and Linguistically Appropriate Services (CLAS) presented by the Office of Minority Health (OMH, 2001) (see *Weblinks* at the end of this chapter for the website). In addition, if planners are not familiar with the culture of those in the priority population we would recommend that they work with indigenous health workers and/or those who are well trained and are bilingual and bicultural.

Table 10.1 Advantages and disadvantages of using internal and external personnel

	Advantages	Disadvantages
INTERNAL PROGRAM PERSONNEL	1. Reduced costs 2. Internal arrangements can be made to free needed personnel from their work schedules. 3. More control over those involved.	1. Limited by the interest and abilities of those on staff. 2. May have to train personnel or be limited by the expertise of those on staff. 3. Might spend more time developing the program than implementing it, thus reaching fewer people.
EXTERNAL PROGRAM PERSONNEL	1. Known expertise. 2. The responsibility for conducting the program becomes the work of another. 3. Can request product (program) guarantees. 4. Sometimes external personnel are more respected than internal personnel just because they are from the outside. 5. Bring global knowledge to the program because they have worked with a variety of entities and cultures (Harris, 2001). 6. Have the resources for sophisticated tools and programs because they can spread the cost across many clients (Harris, 2001). 7. Can reach a priority population that is geographically dispersed (Harris, 2001).	1. Often more costly than using internal resources. 2. Subject to the limitations of any given vendor. 3. Sometimes less control over the program.

Curricula and Other Instructional Resources

When it comes to selecting the **curriculum** and other instructional materials that will be used to present the content of the program, planners can proceed in four ways: (1) by developing their own materials (in-house) or having someone else develop custom materials for them; (2) by purchasing or obtaining various instructional materials from outside sources; (3) by purchasing or obtaining entire "canned" programs from outside vendors; or (4) by using any combination of in-house materials, materials from outside sources, and canned program materials.

Developing **in-house materials** or having someone else develop custom materials has the major advantage of allowing the developers to create materials that match very closely the needs of the priority population. The more "unique" the priority population is, the more important this approach may be—especially if the priority population possesses cultural differences. Materials must be relevant and culturally appropriate to the priority population (Kline & Huff, 1999). However, a serious drawback is the time, money, and effort necessary to develop an original curriculum and other instructional materials. The exact amount of time necessary would obviously depend on the scope of the program and the expertise of those doing the work. No matter who does the work, however, the commitment of time and resources is sure to be considerable. In putting together an in-house program, planners should be aware of several different sources from which they can obtain free or inexpensive materials to supplement the ones they develop. Planners might also find that there is no need to create in-house materials because of the wide array of materials available. For example, most voluntary and official health agencies have up-to-date pamphlets on a variety of subjects that they are willing and eager to give away in quantity. Also, most communities have a public library with a film/video/CD section that includes some health films, videos, and CDs. If the public library does not carry health films/videos/CDs, almost all local and state health departments offer such a service. Planners who are unsure about what sources of information are available in their community can begin by checking the Yellow Pages of the local telephone directory.

Planners need to remember that just because a piece of instructional material exists it may not be appropriate for the priority population with which they are working. To help insure that the materials are suitable for the priority population, we would recommend the use of SAM: a suitability assessment of materials instrument (Doak, Doak, & Root, 1996) (see Figure 10.2). This validated instrument "was originally designed for use with print material and illustrations, but it has also been applied successfully to video- and audiotaped instructions. For each material, SAM provides a numerical score (in percent) that may fall in one of three categories: superior, adequate, or not suitable" (Doak et al., 1996, p. 49). Here are the steps for using SAM (Doak et al., 1996):

1. Read through the SAM factor list and the evaluation criteria.
2. Read the material (or view the video) you wish to evaluate and write brief statements as to its purpose(s) and key points.
3. For short materials, evaluate the entire piece. For long materials, select samples that are central to the purpose of the document to evaluate.
4. Evaluate and score each of the 22 SAM items, rating them as "superior" and assigning a score of two, "adequate" and assigning a score of one, "not suitable" and assigning a score of zero, or marking an item "N/A" if the factor does not apply to the material.
5. Calculate the total suitability score by summing the scores from the rated items and dividing by the total number of items rated. Do not include the items marked N/A. Multiply the score by 100 to get a percentage.

    70–100%   =   superior material
    40–69%   =   adequate material
    0–39%   =   not suitable material

6. Decide on the impact of deficiencies of the material and what action to take about whether to use or not use the material.

Purchasing or obtaining entire canned programs from vendors has become very popular in recent years because of the time and money needed to create programs. A **canned program** is one that has been developed by an outside group and includes the basic components and materials necessary to implement a program. Because some vendors are for-profit groups whereas others are nonprofit organizations, the cost of these programs can range from literally nothing at all to thousands of dollars.

2 points for superior rating
1 point for adequate rating
0 points for not suitable rating
N/A if the factor does not apply to this material

FACTOR TO BE RATED	SCORE	COMMENTS

1. CONTENT

(a) Purpose is evident
(b) Content about behaviors
(c) Scope is limited
(d) Summary or review included

2. LITERACY DEMAND

(a) Reading grade level
(b) Writing style, active voice
(c) Vocabulary uses common words
(d) Context is given first
(e) Learning aids via "road signs"

3. GRAPHICS

(a) Cover graphic shows purpose
(b) Type of graphics
(c) Relevance of illustration
(d) List, tables, etc. explained
(e) Captions used for graphics

4. LAYOUT AND TYPOGRAPHY

(a) Layout factors
(b) Typography
(c) Subheads ("chunking") used

5. LEARNING STIMULATION, MOTIVATION

(a) Interaction used
(b) Behaviors are modeled and specific
(c) Motivation—self-efficacy

6. CULTURAL APPROPRIATENESS

(a) Match in logic, language,
       experience
(b) Cultural image and examples

Total SAM score:_____

Total possible score: _____ , Percent score: _____%

Figure 10.2 SAM scoring sheet

Source: Doak, C. C., Doak, L. G., and Root, J. H., SAM Scoring Sheet, from Teaching Patient With Low Literacy Skills, 2nd edition, J. B. Lippincott & Company, 1996, p. 51. © 1996 Lippincott Williams & Wilkins. Reprinted by permission.

Most canned programs have five major components:

1. A participant's manual (printed material that is easy to follow and read and is handy for participants)

2. An instructor's manual (a much more comprehensive document than the participant's manual, which includes the program content, background information, and lesson and unit plans with ideas for presenting the material)

3. Audiovisual materials that help present the program content (usually including films/video/CDs and audiotapes, overhead transparencies, PowerPoint© presentations charts, or posters)

4. Training for the instructors (a concentrated experience that prepares individuals to become instructors)

5. Marketing (the "wrapping" that makes the program attractive to both the participants and the planners who will purchase it to market to the participants)

The advantages and disadvantages of these canned programs are just the opposite of those for materials developed in-house. No time is spent on development; however, the program may not fit the needs or the demographics of the priority population. For example, using the same canned smoking cessation program with middle-aged adults who realize the long-term hazards of cigarettes and with teenagers who are required to attend a smoking cessation program for disciplinary reasons may not be advisable. Most adults who enter smoking cessation programs are there because they do not want to smoke. Obviously, this is not the case with teenagers who have been caught smoking. The approaches taken with these two programs would have to be very different if both are to be successful. Another example of when use of a canned program would not be advisable is use of a program that was designed for upper-middle-class suburban adults in a program for low-income inner-city populations. The lifestyles of the two groups are just too different for the same program to be appropriate in both situations. Because of the possible mismatch between the needs and peculiarities (i.e., age, culture, ethnicity, norms, race, sex, socioeconomic status) of a particular priority population, planners are urged to move with caution when deciding on the use of a canned program. Make sure there is a good fit.

Canned programs often come attractively packaged and seemingly complete, but this does not mean that they are well conceived and effective programs. Before adopting canned programs for use, planners should consider the following questions:

1. Is the program based on sound theory and tested models? As noted in an earlier chapter, all programs should be based on sound theory and tested models.

2. Does the program include a long-term behavior modification component? There are no "quick fixes" with regard to many health behavior changes. If behavior modification is used, it should be based on sound health behavior practice over an appropriate time frame.

3. Is the program educational? Not only should the program be based on sound psychological and sociological theory but it should also be based on valid educational theory.

4. Is the program motivational? Health behavior change is not easy to accomplish, and so all programs need to include activities that motivate people to get and stay involved.

5. Is the program enjoyable? Planned programs should be enjoyable. Some people like hard work, but it is difficult to sustain hard work for a long time without some enjoyment.

6. Can the program be modified to meet the specific needs and peculiarities of the priority population? As mentioned earlier, not all populations have the same needs, beliefs, traditions, and ways of approaching a problem.

Space

Another major resource needed for most health promotion programs is sufficient space—a place where the program can be held. Depending on the type of program and the intended audience, space may or may not be readily available. For example, an employer may make space available for a worksite program, or a school system may furnish space for a school program. If space is a problem, planners may locate inexpensive space in local schools, colleges, and universities, and in "community service rooms" (rooms that are available free of charge to community groups as a community service) of local businesses. In addition, planners may find educational institutions and local businesses that are willing to cosponsor programs and thus contribute the space necessary to conduct the program. It may also be possible to obtain space by trading for it. For instance, a planner might trade expertise, such as serving as consultant for a program, in return for the use of suitable space. Or it might be possible to trade one space for another, such as trading the use of classrooms for time in the local YMCA/YWCA pool.

Equipment and Supplies

Some programs may require a great deal of equipment and supplies. For example, first aid and safety programs need items such as CPR mannequins, splints, blankets, bandages, dressings, and video equipment. Other programs, such as a stress management program, may need only paper and pencils. Whatever the kinds and amounts of equipment and supplies required, planners must give advance thought to their needs so as to:

1. Determine the necessary equipment and supplies to facilitate the program.
2. Identify the sources where the equipment and supplies can be obtained.
3. Find a way to pay for the needed equipment and supplies.

Financial Resources

To hire the individuals needed to plan, implement, and evaluate a health promotion program and to pay for the other resources required, planners must obtain appropriate financial support. Most programs are limited by the financial support available. In fact, few programs are financed at such a level that planners would say they have all the money they need. Because of this, the planners are often faced with making decisions about how to allocate the funds that are available. Some typical financial questions that planners generally must address are the following:

1. Is it better to run an adequately financed program for a few people or to run a poorly financed program for more people?
2. If funds are limited where is the first place we should cut?
3. Should we start a program knowing that we will be short of funds, or should we wait until we have appropriate funding before we begin?
4. Is it better to have fewer instructors or to make do with fewer supplies?

Programs can be financed in several different ways. Some sources of financial support are very traditional, whereas others may be limited only by the creativity and imagination of those involved. Following are several established ways of financing programs.

Participant Fee

This method of financing a program requires the participants to pay for the cost of the program. Depending on whether the program is offered on a profit-making basis, this fee may be equal to expenses or may include a **profit margin.** Participant fees not only are a means by which programs can be financed but they also help motivate participants to stay involved in a program. If people pay to participate in a program, then they may be more likely to continue to participate because they have made an investment— that is, a commitment. This concept has also been referred to as *ownership.* Many participants who pay a fee feel like they are part "owners" of the program. However, it should be noted that not everyone shares in the ownership concept. There are some participants who still would prefer a free or almost free program that has been paid for by others. An example of the ownership and cost issue is the participant fees associated with smoking cessation programs. If planners were looking for vendors of smoking cessation programs, they would find that the costs of such programs range from zero (i.e., American Cancer Society's *FreshStart* program) to modest (i.e., American Lung Association's *Freedom from Smoking* program) to expensive (i.e., those offered by private health promotion companies).

Deciding to finance a program through a participant fee may sound easy, but planners need to give serious thought to how much they will charge and who will be charged. Often, those most in need of a health promotion program are the least able to pay. Planners do not want to create a barrier to program participation by charging a fee or a setting the fee too high. If a fee is necessary, then planners should consider creating a fee structure on "ability to pay." One form of this is a **sliding-scale fee**— that is, the less one's income, the lower the participant fee. Or, planners may want to consider offering "scholarships" to those unable to pay.

Third-Party Support

Most individuals are familiar with insurance companies acting as third-party payers to cover the costs of health care. Although health insurance companies do not often pay for health promotion programs, others can be third-party payers. Third-party means that someone other than participants (the first-party) or planners (the second-party) is paying for the program. Third-party payers that may cover the cost of health promotion programs are:

1. Employers that pick up the cost for employees, as is often the case in worksite health promotion programs

2. Agencies other than the groups sponsoring the program—for example, when local service or civic groups "adopt" a pet program

3. A professional association or union that financially supports a program

The money used by third-party payers can be generated from a special fund-raising event, from sale of concessions, or with money saved from reduced health care costs, absenteeism, or the remodeling of employee benefit plans.

Cost Sharing

A third means of financing a program is a combination of participant fee and third-party support. It is not unusual to have an employer pay 50% to 80% of a program's costs and let the employee pay the remaining 50% to 20%. Such an arrangement has the advantages of both ownership and a fringe benefit.

Organizational Sponsorship

Many times, the sponsoring organization (health department, hospital, or voluntary agency) bears the cost of the program as a part of its programming or operating budget. For example, the American Cancer Society offers its smoking cessation program free of charge. The program is paid for with the society's community service funds.

Grants and Gifts

Another means of financing health promotion programs is through gifts and grants from other agencies, foundations, groups, and individuals. This source of money is often referred to as **grant money,** external money, or **soft money.** The term *soft money* refers to the fact that grants and gifts are usually given for a specific period of time and at some point will be taken away. This is in contrast to **hard money,** which is an ongoing source of funds that is part of the operating budget of an organization from year to year.

Grant money is becoming more important to planners because of limited resources dedicated to health promotion programming. It thus becomes necessary for planners to develop adequate **grantsmanship** skills. These skills include (1) discovering where the grant money is located, (2) finding out how to get (apply for) the money, and (3) writing a proposal requesting the money.

Locating Grant Money   There are four basic types of grant makers: foundations, corporations, voluntary agencies, and government. These grant makers are found at three different levels: local, state, and national. They are not the only grant makers, however. Planners may also find a variety of local organizations (such as service groups like the Lion's Club or the Jaycees, or a community group like the United Way) that may be willing to support specific local causes through a grant. Philanthropic foundations are not-for-profit organizations that award grants to serve the public interest. There are a number of large national foundations who support health

---

Box 10.1 The Components of a Grant Proposal

1. **Title (or cover) page.** When writing the title, be concise and explicit; avoid words that add nothing.
2. **Abstract or executive summary.** Provides a summary of the proposed project. May be the most important part of the proposal. Should be written last and be about 200 words long.
3. **Table of contents.** May or may not be needed, depending on the length of the proposal. It is a convenience for the reader.
4. **Introduction.** Should begin with a capsule statement, be comprehensible to the informed layperson, and include the statement of the problem, significance of the program, and purpose of the program.
5. **Background.** Should include the proposer's previous related work and the related literature.
6. **Description of proposed program.** Should include the objectives, description of intervention, evaluation plan, and time frame.
7. **Description of relevant institutional/agency resources.** Should identify the resources the proposer's organization will bring to the project.
8. **List of references.** Should include references cited in the proposal.
9. **Personnel section.** Should include the résumés of those who are to work with the program.
10. **Budget.** Should include budget needs for personnel (salaries and wages), equipment, materials and supplies, travel, services, other needed items, and indirect costs.

---

promotion (e.g., Robert Wood Johnson Foundation, Rockefeller Foundation, W. K. Kellogg Foundation), but planners may also find state and local foundations too.

Not all corporations have giving programs, but many do as a part of a community service or public relations program. Planners will need to contact the corporations to "ask who is in charge of charitable giving, what subjects they consider for grants, and how the company giving program operates" (Guyer, 1999, p. 1). Library or Internet searching will possibly help answer these questions.

Voluntary health agencies also have grant programs. Though most grants from voluntary organizations at the national level are specified for research efforts, planners may find the local or state offices of these organizations are willing to provide **seed dollars** (start-up dollars) or **in-kind support** (such as providing free materials or other resources) for local programs.

Government is the largest grant maker. Government, at all three levels—local, state, and federal—make grants for many purposes. With the other three grant makers (foundations, corporations, and voluntary agencies), planners can ask them to fund any project. However, with the government, only grants that are in one of the subjects specified by the government have a chance of being funded (Guyer, 1999).

When looking for grant makers, planners need to look for a pattern in giving by asking key questions: Has this funder made grants in the past for subject areas like mine? In my geographic area? In the amount I need? For the things I need funded?

Income	Amount
Contribution from sponsors	_____
Gifts	_____
Grants	_____
Participant fee	_____
Sale of curriculum material	_____
	Total income _____

Expenses	
Curriculum materials	_____
Equipment	_____
Marketing	_____
Print advertising	_____
Other media	_____
Personnel	_____
For planning	_____
Program facilitators	_____
Clerical	_____
Evaluator(s)	_____
Participants	_____
Postage	_____
Space	_____
Supplies	_____
Travel	_____
	Total expenses _____
	Balance _____

Figure 10.3 Sample budget sheet

(Guyer, 1999). The answers to these questions, often found at Internet websites of the grant makers, will indicate whether it is a good idea to contact the funder. After doing the initial "research," planners should call or write funding sources to ask questions and to obtain any guidelines, grant request forms or applications, and printed material about their grant making. This contact will also help establish a relationship with the funder. Planners not only can obtain needed information but they can also introduce their organization to the funder. This can be done by sending publications about the planners' organization, making personal contacts, and staying in touch (Guyer, 1999).

Planners can identify possible funding sources in a couple of different ways. The first is by networking with others who have been successful in obtaining grant funding in the past. Since seeking grant funding is a competitive process, planners may have to network with others who are not seeking funding from the same grant maker. A second means of identifying funding sources is through library "research." A variety of books on grants may be found in college and university libraries as well as many larger public libraries. For example, there are directories of grant makers for foundations and corporations, and there is usually a directory that lists grant funders that are specific to a state. Most of these books are indexed by subject area.

In looking for a government grant, examine the *Catalog of Federal Domestic Assistance,* which lists the federal grant programs. For each program the *Catalog* shows who is eligible, what the program is about, and an information contact to whom to write for application information. The *Federal Register,* a daily publication, lists the newest grant opportunities. For state and local government grants, there is no one book to use that is comprehensive. You need to call elected officials or appropriate government departments to inquire about what is available. Be persistent in calling around until you find the person who is in charge of grant making. (Guyer, 1999, p. 2)

A third way of identifying funding sources is through the Internet. There are several advantages to using the Internet for seeking grant makers: convenience, time saving, and being able to reach several grant makers at the same time. Planners do not have to leave their office to conduct a search, thus much "leg work" of finding out if a grant maker is a "good fit" with the planner's organization can be found almost instantaneously. In addition, some websites permit an applicant to complete one form for grant consideration at several different funders (Breen, 1999).

The fourth way of identifying grant makers, is the least difficult. Planners should be alert for **requests for proposals,** known as **RFPs.** Many times some funding agency would like to have a project conducted for it, so the group will issue an RFP. If you feel qualified to do the work, you can submit a proposal.

Submitting Grant Proposals   As noted in the previous section, most funding agencies have specific guidelines outlining who is qualified to submit a proposal (perhaps only nonprofit groups can apply, or only practitioners who hold certain certifications) and the format for making an application. Those seeking money can request or apply for the money by writing a proposal. A **proposal** can be thought of as a written document that represents a request for money. A good proposal is one that is well written and explains how the needs of the funding agency can be met by the group wishing to receive the money. To increase their chances of writing a good proposal, planners should call the funding agency first and speak with the grant officer to find out specifically what he or she is looking for and the format desired.

Because there is a great deal of competition for grant money, it is more than likely that proposals will be read by a busy, impatient, skeptical person who has no reason to give any one proposal special consideration and who is faced with many more requests than he or she can grant, or even read thoroughly. Such a reader wants to find out quickly and easily the answers to these questions:

1. What do you want to do, how much will it cost, and how much time will it take?
2. How does the proposed project relate to the sponsor's interests?
3. What will be gained if this project is carried out?
4. What has already been done in the area of the project?
5. How do you plan to do it?
6. How will the results be evaluated?
7. Why should you, rather than someone else, conduct this project?

As noted, funding agencies request proposals in a variety of different forms. However, there are several components that are contained in most proposals no matter what the funding agency. Box 10.1 presents these components.

A Combination of Sources

It should be obvious that planners should not be limited to any single source for financing a health promotion program. In fact, it is more than likely that most programs will be funded via a variety of sources—that is, any combination of the sources listed previously.

Preparing a Budget

Simply put, a budget is a plan that is presented in financial terms using quantitative units such as dollars, pounds, hours, and work force hours (Shim & Siegel, 1994). A budget represents the decision makers' intentions and expectations by allocating funds to achieve desired outcomes (program goals and objectives) (Finkler, 1992; Shim & Siegel, 1994). In financial terms, the budget compares the expected income to the expected expenses in order to estimate the financial results of the program (Finkler, 1992).

A budget can be prepared for any length of time. When programs are planned, budgets are usually created for the entire length of the program. However, when a program is projected to last longer than a year, the overall program budget is typically broken down into 12-month periods.

The purpose of a program has a lot to say about the type of budget created. From a financial standpoint, programs can make money (a profit), lose money, or break even. If a program must make money, the income will have to be greater than the expenses, and the intended profit (profit margin) will need to be included in the budgeting process. No matter what the desired bottom line is in a budget, the budget should be put together in sufficient detail that all income and expenses are accounted for. Figure 10.3 presents a sample budget sheet that lists some line items that are typically included in a health promotion program budget.

SUMMARY

This chapter identified and discussed the most often used resources for health promotion programs: personnel, curriculum and other instructional materials, space, equipment and supplies, and funding. In addition, typical questions were covered regarding how to secure and allocate resources and how to obtain funding.

REVIEW QUESTIONS

1. What are the major categories of resources that planners need to consider when planning a health promotion program?
2. What are the advantages and disadvantages of using internal resources? External resources?
3. Define the terms *ownership, flex time, vendor,* and *canned programs.*
4. What are some key questions that planners should ask vendors when they try to sell their product?
5. How might program planners obtain free or inexpensive space for a program?
6. What is the SAM? What is it used for?
7. List and explain the different means by which health promotion programs can be funded.
8. What is meant by the term *profit margin?*

ACTIVITIES

1. Identify and describe the resources you anticipate needing to carry out a program you are planning. Be sure to answer the following questions that apply to your program:
   a. What personnel will be needed to carry out the program? List the individuals and the duties to be carried out.
   b. What curriculum or educational materials will you use in your program? Why did you select it or them?
   c. What kind of space allocation will your program require? How will you obtain the space? How much will it cost?
   d. What equipment and supplies do you anticipate using? How will you obtain them?
   e. How do you anticipate paying for the program? Why did you select this method?

2. Visit the local office of a voluntary agency and find out what type of resources it makes available to individuals planning health promotion programs. Ask for a sample of the materials. Also, ask if the agency offers any canned programs. If it does, find out as much as you can about the programs and ask for any available descriptive literature.

3. Collect information on a single type of canned health promotion program (for example, smoking cessation or stress management) from vendors. Then compare the strengths and weaknesses of the programs.

4. Through the process of networking and using the local telephone book, find where in your community there is free or inexpensive space available for health promotion programs.

5. Call three different voluntary agencies and one hospital in your community and find out if they have a speaker's bureau. If they do, find out how to use the bureaus and what topics the speakers can address.

6. Prepare a mock grant proposal for a program you are planning. Make sure it includes all the components noted in Box 10.1.

7. Outline the major sources of income and expenses that would be associated with the program you are planning by preparing a budget sheet.

WEBLINKS

Note to readers: Because this chapter focuses on the resources necessary to conduct a program additional *Weblinks* are provided.

1. **http://www.cancer.org/**
   American Cancer Society (ACS)

   This is the home page for ACS. The site presents the most up to date information on cancer including treatment and prevention. The site also provides information about the ACS and the resources it can provide for cancer survivors and program planners.

2. **http://www.americanheart.org**
   American Heart Association (AHA)

   This is the home page for the AHA. It provides planners with a wealth of information and materials about many of the cardiovascular diseases and stroke.

3. **http://www.lungusa.org**
   American Lung Association (ALA)

   This is the home page for the ALA. It provides a variety of information about various lung diseases including asthma, chronic obstructive pulmonary disease (COPD), and lung cancer.

4. **http://www.plannedparenthood.org**
   Planned Parenthood Federation of America, Inc.

   This is the home page for the Planned Parenthood. It is the world's largest voluntary reproductive health care organization. Planners working on programs aimed at reproductive health should find it useful.

5. **http://www.welcoa.org**
   The Wellness Councils of America (WELCOA)

   This is the home page for the WELCOA. This site provides a variety of resources for those interested in worksite wellness programs.

6. **http://www.aarp.org**
   AARP

   This is the home page of the AARP. AARP is a nonprofit membership organization dedicated to addressing the needs and interests of persons 50 and older. This site has a lot of information that would be applicable to those planning programs for seniors. This site also has a special section on health and wellness.

7. **http://www.nationaldairycouncil.org**
   National Dairy Council (NDC)

   This is the home page for the NDC. The site provides a wealth of information about nutrition and weight management.

8. **http://www.nih.gov/**
   National Institutes of Health (NIH)

   This is the home page of the NIH. It not only includes information about NIH and links to all the institutes, centers, and offices, but it also includes health information, grant opportunities, and scientific resources.

9. **http://www.cdc.gov/**
   Centers for Disease Control and Prevention (CDC)

   This is the home page of the CDC. It includes information for the lay public (i.e., traveler's health, and emergency preparedness) as well as information to assist health promotion planners (i.e., health topics A-Z, CDC recommendations, MMWR, and special funded initiatives).

10. **http://www.healthfinder.gov/**
    healthfinder®

    This is the home page of healthfinder®. Of all the *Weblinks* provided in this chapter, this one includes information on the greatest variety of health topics. It includes information on prevention, wellness, diseases, health care, and alternative medicine. It also includes medical dictionaries, an encyclopedia, journals, and more.

11. **http://cdcnpin.org/scripts/index.asp**
    CDC National Prevention Information Network (NPIN)

    This is the home page for the NPIN. This site houses the nation's largest collection of information and resources on HIV/AIDS, STD, and TB prevention.

12. **http://www.cfda.gov/public/cat-howtouse.htm**
    The Catalog of Federal Domestic Assistance (CFDA)

    This is the web page for the CFDA that provides information on Federal grants. The site deals with all types of assistance, not just financial aid. The site uses "Assistance Program" as a generic term rather than speaking specifically about grant, loan, or another sort of program.

13. **http://www.grants.gov**
    Grants.gov

    This site allows planners to electronically find and apply for competitive grant opportunities from all Federal grant-making agencies. The site provides all the information planners need to apply for a grant and walks them through the process, step by step.

14. **http://www.gpoaccess.gov/fr/index.html**
    Federal Register (FR)

    This is the main page of the FR. Published by the Office of the Federal Register, National Archives and Records Administration (NARA), the FR is the official daily publication for rules, proposed rules, and notices of Federal agencies and organizations, as well as executive orders and other presidential documents.

15. **http://www.omhrc.gov/clas/ds.htm**
    Office of Minority Health (OMH)

    This is a web page of the OMH where the National Standards on Culturally and Linguistically Appropriate Services (CLAS) in Health Care Final Report can be found. The CLAS was completed in March 2001. The final report describes 14 individual standards and outlines the development, methodology, and analysis undertaken to create the national standards.

16. **http://www.omhrc.gov/cultural/index.htm**
    Office of Minority Health (OMH)

    This is a web page of the OMH that presents information on cultural competence. The OMH was mandated by the U.S. Congress in 1994, via P.L. 101-527, to develop the capacity of health care professionals to address the cultural and linguistic barriers to health care delivery and increase access to health care for limited English-proficient people. This site provides many different resources including, but not limited to, standards, materials, and links to other websites to assist health professionals to become more culturally competent.

CHAPTER 11

Marketing
Making Sure Programs Respond to the Wants and Needs of Consumers

---

Chapter Objectives

After reading this chapter and answering the questions at the end, you should be able to:

- Define *market, marketing,* and *social marketing.*
- Explain the diffusion theory.
- Explain how the diffusion theory can be used in marketing a health promotion program.
- Identify the functions involved in the marketing process as outlined by Syre and Wilson (1990).
- Explain the relationship between a needs assessment and a marketing program.
- Explain the four Ps of marketing.
- Define *marketing mix.*
- Name techniques for motivating program participants to continue in a program.

Key Terms

audience segmentation	intangible	price
contingencies	internal advertising	product
diffusion theory	laggards	promotion
early adopters	late majority	segmentation
early majority	market	social marketing
external advertising	marketing	social support
incentives	marketing mix	tangible
innovators	place	

In Chapter 2, you read about social marketing, the SMART model and other marketing concepts. While social marketing attempts to change behavior for improved health or social outcomes, commercial marketing is concerned with financial profit. Regardless of the intended outcome, the key to success in either social marketing or commercial marketing is a continual focus on the wants and needs of consumers in a predetermined priority population.

However, often in health promotion programs canned programs are purchased or borrowed because they were previously successful in other locations. Many times programs are developed from top to bottom by planners themselves, and while any of these approaches may be acceptable it is not appropriate to call them "marketing" since they are based primarily on the preferences of planners rather than consumers. In these instances the process of promoting, spreading the word or gaining community support is better termed "advertising." On the other hand marketing as it is used in this chapter is synonymous with consumer-orientation.

After investing so much time and energy in identifying consumer preferences, planners hope the priority population will participate in the program until the desired outcomes are achieved. But this takes expertise in not only marketing, but social psychology and population dynamics as well. These skills often distinguish successful programs from mediocre or failed programs.

Market and Marketing

For the purposes of program planning, the people in the priority population make up the market. Kotler and Clarke (1987, p. 108) define **market** as "the set of all people who have an actual or potential interest in a product or service." A key to getting and keeping these people involved in a health promotion program is to be able to market the program effectively. The process of **marketing** operates on the underlying concept of the exchange theory.

> Marketing is the planned attempt to influence the characteristics of voluntary exchange transactions—exchanges of costs and benefits by buyers and sellers or providers and consumers. Marketing is considerably different from selling in that selling concentrates on the needs of the producer (to sell more products), whereas marketing, which may have the same ultimate objective, concentrates necessarily on the needs of the buyer or the public. (Pickett & Hanlon, 1990, p. 231)

"Strip away all the fancy language, and marketing comes down to offering benefits that an identified group of potential customers will pay a price for and be satisfied with" (Novelli, 1988, p. 7).

Applying the definition of marketing to health promotion suggests that planners would like to exchange costs and benefits with those in the priority population. That is to say, planners would like to exchange the benefits of participation in health promotion programs (the objectives or outcomes of the programs they planned), such as "a longer healthier life, looking and feeling better, and having fewer but healthier children" (Novelli, 1988, p. 6) for the costs of the program, which come from the participants. The cost to the participant may be financial, but often with health promotion programs, the costs are something other than financial. Consumers may pay a price in terms of the time and energy they spend acquiring new information or in developing a new personal habit. Another price may be pain or discomfort related to behavior change, or missing out on favorite activities such as hobbies or watching television (Weinreich, 1999).

For this exchange to take place, planners must have an understanding of marketing principles. Unfortunately, many health promotion planners have had to learn the hard way—by planning a program and then not have anyone sign up to participate. The principles of marketing are not difficult to learn, but their application can be challenging. Applying marketing principles to health promotion programs is not as easy as

---

Box 11.1 Marketing a Tangible versus an Intangible

Concern	Tangible	Intangible
Success	Increase sales 3–5%	Great enough to be cost effective
Changes	One-time sales	Lasting a lifetime
Priority population	Most likely to respond	Least likely to respond

---

applying them to the latest model of a car or a new line of clothing. Health promotion programs are social programs; as such, they do not have material objects to market, but instead must market awareness, knowledge, skills, and behavior. As discussed previously, this is social marketing.

Thus in social marketing, the exchange may come down to exchanging an intangible for another intangible, such as the effort to accept a new idea and discard an old custom, or adopt a new behavior and give up a habit (Lefebvre, 1992). Box 11.1 compares the marketing of a **tangible** (product) and an **intangible** (a program that will improve the quality of life).

Marketing and the Diffusion Theory

One approach that is useful in understanding the importance of marketing principles is **diffusion theory** (Rogers, 1962). The theory provides an explanation for the diffusion of innovations (something new) in populations; stated another way, it provides an explanation for the pattern of adoption of the innovations. If one thinks of a health promotion program as an innovation, the theory describes a pattern the priority population will follow in adopting the program. The pattern of adoption can be represented by the normal bell-shaped curve (Rogers, 2003) (see Figure 11.1). Therefore those individuals who fall in the portion of the curve to the left of minus 2 standard deviations from the mean (this would be between 2% and 3% of the priority population) would probably become involved in the program just because they had heard about it and wanted to be first. These people are called **innovators.** They are venturesome, independent, risky, and daring. They want to be the first to do things, though they may not be respected by others in the social system.

The second group of people to adopt something new are those represented on the curve between minus 2 and minus 1 standard deviations. This group which composes about 14% of the priority population, is called **early adopters.** These people are very interested in the innovation, but they are not the first to sign up. They wait until the innovators are already involved to make sure the innovation is useful. Early adopters are respected by others in the social system and looked upon as opinion leaders.

The next two groups are the **early majority** and the **late majority.** They fall between minus 1 standard deviation and the mean and between the mean and plus 1 standard deviation on the curve, respectively. Each of these groups comprises about 34% of the priority population. Those in the early majority may be interested in the health promotion program, but they will need external motivation to become

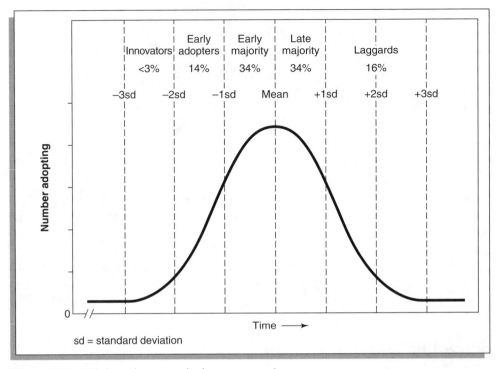

Figure 11.1 Bell-shaped curve and adopter categories

involved. Those in the early majority will deliberate for some time before making a decision. It will take more work to get the late majority involved, because they are skeptical and will not adopt an innovation until most people in the social system have done so. Planners may be able to get them involved through a peer or mentoring program, or through constant exposure about the innovation.

The last group, the **laggards** (16%), are represented by the part of the curve greater than plus 1 standard deviation. They are not very interested in innovation and would be the last to become involved in new health promotion programs, if at all. Some would say that this group will not become involved in health promotion programs at all. They are very traditional and are suspicious of innovations. Laggards tend to have limited communication networks, so they really do not know much about new things.

Figure 11.2 presents an *s*-shaped curve showing the cumulative prevalence of adopters at successive points in time. At first, only a few people adopt (innovators). However, over time, the curve begins to climb as additional individuals decide to adopt the innovation (early adopters, early majority, and late majority). The curve then levels off as adoption of the innovation ceases, leaving a few who have not adopted (laggards) (Goldman, 1998; Rogers, 2003).

The real advantage of using the diffusion theory when trying to market a health promotion program is that "the distinguishing characteristics of the people who fall

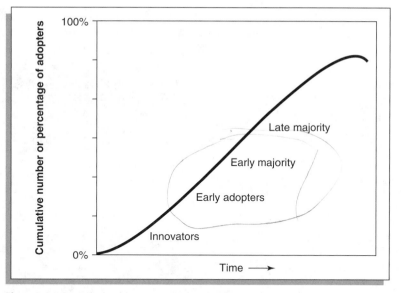

Figure 11.2 *S*-shaped curve and cumulative adoption

into each category of adopters from 'innovators' to 'early adopters' to middle majority categories to 'late adopters' [laggards] tend to be consistent across a wide range of innovations" (Green, 1989). Therefore different marketing techniques can be used depending on the type of people the planners are trying to attract to a program. For example, program planners want rapid diffusion of innovations. They know that although **innovators** will adopt the program or product first, the key subgroups of the priority population are the **early adopters** and **early majority.** It is especially important to identify the early adopters (opinion leaders) as soon as possible in the implementation process since, according to diffusion theory, the sooner they adopt the innovation the sooner the rest of the population will follow. The challenge is how to identify and reach the early adopters. Box 11.2 lists some generalizations drawn from the work of various researchers on innovations and reported in Rogers (2003).

The application of the diffusion theory to health promotion programs is quite common now. To learn more about the concept and its application to health promotion programs review some of the following references to see how they have applied the concept in a variety of health promotion and health education settings (Backer & Rogers, 1998; Berwick, 2003; Borras, Fernandez, Schiaffino, Borrell, & La Vecchia, 2000; Ferrence, 1996; Goldman, 1998; Hallfors & Godette, 2002; Rogers, 2002; Ruof, Mittendorf, Pirk, & von der Schulenberg, 2002; Svenkerud & Singhal, 1998; Taylor, Elliott & Riley, 1998).

One of the more interesting uses of the diffusion theory has been its use to "conceptualize the transference of health promotion programs from one locale to another" (Steckler et al., 1992). Steckler and colleagues (1992) developed a series of six questionnaires to measure the extent to which health promotion programs are successfully

Box 11.2 Generalizations about Selected Variables and Innovation

Socioeconomic Characteristics

1. Earlier adopters have more years of education than later adopters.
2. Earlier adopters are more likely to be literate than are later adopters.
3. Earlier adopters have higher social status than do later adopters.
4. Earlier adopters have a greater degree of upward social mobility than do later adopters.
5. Earlier adopters are more likely to have a commercial (rather than a subsistence) economic orientation compared with later adopters.

Personality Variables

1. Earlier adopters have a greater ability to deal with abstractions than do later adopters.
2. Earlier adopters have a more favorable attitude toward change than later adopters have.
3. Earlier adopters are more able to cope with uncertainty and risk than are later adopters.
4. Earlier adopters have a more favorable attitude toward education than do later adopters.
5. Earlier adopters have a more favorable attitude toward science than do later adopters.
6. Earlier adopters have higher levels of achievement motivation than do later adopters.
7. Earlier adopters have higher aspirations (for education, occupations, and so on) than later adopters have.

Communication Behavior

1. Earlier adopters have more social participation than do later adopters.
2. Earlier adopters are more highly interconnected in the social system than are later adopters.
3. Earlier adopters are more cosmopolitan than later adopters.
4. Earlier adopters have more change agent contact than do later adopters.
5. Earlier adopters have greater exposure to mass media communication channels than do later adopters.
6. Earlier adopters have greater exposure to interpersonal communication channels than do later adopters.
7. Earlier adopters have a higher degree of opinion leadership than later adopters.
8. Earlier adopters are more likely to belong to highly interconnected systems than are later adopters.

disseminated. Planners should refer to this work if they are interested in using and measuring diffusion.

The Marketing Process and Health Promotion Programs

If everyone in a given population were an innovator or early adopter, there would be no need for marketing or advertising plans. Since that is not the case, there is a need for planners to understand the marketing process and be able to apply its principles.

Syre and Wilson (1990) have identified five distinct functions of the marketing process as they relate to the health care field:

1. Using marketing research to determine the needs and desires of the present and prospective clients from the priority population.

2. Developing a product that satisfies the needs and desires of the clients.

3. Developing informative and persuasive communication flows between those offering the program and the clients.

4. Ensuring that the product is provided in the appropriate form, at the right time and place, and at the best price.

5. Keeping the clients satisfied and loyal after the exchange has taken place.

Next, each of these functions will be discussed.

Using Marketing Research to Determine Needs and Desires

This particular function involves conducting formative research as discussed in Chapter 2. Since the needs assessment process was discussed in detail in Chapter 4, that discussion will not be repeated here. However, the focus of formative research as performed in social marketing is a bit different than that of a traditional needs assessment for a program. The types of data planners try to uncover in formative research are, as described in the SMART Model, related to consumer analysis (wants, needs and preferences of the priority population), market analysis (defining the market mix, described later in this chapter, and identifying competing behaviors, messages and programs) and channel analyses (communication and promotion strategies). Some formative research can be conducted as part of a regular needs assessment, such as collecting information that would help segment the market (see the next section for a discussion of market segmentation) or finding out how best to position a program for a specific audience. Still other components, such as pretesting and pilot tests are also considered formative research techniques.

If planners want to conduct formative research as part of primary data collection for a program needs assessment, they may want to consider questions such as:

1. What type of health promotion programs would the priority population participate in if they were offered in the community?

2. Where would the priority population like the program offered?

3. On what days of the week would the priority population like the program offered?

4. At what time of the day would the priority population like the program offered?

5. Would the priority population prefer individual attention or small group participation?

6. How much would the priority population be willing to pay to attend the program?

7. What is the best way to communicate information to the priority population about the program?

8. Does the priority population think other members of their family would like to attend these programs? If yes, which members?

Developing a Product That Satisfies the Needs and Desires of Clients

The steps involved in developing a high-quality, marketable product (health promotion program) were discussed in earlier chapters. One key to developing a marketable product is knowing as much as possible about the priority population (i.e., conducting formative research). The more they know about a population, the better planners can describe the population. By describing the population, planners are then able to divide the population based on certain characteristics, a process called **segmentation.** Figure 11.3 shows the concept of **audience segmentation,** identifying African-American teenagers for a dietary excess intervention. This figure illustrates that the

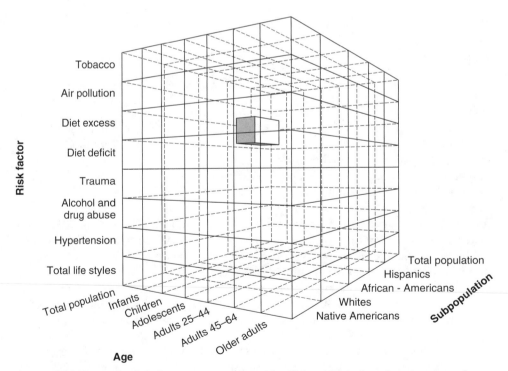

Figure 11.3 Example of audience segmentation, identifying African-American teenagers for a dietary intervention

Source: U.S. Dept. of Health and Human Services (1986a), p. 41.

priority population, African-American teenagers, is a unique but potentially small segment when considering the total population and all of its health problems. Yet, segmenting a priority population is critical in order to deliver programs to individuals who need them most. Audience segmentation has two major goals: (1) define homogeneous or similar subgroups for message and product design purposes, and (2) identify segments within the subgroup that will be the target for distribution and communication channel strategies (Lefebvre & Flora, 1988). Segmentation permits planners to develop programs that will meet the specific needs and desires of the priority population, thus greatly increasing the chances for an exchange between the two parties. For example, there are certain employee segments that are more likely than others to read health newsletters distributed by their company (Davis, 1990; Golaszewski et al., 1989; Miller & Golaszewski, 1992). Segmentation is especially useful when trying to reach "high-risk" and "hard-to-reach" groups.

Planners can carry out the segmentation of groups of people before surveying them (a priori) by examining demographic variables—such as age, gender, income, marital status, occupation, religion, ethnicity, and socioeconomic status—or on the basis of a relevant model or theory. Or planners can conduct segmentation after surveying (a posteriori) the priority population and collecting data, such as psychographics (attitudes, values, and lifestyle), risk factors, health history, or personal health behaviors. For example, the National Cancer Institute (NCI) used attitudes and lifestyle to identify different segments of the priority population for communications about cancer. They found that one group, which they called the naive optimists, were generally optimistic, self-involved, and complacent about their health. They did not make any effort to stay healthy or seek health information and did not worry about their health. This group of people was young with high incomes and made up about 12% of the population (Freimuth & Mettger, 1990). Segmentation could thus be most helpful in developing a market plan for this group of people.

Kotler and Clarke (1987, p. 236) indicate that "there is no one, or right, way to segment a market." Demographic segmentation has been the most common means of segmentation in commercial marketing (Hertoz et al., 1993). However, it may not be the most efficient for social marketing. Planners will need to experiment with several variables to determine what works best for them. Box 11.3 includes many of the major segmenting variables identified by several different authors (Hertoz et al., 1993; Kotler & Clarke, 1987; Romer & Kim, 1995; Williams & Flora, 1995).

It should also be noted that segmentation need not be limited to just individuals. In situations when planners are trying to influence the priority population at the organizational/institutional, community, or public policy levels, the segmentation process can be categorized by social systems.

> Social systems are easily divided into sector "segments"—educational, industry, government, health, etc. These sectors can be further segmented by location (e.g., urban vs. rural health departments), membership size of composite units (e.g., larger school districts vs. smaller ones), type of business (e.g., service industries vs. manufacturing vs. agricultural), current practices (e.g., businesses with active health promotion programmes [sic] for employees), organizational factors (e.g., innovativeness, leadership style, employee participation, community involvement), characteristics associated with organizational innovativeness (e.g., centralization, complexity, formalization, interconnectedness, organizational slack, size: Rogers, 1983), and many other variables. (Lefebvre, 1992, p. 159)

Box 11.3 Segmentation Categories and Variables

1. Geographic segmentation
   a. Nations
   b. States
   c. Regions
   d. Service areas
   e. Counties
   f. Cities, towns, villages
   g. Neighborhoods
2. Demographic segmentation
   a. Age
   b. Stage of life cycle
   c. Disease or diagnostic category
      - Health history
      - Risk factors
   d. Gender
   e. Health insurance
   f. Income
   g. Education
   h. Religion
   i. Race/ethnicity
3. Psychographic segmentation
   a. Social class
      - Upper upper (less than 1% of population)
      - Lower upper (2%)
      - Upper middle (12%)
      - Lower middle (30%)
      - Upper lower (35%)
      - Lower lower (20%)
   b. Lifestyle
   c. Attitudes
   d. Values
   e. Personality
      - Self-image
      - Self-concept
4. Behavioral segmentation
   a. Purchase occasion
   b. Benefits sought

(Box 9.3 *continues*)

(Box 9.3 *continued*)

      c. User status
      d. Usage rate
      e. Loyalty status
      f. Stages of buyer readiness
      g. Health behavior
  5. Multivariable segmentation (i.e., males age 42 living in Indiana)
  6. Constructs of behavior theories

Developing Informative and Persuasive Communication Flows

The third function of marketing is developing informative and persuasive communication flows; that is, what avenues will planners use to get the "message" out about their product, and how can they frame the "message" in such a way that will make the product (the health promotion program) appealing to the priority population? This requires planners to identify appropriate channels to communicate messages and promote their programs. As described earlier, channels may include interpersonal, small group, organizational, community, and mass media outlets. But to select the right channel or combination of channels, planners must understand the tendencies and preferences of the priority population as identified in formative research. In order to frame the message appropriately, planners must know what may be motivating the priority population.

For example, after performing formative research related to diet and physical activity among a group of public employees, planners learned that preferences for message content included, "helping employees understand that the desired changes could be inexpensive, fun and easy, and that changes would require only a minimal amount of time." Based on these preferences, messages through electronic mail, public announcements, posters, and direct supervisor contacts (all preferred channels), were successfully used to recruit a large group of participants in a successful intervention (Neiger et al., 2001). Several authors (Kline & Huff, 1999; Lefebvre & Flora, 1988, Rice & Atkin, 1989) have made suggestions on items that planners should consider when developing the communication message and flow:

1. What are the media habits of the priority population?

2. What medium (electronic or print, visual or auditory, combination of several) should be used?

3. What are the costs of each medium versus the benefits?

4. Can the medium's capability build on or multiply the effects of another medium?

5. Will the message reach a significant portion of the priority population?

6. Can the message be sent through several different channels?

7. Is the message culturally appropriate?

8. Through how many intermediaries must the message travel to reach the priority population?

9. How frequently should the message be delivered?

10. Can a medium be overused to the point that it will "turn off" the priority population to the message?

Ensuring That the Product Is Provided in an Appropriate Manner

The fourth marketing function outlined by Syre and Wilson (1990) can best be explained by marketing's traditional four Ps: product, price, place, and promotion. The particular blend of these four marketing variables that planners use to achieve their objective(s) is referred to as the **marketing mix.**

Product   **Product** refers to the actual program you are planning. Hence, the program is your product. A goal for all planners is to develop the best product possible with the resources available. In Chapter 8, it was indicated that a health promotion program can be comprised of a variety of intervention strategies and thus take many different forms. Lefebvre (1992) developed a three-tiered classification system for health promotion products. The first is *messages,* or the *communication of information.* These are the most common products since "the dissemination of 'information products' comprises the major thrust of public information, or health communication, campaigns. The creation of messages that are both scientifically sound in content and possess the creative ability to capture attention and reliably communicate the content to the desired audience are necessary features of social marketing programmes [sic]" (p. 163).

The second category of health promotion products is *tangible products.* "These products might range from condoms in family planning projects to school curricula for AIDS education to self-help materials for smoking cessation in various formats (print, electronic video)" (Lefebvre, 1992, p. 164). The third type of health promotion product is *service delivery,* which can include screening, counseling, education programs, self-help and support groups, telephone hotlines, health care, and social welfare assistance to name a few.

As noted in Chapters 2 and 8, the CDCynergy planning model uses a similar classification as Lefebvre (1992) for describing a product. However, in CDCynergy the categories are labeled *health communication/education, health-related community services, health engineering,* and *health policy/enforcement.*

Price   "Prices can be thought of in a variety of ways; in addition to economic reasons, there are social, behavioral, psychological, temporal, structural, geographic, and physical reasons for exchanging or not exchanging" (Lefebvre & Flora, 1988, p. 307). In other words, price is the sum of costs the consumer must accept to engage in the exchange process (Neiger, 1998). From an economic standpoint, **price** refers to charging the appropriate amount for the product (program) being provided. As was mentioned in Chapter 10, there are many ways to finance a program. If you are "selling" participation in the program, then the price must match the participants' ability and willingness to pay. When considering the amount to be charged for a product (program), planners should determine:

1. Who are the clients?

2. What is their ability to pay?

3. Are copayers involved?

4. Is the program covered under an insurance program?

5. What is the mission of the planner's agency?

6. What are competitors charging?

7. What is the demand for the program?

The price of a program and who pays for it help determine how a program should be marketed. Whether the program is intended to make a profit will have a great impact on the price. Does the program have to make money? Break even? Or can it lose money? It is a real art not to overprice or underprice the program. Demand and location (*place*) will also influence price. If a program is in high demand, obviously the price can be raised. For example, a stress-management program in a large metropolitan area may be able to command a higher price than one located in a small rural area.

Not only do the demand and the location influence the amount one might charge for a program, but so can the psychological mindset of those in the priority population. There are some individuals who would not participate in a free or inexpensive program because they question how such a program could be any good. Some people believe they have to spend a lot of money to get anything of worth. Also, sometimes when programs are offered free of charge, people may be less likely to attend regularly because they have not "invested" financially in the program. On the other hand, there are some people who, if given the choice of a free program versus one with a cost, will always take the free program, even if they are financially able to pay. Being able to segment the priority population with regard to these economic issues can help set the right price. Box 11.4 provides several examples of "price," other than economic, that the priority population may face when participating in a health promotion program.

Place   The third marketing variable is **place,** which can be thought of as where and how the product is received or delivered. Where is the best place to offer the program? How large is the service area? How many distribution points should there be? A good example of the importance of placement is worksite health promotion programs. The advantages of providing health promotion programs in this setting include the following:

1. Access to a large portion of the adult population

2. An effective internal communication channel to employees

3. Stable social support

4. Opportunity to create environments that support healthy behaviors

5. Convenient access for employees (O'Donnell, 1992; O'Donnell & Ainsworth, 1984; Sciacca et al., 1993; Sloan, Gruman, & Allegrante, 1987)

In placing a program, it is also important to avoid areas where people do not normally go or places where they would not feel comfortable or safe.

The timing of a program is closely associated with its place. When is the program best offered? If a worksite program was offered in the evenings, so that the workers had to return to the worksite after dinner, that probably would not be much different

> ## Box 11.4 Other Prices of Participation in a Health Program
>
> *Behavioral*
>> What can I do to replace my old behavior/habit? What will I do when confronted with a high-risk (potential relapse) situation?
>
> *Geography*
>> Is the place where the program is offered convenient? Is it safe?
>
> *Physical*
>> Will I physically hurt when I make the change? Will it be painful?
>
> *Psychological*
>> What if I am not successful with the change? Will the change be worth all I have to go through to achieve it?
>
> *Social*
>> Will my peers pressure me not to change my behavior? Will there be social support for my change? How will my friends react to my change? Will my spouse/mate support me?
>
> *Structural*
>> Will I be able to make the change in the environment in which I work? Recreate? Eat?
>
> *Temporal*
>> Is the timing right for this change? Would it be better to wait until _____ to make change?
>
> *Source:* Adapted from Figure 11.6, by Lefebvre, in *Health Promotion: Discipline and Diversity* by R. Bunton & G. MacDonald, 1992, pp. 153–181, published by Routledge. Used by permission of the publisher. Bensley, "Schoolsite Health Promotion: Ways of Sustaining Interest," *Journal of Health Education,* 22 (2), 1989, pp. 86–89. Reprinted by permission of the American Association for Health Education.

from driving across town from work to attend a program. Offering a program right after a shift or on a lunch hour would be much more appealing to most workers. Obviously, planners should be concerned about placing their program in a desirable locale (where they are wanted and needed) at the best possible time.

Promotion   The fourth marketing variable is **promotion.** "Promotion consists of the integrated use of advertising, public relations, media advocacy, personal selling and entertainment vehicles. The focus is on creating and sustaining demand for the product" (Weinreich, 1999, p. 1). This means taking the necessary steps to make people aware that you have a product (program) in which they would be interested. Such communication should be both informative and persuasive. The choice of a program name is an important element in its promotion, since the name can make a difference in whether someone from the priority population will be interested in the program. Creating a name is part of the marketing process used to develop informative and persuasive communication flows between the providers of a program and those in the priority population. More likely than not, a program name will be the first contact that someone in the priority population will have with the product (health promotion program). A program name is analogous to the headline of a newspaper article. When most people read a newspaper, they do not read every article; rather, they skim the headlines of the articles and then read those articles that appeal to them. It is the headlines that grab their attention. The same concept applies in advertising a product. A good headline ought to compel members of the priority population to read the rest of the message (Granat, 1994), or, in the case of a health promotion program, create enough interest that those in the priority population want to find out more about the program.

In addition to creative names, acronyms are useful in bringing attention to a program. For example, Foldcraft, a company in Minnesota, uses the acronym H.E.A.L.T.H. as the name of its health program. It stands for "Hey Everyone Always Learns The Hardway." Program titles and acronyms seem to be limited only by the planners' creativity. Box 11.5 shows additional examples of program names.

Box 11.5 Sample Program Names

Title (topic)	Organization/Company
A Plan for Life (general health)	IBM
Awakening the Spirit (diabetes program for Native Americans)	American Diabetes Association
Freedom from Smoking (smoking cessation)	American Lung Association
FreshStart (smoking cessation)	American Cancer Society
Health e Strategies (e-health)	Wellness Councils of America
Health Track (general health)	Union Pacific
Heart at Work (cardiovascular health)	American Heart Association
Hey everyone always learns the hardway	Foldcraft (Minnesota)
Live for Life (general health)	Johnson & Johnson
Live Well—Be Well (general health)	Quaker Oats
STEPS to a Healthier U.S.	U.S. Department of Health and Human Service
Time Out for Life (general health)	Colonial Life and Accident Insurance Company
Total Life Concept (general health)	AT&T
United Way at Work (general health)	United Way
StayWell (general health)	Control Data
Up with Life (general health)	Dow Chemical

Promotion can be thought of as advertising the program. As with product development, planners should consider the segmentation of the priority population when promoting the program. For example, advertising for a program to reach high-risk new mothers would be very different from one intended for all new mothers. Depending on the type of program planned and the setting for the program, the techniques of advertising the program will vary. If the program is being promoted through **internal advertising**—that is within an organization, say for the employees of a business or for the faculty and staff of a school—promotion might include such elements as posters, bulletin boards, brochures, displays, table tents, newsletters, envelope stuffers, and announcements made through groups that represent the priority population, such as unions or professional organizations. If the program is being promoted through **external advertising**—that is, not within an organization but in a community at large—some of the same techniques can be used. Posters, bulletin boards, brochures, and displays are also useful when trying to attract members of a larger community. Other useful techniques for external advertising might include the following:

1. Advertising through the mass media (newspapers; television, including the use of message boards that run across the bottom of a television screen on cable stations; radio; and billboards; etc.)

2. Direct contact with specific groups that might be at high risk and in need of the programs (contacting recent heart attack patients about a program on the need to eat in a "heart healthy" manner)

3. Contact with specific professionals who would be in a position to make referrals to your program

Of these techniques, the first, advertising through the mass media, requires a special set of skills in order to be used effectively. High on the list of these skills is the ability to interact with media representatives (newspaper reporters and television or radio journalists, and advertising staff). Before a program is ready to be marketed, planners should meet with the advertising staff, the health editor and/or writers, and the health/consumer reporters. These people can provide insight into the type of advertising to be used. They know what attracts their readers, listeners, and viewers to an advertisement. They can also provide additional insight into how to prepare news releases and stage newsworthy activities that can lead to stories and articles in the media. Such stories can be thought of as free advertising, since the space or time is not paid for.

Other techniques that can be useful in promoting a program either internally or externally are as follows:

1. Providing incentives for people to become involved, such as free tee-shirts, extra vacation time, a free introductory offer, free health appraisal, flex time, or money (see Chapter 8 for more incentives)

2. Gaining the endorsement of key people in an organization (those who are admired, a supervisor or the boss) or a famous person or someone well known in the community

3. Distributing mailbox stuffers or door-to-door flyers

4. Making a personal contact with an individual, such as a friend or a superior or boss who is already involved

5. Setting up a mentoring program where someone already in the program works with a beginner

6. A special kickoff, countdown, ribbon-cutting, or health party to get a program started

Keeping Clients Satisfied and Loyal

Keeping clients satisfied and loyal involves two key concepts. The first is that satisfied and loyal clients can add much to future marketing efforts by providing word-of-mouth advertising. They can provide a lot of favorable advertising, free of charge. Second, and more important, is the value of keeping those in the priority population involved in the health-enhancing behavior that they began as a result of being involved in the health promotion program. Becoming involved in a program is important, but maintaining a health-enhancing behavior is a more important objective. There is strong evidence that people are not very likely to maintain health behavior change over a long period of time. The problem of recidivism to past behaviors, such as substance abuse, has been known for quite a while (Hunt, Barnett, & Branch, 1971). In addition, researchers have warned health education and health promotion program planners of recidivism and dropout problems associated with exercise (Dishman, Sallis, & Orenstein, 1985; Horne, 1975), weight loss (Stunkard & Braunwell, 1980), and smoking cessation (Leventhal & Cleary, 1980; Marlatt & Gordon, 1980). (Further discussion of relapse can be found in Chapter 7.)

Why do people behave the way they do? Why do some people begin and continue with health promotion programs, whereas others make a strong start but drop out, and still others never begin? Research has shown that the reasons are many and varied. Participation in health promotion programs may be influenced by a variety of factors—including demographic, behavioral, and psychosocial variables—and program structure. "Lack of time, failure to recognize significance of participation, inconvenience to the participant, failure to achieve personal goals, and lack of enjoyment of participation are some of the reasons why individuals drop out of wellness [health promotion] programs" (Bensley, 1991, p. 89). Proper motivation is one way of preventing dropouts.

Motivation A key element for initial involvement and continued participation in a health promotion program seems to be motivation, which has been described as a concept that is both simple and complex. "The concept of motivation . . . is simple because the behavior of individuals is goal-directed and either externally or internally induced. It is complex because the mechanism which induces behavior consists of the individual's needs, wants, and desires and these are shaped, affected, and satisfied in many different ways" (Rakich, Longest, & O'Donovan, 1977, p. 262). Feldman (1983) suggests a variety of ways in which participants may be motivated to adopt a new health behavior. These means are seldom independent of each other, but from a planning standpoint, they are usually viewed separately. The key to motivation is matching the means of motivating with those things that seem to reinforce the individual program participants. What motivates one individual may not be motivating to another individual, and vice versa.

Two approaches are commonly used. The first is to include questions about motivation as part of a needs assessment when planning the program. For example, if the planners are surveying a priority population regarding their needs, they could include questions on reinforcers, such as "What incentives would entice you to participate in the exercise program?" or "What would it take to get you to participate in this program?" or "What would it take to keep you involved in a program?" The responses to these questions should provide some direction concerning the type of reinforcers that would be most useful for the priority population. The second is the "shotgun" approach based on a planner's previous experience or the experience reported by others. Using the shotgun approach, a program planner would offer a variety of reinforcers to meet the needs of a large percentage of the program's priority population. The former approach is recommended in most cases, but sometimes motivation is not considered when a needs assessment is completed. In such a case, the latter approach is used. The remaining portions of this chapter provide ideas for motivating program participants.

Using Contracts to Motivate.   A *contract* is an agreement between two or more parties that outlines the future behavior of those parties. Contracts are a common part of everyday living. People enter into contracts when they sign a lease for an apartment or a residence hall agreement, take out an insurance policy, borrow money, or buy something over a period of time. The same concept can be applied to getting and keeping people motivated in health promotion programs. Each program participant would enter into a contract with another person (the program facilitator, a significant other, or a fellow participant) and then work toward an objective or agreement specified in the contract. The contract would also specify **contingencies**— that is, what happens as a result of the contract's either being met or not being met.

For an exercise program, this system might work as follows. The program participant and program facilitator would draw up a contract based on the participant's present status in the program (e.g., exercising for 30 minutes once a week) and on what would be a reasonable goal for the near future (e.g., eight weeks). Thus the contract might state that the participant will exercise for 30 minutes twice a week for the first week, 30 minutes three times a week for the second week, and so forth, building up gradually to the final goal of exercising for 60 minutes most days of the week at the end of eight weeks. The outcome should focus on a behavior that can be maintained at the end of the contract period. For a weight loss program, the goal might be written as eliminating snacking in the evening, increasing fruits and vegetables in the diet to five servings per day, and walking for 30 minutes three times a week. These are behaviors that can reasonably be maintained after the weight loss.

The parties to the contract then decide on what the contingencies will be. Thus the participant might offer to make a contribution to some local charity or state that she will continue in the program for another eight weeks if she does not meet the contract goal. The facilitator might promise the participant a program tee-shirt if she fulfills the contract during the specified eight-week period. Other ideas for contingencies might include granting a kickback on fees for completing a certain percentage of the classes, or earning points towards products or services. No matter what the contingencies are, it seems to help if the contract is completed in writing. A sample contract is presented in Appendix D.

Using Social Support to Motivate.   It has long been recognized that whatever the behavior may be, it is almost always easier to do if people have the support of those around them. Long-standing examples of the concept of **social support** in the area of health promotion are programs such as Weight Watchers and Alcoholics Anonymous. They are based on the support of others who are experiencing the same behavior change. One of the key reasons why worksite health promotion programs are so effective is that the working environment lends itself to social support. Being around other individuals who are engaging in the same behavior change provides a good support system.

Another means of helping program participants develop the necessary support system might be to pair them with other participants in a "buddy" arrangement. People find it harder to let others down than to disappoint themselves. Another technique that is being used increasingly is to incorporate the help of family members or significant others to provide the needed motivation. It is easier for someone to quit smoking if all members in the household try quitting at the same time, than to "go it alone" while others in the household continue to smoke.

Using Media to Motivate.   Another technique for keeping people motivated to continue in a health promotion program is to recognize them publicly through some medium available to those in the program. Examples of such media include organization newsletters or newspapers, community newspapers, local television and radio stations, bulletin boards at the location where the program is being offered or public bulletin boards elsewhere, and letters sent to the significant others of the participants (family members, job superiors, etc.) noting the participants' progress in the program.

It is important for planners to exercise caution when recognizing people through the different types of media. Not everyone likes to see their name publicized. Before you publicly acknowledge individual participants, make sure they do not mind if you do so.

Using Incentives to Motivate.   In Chapter 8, **incentives** were discussed as an intervention strategy, but they are also useful in keeping people involved in programs (Jason et al., 1990). Dunbar, Marshall, and Howell (1979) state that reinforcement may be any consequence that would increase the probability of a behavior's being repeated. Wilson (1990, p. 33) defines incentive as "some reward for achieving a level of performance or goal." It has been reported (Frederiksen, 1984) that incentives seem to be most effective if they are provided in small quantities, are frequent in nature, are tailored to those in the priority population, address behaviors over which the individual has control, and do not conflict with any organizational policies.

Competition as a Means of Motivating.   Wilson (1990, p. 33) reports that competitions have been a useful means of "introducing and promoting health promotion programs and achieving significant initial participation rates." A *competition* can be described as a contest between two teams (groups) or individuals in which the object is to try to out-perform the other competitor. In a health promotion context, this could mean competing to lose the most pounds, smoke the fewest cigarettes, walk the most miles, swim the most laps, or plan the most nutritious meals. Competitions are a good method of introducing a health promotion program, but they are probably not useful as an ongoing recruitment tool (Wilson, 1990).

Final Comment on Marketing

Planners who intend to use a canned program should be sure to ask the vendor if there is a marketing plan that goes along with the program. The good programs will usually include some useful marketing strategies, if not an entire plan. A word of caution about the marketing materials: Like the canned programs themselves, they are usually aimed at a general population, not one that has been segmented. Therefore they may have to be tailored to meet local needs.

SUMMARY

An important aspect of any health promotion program is being able to attract participants initially and to keep them involved once they have started the program. An understanding of the diffusion theory is helpful in determining strategies for marketing a program. The actual marketing mix for a program should take into account the four Ps of marketing: product, price, place, and promotion. Special attention should be given to segmenting the priority population. Once people are enrolled in a program, they need to be motivated to remain involved. Strategies of contracts, social support, media recognition, incentives, and competition can be most helpful in motivating people to continue their participation in a program.

REVIEW QUESTIONS

1. Define the following terms: *market, marketing,* and *social marketing.*
2. What is the relationship between marketing and needs assessment?
3. How does the diffusion theory relate to marketing a program?
4. What are the five different groups of people described in the diffusion theory? When would each group most likely join a health promotion program?
5. What is the difference between marketing a tangible product and an intangible product?
6. What are the four Ps of marketing? Explain each one.
7. What is meant by *marketing mix?*
8. What are five techniques for motivating people to stay involved in a health promotion program?

ACTIVITIES

1. Respond to the following statements/questions with regard to a program you are planning:
   a. Describe your product.
   b. Describe your segmented population.
   c. How much will you charge for the program? Explain the rationale on which you based your decision. What other "prices" do you see for this program?
   d. Where will you place your program (location, days, and time)? Why are you placing it this way?
   e. How will you promote your program? How, when, and where will you advertise?

2. Create a one-page advertisement that could be used as a table tent, a newspaper ad, or a flyer for your program. This advertisement should include both text and graphics.

3. Give an example of how you could use each of the four methods described in the chapter for motivating program participants to stay in a program.

WEBLINKS

1. **http://www.aed.org/**
   Academy for Educational Development

   The Academy for Educational Development has done extensive work in social marketing, particularly as it relates to development and health in global settings. This website is a good resource for social marketing, health communications, and health promotion in general.

2. **http://www.mapnp.org/library/mrktng/mrktng.htm**
   All About Marketing

   This site provides an overview of program design and marketing for nonprofit organizations. It includes valuable insight into marketing in general, market planning, positioning programs, pricing, naming and branding, advertising and promotions, and public and media relations.

3. **http://www.marketingpower.com/welcome.php**
   American Marketing Association

   The American Marketing Association is one of the largest professional associations for marketers. This site provides best practices related to marketing strategies including marketing tools and templates and marketing services directories.

4. **http://ctb.ku.edu/**
   Community Tool Box

   The site provides excellent resources on promoting participation and social marketing. Topic sections include step-by-step instruction, examples, checklists, and related resources.

5. **http://www.social-marketing.org/index.html**
   Social Marketing Institute

   The mission of the Social Marketing Institute is to advance the science and practice of social marketing. This site provides a comprehensive library of success stories in social marketing, papers, conferences, employment listings, and related sites.

6. **http://www.hc-sc.gc.ca/english/socialmarketing/index.html**
   Social Marketing Network

   This site provides the latest information on social marketing and lessons learned by Health Canada's Marketing and Creative Services Division. Current case studies provide step by step instructions for the marketing process.

7. **http://www.sophe.org/**
   Society for Public Health Education

   Under the link, Publications and Journals, view, *Social Marketing Resource Guide*. This guide provides information on social marketing in general, audience segmentation, message development, planning tools, and health communications.

CHAPTER 12

Implementation
Strategies and Associated Concerns

Chapter Objectives

After reading this chapter and answering the questions at the end, you should be able to:

- Define *implementation.*
- Identify the different phases for implementing health promotion programs.
- List the concerns that need to be addressed before implementation can take place.

Key Terms

acts	informed consent	PERT
anonymity	key activity chart	phased in
beneficence	liability	pilot testing
confidentiality	logistics	program launch
commission	management	program rollout
critical path method	negligence	prudent
Gantt chart	news hook	sustainability
HIPAA	nonmaleficence	Task Development Time Line
implementation	omission	(TDTL)

In Chapters 1–10 of this book we discussed the steps necessary to plan a solid health promotion program. In Chapter 11, we presented information that would assist planners in marketing the program they planned. As a part of the marketing process we presented information on the process of program adoption using the diffusion theory (Rogers, 2003). It is the adoption of a program (or stated differently, the decision to participate) by those in the priority population that is the beginning of the program implementation process. Yet there are many other things that need to be considered in the implementation process that are critical to a successful program. The eventual impact of a program will be judged not only by the effectiveness of the interventions but also by the quality of the implementation (Parcel, 1995). In fact, Timmreck (2003) has stated "implementation is the most critical part of the planning process; a plan that is not implemented is no plan at all" (p. 171). In this chapter, we present the key phases in implementing a program and identify the many concerns that must be addressed as implementation unfolds.

Defining Implementation

In the simplest terms, implementation means to carry out. Timmreck (1997) defined **implementation** as the "the act of converting planning, goals, and objectives into action through administrative structure, management activities, policies, procedures, regulations, and organizational actions of new programs" (p. 328). Keyser and colleagues (1997) summarize implementation as the setting up, managing, and executing of a project. While Bartholomew, Parcel, Kok, and Gottleib (2001) indicate that implementation is one of the three stages of program diffusion with the other two being adoption and **sustainability** ["the maintenance and institutionalization of a program or its outcomes" (p. 292.)]. Let's look now at the phases in the implementation process.

Phases of Program Implementation

The phases of implementation that we present here are a combination of some of our own ideas with those of Parkinson and Associates (1982), Hayden (2000), and Bartholomew and colleagues (2001). It should be noted that the resulting generic phases presented are flexible in nature and can be modified to meet the many different situations and circumstances faced by planners.

Phase 1: Adoption of the Program

Since the adoption process was presented at length in Chapter 11, it will not be repeated here. However, we do want to remind planners that great care must go into the marketing process to ensure that a relevant product (i.e., the health promotion program) is planned so that those in the priority population will want to participate in it.

Phase 2: Identifying and Prioritizing the Tasks to be Completed

In order for a program to be implemented, planners will need to identify and prioritize a number of smaller tasks. Even though many of these tasks are small in nature, they cannot be overlooked if planners want a smooth implementation. Many of these tasks are often referred to as program **logistics,** defined as the procurement, maintenance, and transportation of materials, facilities, and personnel (Woolf, 1979). Reserving space where the program is to be held, making sure audiovisual equipment is available when requested, ordering the correct number of participant education packets or manuals, and arranging for interpreters when working a diverse population are examples of program logistics that are important to the success of a program. Other logistical issues are presented later in this chapter in the section titled "Concerns Associated with Implementation."

To assist planners in identifying and prioritizing these tasks, it is recommended that the planners use some form of a planning timetable or timeline. Planning timetables can assist in "the defining of tasks, the laying out of plans over the life of the project, and the monitoring of progress so that midcourse corrections can be made, if needed" (McDermott & Sarvela, 1999, p. 72). Planning timetables that are commonly used include: key activity charts, (McDermott & Sarvela, 1999), Task Development Time Lines (TDTLs) (Anspaugh, Dignan, & Anspaugh, 2000), Gantt charts, PERT charts, and the critical path method (CPM). A **key activity chart** may be the simplest of the tools. It includes three components, a listing of all the key activities or tasks to be carried out, an estimate of the dates when the activities will take place, and the time allocated to complete the activities.

Task Development Time Lines and Gantt charts all are very similar. They are both comprised of rows and columns. The rows on the left-hand side of the chart represent the tasks or activities to be completed, while the columns represent periods of time. In the examples presented in Figures 12.1 and 12.2, the columns represent months, but they could just as easily represent weeks or for that matter hours if the chart were being used for a short-term project. The major difference between a TDTL and a Gantt chart is in the detail presented. A **Task Development Time Line** identifies the tasks that need to be completed and the time frame in which the tasks will be completed (Anspaugh et al., 2000) using "Xs" or "√s" (see Figure 12.1). A **Gantt chart**

Tasks Year 1	Months											
	J	F	M	A	M	J	J	A	S	O	N	D
Develop program rationale	✔	✔										
Conduct needs assessment			✔									
Develop goals and objectives				✔								
Create intervention					✔							
Conduct formative evaluation						✔						
Assemble necessary resources						✔						
Market program						✔	✔					
Pilot test program								✔				
Refine program									✔			
Phase in intervention #1										✔		
Phase in intervention #2											✔	
Phase in intervention #3												✔

Figure 12.1 Sample task development time line *(Figure 12.1 continues)*

Tasks Year 2	Months											
	J	F	M	A	M	J	J	A	S	O	N	D
Phase in intervention #4	✔											
Total implementation		✔	✔	✔	✔	✔	✔	✔	✔	✔	✔	✔
Collect and analyze data for evaluation			✔									
Prepare evaluation report				✔								
Distribute report					✔							
Continue with follow-up for long-term evaluation						✔	✔	✔	✔	✔	✔	✔

Figure 12.1 *(continued)*

Date
√

	Mar.	April	May	June	July	Aug.	Sept.	Oct.	Nov.	Dec.
Develop rationale										
Needs assessment										
Create goals & objectives										
Create intervention										
Assemble resources										
Market program										
Implement program										
Evaluate program										
Write final report										

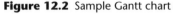 = planned time frame
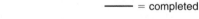 = completed

Figure 12.2 Sample Gantt chart

does the same plus provides an indication of the progress made toward completing the task by using different size lines to distinguish between the projected time frame for a task and the progress toward completing the task. In addition, a Gantt chart uses a marker above the columns to indicate the current date (Timmreck, 2003) (see Figure 12.2). Thus if using a Gantt chart, planners would update their progress regularly on the chart.

PERT is an acronym for program evaluation and review technique. PERT charts are more complex than Gantt charts and thus have not been used as much with health promotion programs (Timmreck, 2003). PERT charts are comprised of two components, a diagram and a timetable (Breckon, 1997). The diagram presents a visual representation of the relationship between and among the tasks to be completed. The diagram also indicates the order by sequentially numbering the tasks to be completed. The timetable of a PERT chart is similar to the key activity chart but also includes three estimates of time for each task. Included in the estimates are an optimistic, pessimistic, and a probabilistic timeframe. The complexity of PERT puts a detailed explanation beyond the scope of this textbook. If readers are interested in learning more about it, we recommend referring to business management textbooks.

The last planning timetable to be presented is the **critical path method** (CPM). Critical Path Method (CPM) charts are similar to PERT charts and are sometimes known as PERT/CPM (Modell, 1996). The CPM focuses on the total time to complete the tasks. In a CPM chart, the critical path is indicated and consists of the set of dependent tasks (each dependent on the preceding one) which together take the longest time to complete (Modell, 1996). More specifically, the CPM

> analyzes what activities have the least amount of scheduling flexibility (i.e., are the most mission-critical) and then predicts project duration schedule based on the activities that fall along the 'critical path.' Activities that lie along the critical path cannot be delayed without delaying the finish time for the entire project (Webopdia, 2003, ¶1).

Like some of the other planning timetables presented here the CPM provides a graphical view of the project and predicts the time required to complete the project. But what is unique to CPM is that it shows which activities are critical to maintaining the planning schedule and which are not (NetMBA, 2003).

Phase 3: Establishing a System of Management

Once all the tasks have been identified and the timetable for completing them have been developed, planners need to turn their attention to how the program will be managed. "The efficient, satisfactory management of a health promotion program is vital to its long-term success" (Anspaugh et al., 2000, p. 124). **Management** has been defined as "the process of achieving results through controlling human, financial, and technical resources" (Breckon, 1997, p. 313). Depending on the type of program being planned, the management process could range from consuming a small portion of a single planner's time and resources, such as when a smoking cessation program is being planned for 10 people, to needing several people working full-time to manage a large community-wide program. Many of the tasks associated with the phase of implementation are presented later in this chapter. However, because of the complexity of principles associated with establishing a system of management we recommend readers refer to a management textbook (e.g., Breckon, 1997) for more information on management techniques.

Phase 4: Putting the Plans into Action

Parkinson and Associates (1982) suggest three major ways of putting plans into action: by using a piloting process; by phasing it in, in small segments; and by initiating the total program all at once. These three strategies are best explained by using an inverted triangle, as shown in Figure 12.3. The triangle represents the number of people

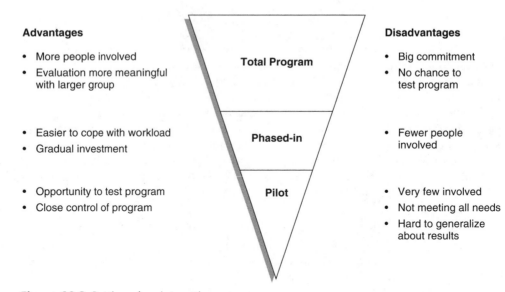

Advantages

- More people involved
- Evaluation more meaningful with larger group

- Easier to cope with workload
- Gradual investment

- Opportunity to test program
- Close control of program

Disadvantages

- Big commitment
- No chance to test program

- Fewer people involved

- Very few involved
- Not meeting all needs
- Hard to generalize about results

Total Program

Phased-in

Pilot

Figure 12.3 Putting plans into action

from the priority population who would be involved in the program based on the implementation strategy chosen. The wider portion of the triangle at the top would indicate offering the program to a larger number of people than is represented by the point of the triangle at the bottom.

These three different implementation strategies exist in a hierarchy. It is recommended that all programs go through all three of the strategies, starting with piloting, then phasing in, and finally implementing the total program. However, keep in mind that limited time and resources may not always allow planners to work through all three strategies.

Pilot Testing   **Pilot testing** (or piloting or field testing) the program is a crucial step. Even though planners work hard to bring a program to the point of putting it into action, it is important to try to identify any problems with the program that might exist. Pilot testing allows planners to work out any bugs before the program is offered to a larger segment of the priority population, and also to validate the work that has been completed up to this point. For the most meaningful results, a newly developed program should be piloted in a similar setting and with people like those who are eventually to use the program. Use of any other group may fail to identify problems or concerns that would be specific to the priority population. As an example of the piloting process, take the case of a hospital developing a worksite health promotion program that will be marketed to outside companies. It would be best if the program were piloted on a worksite group before it was marketed to worksites in the community. The hospital could look for a company that might want to serve as a pilot group, or it might use its own employees.

As part of piloting the program, planners should check on the following:

1. The intervention strategies were implemented as planned.
2. The intervention strategies worked as planned.

3. Adequate resources were available to carry out the program.

4. Those participants in the pilot group had an opportunity to evaluate the program.

It is important to have the program participants critique such aspects of the program as content, approaches used, facilitator's effectiveness, space, accommodations, and other resources used. Such feedback will give planners insight into how to revise the program. If many changes are made in the program as a result of piloting, planners may want to pilot it again before moving ahead. This evaluation process during the piloting phase is part of formative evaluation and will be discussed further in Chapter 13.

Phasing In   Once a program has been piloted and revised, the program should, if applicable, be **phased in** rather than implemented in its entirety. This is especially true when there is a very large priority population. Phasing in allows the planners to have more control over the program and helps to protect planners and facilitators from getting in over their heads. There are several ways in which to phase in a program:

1. By different program offerings
2. By a limit on the number of participants
3. By choice of location
4. By participant ability

Say a comprehensive health promotion program was being planned for Blue Earth County, Minnesota. To phase in the program by different offerings, planners might offer stress-management classes the first six months. During the next six-month period, they could again offer stress management but also add smoking cessation programs. This process would continue until all offerings are included.

If the program were to be phased in by limiting the number of participants, planners might limit the first month's enrollment to 25 participants, expand it to 35 the second month, to 45 the third month, and so on, until all who wanted to participate were included. To phase in the program by location, it might initially be offered only to those living in the southwest portion of the county. The second year, it might expand to include those in the southeast, and continue in the same manner until all were included. A program planned for a college town might be offered first on campus, then off campus to the general public. A program phased in by participant ability might start with a beginning group of exercisers, then add an intermediate group, and finally include an advanced group.

Total Implementation   Implementing the total program all at once would be a mistake. Rather, planners should work toward total implementation through the piloting and phasing-in processes. The only exceptions to this might be "one-shot" programs, such as programs designed around a single lecture, and possibly screening programs, but even then piloting would probably help.

First Day of Implementation

No matter what program is being planned, there will be a "first day" for the program. The first day of the program, also referred to as the **program launch** or **program rollout,** is just an extension of the fourth P of marketing: Promotion (see Chapter 11).

The focus of promotion is on creating and sustaining demand for the product (Weinreich, 1999). The creation of the demand for the product leads to the initiation of the program. As such, some special planning needs to take place for the first day of implementation. First, decide on a day when the program is to be rolled out. Consider launching the program to coincide with other already occurring events or special days that can help promote the program. Examples include: starting a weight loss program at the beginning of the calendar year to coincide with New Year's resolutions; beginning a smoking cessation program on the third Thursday of November (the day each year for the American Cancer Society's Great American Smokeout); having immunization programs and physical examinations for children prior to the beginning of a new school year; launching a skin cancer prevention program on a college campus prior to the annual spring break; or rolling out the community-wide exercise program at the beginning of February, Heart Health month.

Second, consideration should be given to obtaining news coverage (print and/or broadcast) for the first day to further publicize the program. If it is decided to seek such coverage, you should (CDC, 2003):

- inform appropriate media representatives of your plans
- make arrangements to meet the media representatives at the designated time and place
- prepare the following and have them ready for the day:
    —press releases
    —video news releases
    —spokespersons trained to respond to inquires from media representatives

Because many health promotion programs are not newsworthy in their own right, it might be necessary to use a **news hook** to interest the media in the program being launched. By news hook, we mean something that would make the media want to cover the launch. The planners' organization may have newsworthy data or information related to the health problem being targeted by the program, or there may be a related news event that is receiving media attention, that would help bring attention to the new program (CDC, 2003). For example, if the new program is aimed at reducing teen pregnancy and new state legislation has been proposed to assist in such efforts or an event related to teen pregnancy is currently an important news item, then linking the new program with those timely events can make it more newsworthy (CDC, 2003). Planners should even consider linking the launch of the program with some important date in history to make it newsworthy. Linking the influenza epidemic of 1918 to launch the county-wide flu shot program may make it more newsworthy.

And finally, short of having a newsworthy program, planners need to consider having a first day that includes some special event, such as a ribbon cutting, appearance by a celebrity, or some other event that starts off the program on a positive note. Celebrities need not be individuals with national or international recognition, but may be individuals such as the chief executive officer (CEO) of the company, a supervisor, a visible or well-known person (Anspaugh, Hunter, & Savage, 1996) in the community (i.e., the mayor or a coach), or a common person who has been affected by the health problem.

Phase 5: Ending or Sustaining a Program

The final phase of the implementation process is to determine how long to run a program. For some programs the answer will be simple; if the program met its goals and objectives and the priority population has been served to the fullest extent necessary, then the program can be ended. For example, a worksite health promotion may have a goal to certify 50% of the workforce in CPR. If that goal is reached, then the program's resources could be used on other health promotion programming. However, a greater concern facing most planners is how to sustain a needed program for a longer period of time when the goals and objectives have not been met (i.e., only half of those who were expected to get flu shots got them), or goals and objectives of the program are long-term in nature (i.e., providing food and shelter for the homeless). This is especially difficult when original program funding and other types of resources and support may end or be withdrawn. In Chapter 11, we presented information on how to maintain interest in program participants, but here we are referring to the maintenance and institutionalization of a program or its outcomes. Techniques that have been used by planners to sustain programs include: a) working to institutionalize the program (see Chapter 3, Goodman & Steckler, 1989, and Goodman et al., 1993), b) advocating for the program (see Chapter 8 for a discussion of advocacy), c) partnering with other organizations/agencies with similar missions to share resources and responsibilities, and d) by revisiting and revising the rationale used to create the program initially (see Chapter 3).

Concerns Associated with Implementation

There are many matters of detail to be considered before and during the implementation process. The exact order in which they are considered is not as important as just making sure that they have been taken care of. Therefore, we present and describe these items in no specific order.

Legal Concerns

Liability is on the mind of many professionals today because of the concern over lawsuits. With this in mind, all personnel connected with the planned health promotion program, no matter how small the risk of injury to the participants (physical or mental), should make sure that they are adequately covered by liability insurance. In addition, program personnel should have an understanding of informed consent, negligence, and approval of appropriate professional groups. (See Chapter 8 for information about guidelines from professional groups.)

Informed Consent   Individuals should not be allowed to participate in any health promotion program without giving their informed consent. **Informed consent** has been defined as:

> the voluntary agreement of an individual, or his or her authorized representative, who has the legal capacity to give consent, and who exercises free power of choice, without undue inducement or any other form of constraint or coercion to participate in research [the program]. The individual must have sufficient knowledge and understanding of the nature of the proposed research [program], the anticipated risks and potential benefits, and the requirements of the research [program] to be able to make an informed decision (Levine, 1988, as stated in NIH, n.d., p. 1).

As a part of the process of obtaining informed consent from participants, program facilitators should:

1. Explain the nature and purpose(s) of the program.

2. Inform program participants of any inherent risks or dangers associated with participation and any possible discomfort they may experience.

3. Explain the expected benefits of participation.

4. Inform participants of alternative programs (procedures) that will accomplish the same thing.

5. Indicate to the participants that they are free to discontinue participation at any time.

In addition, planners must ask if the participants "have any questions, answer any such questions, and make it clear they should ask any questions they may have at any time during the program. Informed consent forms should be signed by participants before they enter the program" (Patton et al., 1986, p. 236).

Program planners must be aware that informed consent forms (sometimes called *waiver of liability* or *release of liability*) do not protect them from being sued. There is no such thing as a waiver of liability. If you are negligent, you can be found liable. However, informed consent forms do make participants aware of special concerns. Further, because people must sign the forms, they may not consider legal action even if they have a case, feeling that they were duly warned. Appendix E provides a sample consent form.

Negligence   **Negligence** is failing to act in a **prudent** (reasonable) manner. If there is a question whether someone should or should not do something, it is generally best to err on the side of safety. Negligence can arise from two types of **acts: omission** and **commission.** An act of *omission* is not doing something when you should, such as failing to warn program participants of the inherent danger in participation. An act of *commission* is doing something you should not be doing, such as leading an aerobic dance program when you are not trained to do so.

Reducing the Risk of Liability   The real key to avoiding liability is to reduce risk by planning ahead. Patton and colleagues (1986, p. 236) offer the following tips for reducing legal problems in exercise programs; however, similar advice would apply to all types of health promotion programs:

1. Be aware of legal liabilities.

2. Select certified instructors [in the activity and emergency care procedures] to lead classes and supervise exercise equipment [and for that matter all types of equipment].

3. Use good judgment in setting up programs and provide written guidelines for medical emergency procedures.

4. Inform participants about the risks and danger of exercise [or other activities] and require written informed consent.

5. Require that participants obtain medical clearance before entering an exercise program [or other strenuous programs].

6. Instruct staff not to "practice medicine," but instead to limit their advice to their own area of expertise.

7. Provide a safe environment by following building codes and regular maintenance schedule for equipment.

8. Purchase adequate liability insurance for all staff.

With regard to item 8 in the preceding list, planners should check on the availability of liability insurance through (1) their employer, (2) their homeowner's or renter's policy, or (3) special coverage from a professional organization.

Medical Concerns

Does the program put the participants at any special medical risk so that they would need medical clearance (for example, cardiovascular exercise programs)? If so, the necessary steps need to be taken so that the participants can provide proof of clearance. Appendix F presents an example of a medical clearance form.

Program Safety

Necessary steps must be taken to ensure the health and safety of those participating in the program and all staff members. Providing a safe environment includes finding a safe program location (e.g., low-crime area), ensuring that classrooms and laboratories are free of hazards, providing qualified facilitators, supplying first-aid equipment, and developing an emergency care plan. Box 12.1 provides a checklist of items that should be considered when creating an appropriate emergency care plan.

Program Registration and Fee Collection

If the program you are planning requires people to sign up and/or pay fees, you will need to establish registration procedures. Program registration and fee collection may take place before the program (preregistration), by mail, in person, via an indirect method like payroll deduction, or at the first session. Planners should also give thought to the type of payment that will be accepted (cash, credit card, or check) and plan accordingly. Though it may seem obvious, some thought also must be given to the security of the money received. That is, how it will be handled, transported, and deposited or otherwise secured.

Procedures for Recordkeeping

Almost every program requires that some records be kept. Items such as information collected at registration, medical information, data on participant progress, and evaluations must be accounted for. The importance of privacy for those planners working in health care settings was further emphasized in April 2003 with the enactment of the *Standards for Privacy of Individually Identifiable Health Information* section (The Privacy Rule) of the Health Insurance Portability and Accountability Act of 1996 (officially known as Public Law 104-191 and referred to as **HIPAA**). The Rule sets national standards that health plans, health care clearinghouses, and health care providers who conduct certain health care transactions electronically must implement to protect and guard against the misuse of individually identifiable health information. Failure to implement the standards can lead to civil and criminal penalties (USDHHS, 2003).

Box 12.1 Checklist of Items to Consider when Developing an Emergency Care Plan

_____ 1. Duties of program staff in an emergency situation are defined.

_____ 2. Program staff are trained (CPR and first aid) to handle emergencies.

_____ 3. Program participants are instructed what to do in an emergency situation (e.g., medical, natural disaster).

_____ 4. Participants with high-risk health problems are known to program staff.

_____ 5. Emergency care supplies and equipment are available.

_____ 6. Program staff has access to a telephone.

_____ 7. Standing orders are available for common emergency problems.

_____ 8. There is a plan for notifying those needed in emergency situations.

_____ 9. Responsibility for transportation of ill/injured is defined.

_____ 10. Accident report form procedures are defined.

_____ 11. Universal precautions are outlined and followed.

_____ 12. Responsibility for financial charges incurred in the emergency care process are defined.

_____ 13. The emergency care plan has been approved by the appropriate personnel.

_____ 14. The emergency care plan is reviewed and updated on a regular basis.

The two techniques that are used to protect the privacy of participants are anonymity and confidentiality. **Anonymity** exists when no one, including the planners, can relate a participant's identity to any information pertaining to the program (Dane, 1990). Thus information associated with a participant may be considered anonymous when such information cannot be linked to the participant who provided it. In applying this concept, planners need to ensure that collected data had no identifying information attached to them such as the participant's name, social security number, or any other less common information.

Confidentiality exists when planners are aware of the participants' identities and have promised not to reveal those identities to others (Dane, 1990). When handling confidential data, planners need to take every precaution to protect the participants' information. Often this means keeping the information "under lock and key" while participants are active in a program, then destroying (i.e., shredding) the information when it is no longer needed.

Moral and Ethical Concerns

There are times when certain behavior is legal but not moral or ethical. Program planning and evaluation provide planners with almost daily opportunities to make decisions that affect other people. Some of these decisions are easy to make; others raise the question of what is the right or wrong decision. In other words, because of the nature of health promotion, planners are confronted with many moral and ethical decisions.

Who is to judge what is right and wrong? Most often, these decisions are compared to a standard of practice that has been defined by other professionals in the same field. For health promotion planners, the standard of practice is outlined in the Code of Ethics for the Health Education Profession developed by the Coalition of National Health Education Organizations, USA (CNHEO) (see Appendix G). However, even a code of ethics cannot spell out all the rights and wrongs of the many decisions that must be made. The interpretation of the code still creates some gray areas. Although the purpose of this section is not to say what is right or wrong, planners should be alerted to some of the more common ethical issues that they will face.

The first is respect. Even though one may not agree with the values, behavior, and goals of others, it is important to respect them. The planner's role is not to judge but to facilitate. Fennell and Beyrer (1989) have written a thought-provoking article on some ethical issues concerning AIDS and the health educator.

Autonomy is another issue with which planners must deal. Should letting people voluntarily adopt health behavior be the guiding principle? Or is there a place for manipulation and coercion in health promotion? Box 12.2 presents a hierarchy of autonomy.

A third issue concerns informed consent. Although this was discussed earlier with regard to legal concerns, it is often also an ethical concern. Planners are faced with questions such as these: Even though the benefits outnumber the risks, do we scare people away by telling them the risks? Is it okay to withhold information if it could affect the results of an evaluation?

Planners also have to consider the concept of **nonmaleficence**—not causing harm or not doing evil. For example, is it permissible to use an aversive behavior technique to get someone to stop smoking? Which is worse, smoking cigarettes or receiving some physical punishment for doing so?

The concept of **beneficence**—that is, bringing about or doing good—can also be related to ethical issues. Can there be any question whether it is right to do good? If the good comes at the expense of another, then it raises ethical concerns.

Justice and fairness are also involved in ethical issues. For example, the question of fairness might arise in pricing a program. The program needs to show a profit, but

---

Box 12.2 Hierarchy of Autonomy

1. *Facilitation:* Assist in achieving objectives set by a priority group. Examples: putting safety belts in cars or teaching people the skills necessary to perform CPR.
2. *Persuasion:* Argue and reason. Examples: tell people about the importance of wearing safety belts or taking blood pressure medicine.
3. *Manipulation:* Modify the environment around a person or the psychic disposition of the person. Example: automatic safety belts.
4. *Coercion:* Threat of deprivation. Example: safety belt or motorcycle helmet laws and fines for breaking the laws.

the clients cannot afford the price that would be necessary to achieve a profit. (Legal concerns can enter into this area, too.) Issues of sexism, racism, and other cultural biases also involve concepts of justice and fairness.

Finally, the concepts of confidentiality and privacy are involved in ethical issues. Should a program planner be barred from releasing information about a person without his or her consent, even though it will benefit that person? Consider a high school sophomore who approaches the health teacher with confidential information that she is pregnant. Should the health teacher tell anyone else, such as the girl's parents?

The opportunities for dealing with ethical issues are many, and planners need to be prepared to handle them.

Procedural Manual and/or Participants' Manual

Depending on the complexity of a program, there may be a need to develop manuals or to purchase them from a vendor. Manuals may outline procedures for program facilitators; some refer to these as *training manuals*. Manuals may also provide the participants with detailed information. Developing either type of manual in-house would be a major task; therefore, adequate resources and time need to be given to developing manuals.

Training for Facilitators

If a program that is being planned needs a specially qualified person (certified or licensed) to facilitate it, every effort should be made to secure such a person. This may mean having to hire a vendor to provide such a service. If funds to hire one are not available, others will need to be selected, trained, supported, and monitored appropriately. This may mean running your own training program or sending people to other training classes to become qualified facilitators.

Dealing with Problems

With the program up and running, the task of the planners is to anticipate and deal with problems that might arise and to do so in a constructive manner. Even if a program has been piloted, problems can still arise. Astute and effective planners must anticipate the possibility of things going wrong (Timmreck, 2003). "If problems are anticipated, they can be resolved more easily should they occur in the implementation process" (Timmreck, 2003, pp. 182–183). The problems that could be encountered can range from petty concerns to matters of life and death. Problems might involve logistics (room size, meeting time, or room temperature), participant dissatisfaction, or a personal or medical emergency. Whatever the problem, it should be worked out as much as possible to the satisfaction of all concerned. If there is a question of whether to accommodate a program participant or the program personnel, 99% of the time the participants should be satisfied. They are the lifeblood of all programs. As a part of this implementation concern, it might be a good idea to conduct a one-month evaluation asking questions similar to the ones asked in the piloting evaluation.

Reporting and Documenting

Planners need to give attention to reporting or documenting the ongoing progress of the program to interested others (Ross & Mico, 1980). Planners should keep others informed about the progress of the program for several different reasons, including

(1) accountability, (2) public relations, (3) motivation of present participants, and (4) recruitment of new participants. The exact nature of the reporting or documenting will vary, but it is important for planners to keep all stakeholders informed.

Summary

A great deal of work goes into developing a program before it is ready for implementation. The process used to implement a program may have much to say about its success. This chapter presents five phases planners can follow in implementing a program; 1) adoption of the program, 2) identifying and prioritizing the tasks to be completed, 3) establishing a system of management, 4) putting the plans into action, and 5) ending or sustaining a program. Also presented in this chapter are matters that need to be considered and planned for prior to and during implementation.

Review Questions

1. What is meant by the term *implementation?*
2. Name and briefly describe the five phases of implementation presented in this chapter.
3. Briefly describe how each of the following planning timetables can be used:
   a. key activity chart
   b. Task Development Time Line (TDTL)
   c. Gantt chart
   d. PERT chart
   e. critical path method (CPM)
4. What are three strategies from the modified model of Parkinson and Associates (1982) for implementing health promotion?
5. What are some techniques planners can use to enhance the first day of implementation?
6. What is meant by the term informed consent?
7. What implications does HIPAA have for planners?
8. What are the legal concerns planners need to be aware of when implementing a program?
9. What are logistics and why are they important to program planners?
10. What is the difference between an act of omission and an act of commission?
11. What role does autonomy play in the ethical decisions a program planner must make?

Activities

1. Explain how you would implement a program you are planning, using a pilot study, phasing in, and total implementation. Also explain what you plan to do to "kick off" the program.
2. Develop an informed consent form that outlines the risks inherent in a program you are planning. Make sure the form includes a place for signatures of the participant and a witness and the date.
3. In a one-page paper, identify what you see as the biggest ethical concern of health promotion programming, and explain your choice.

4. Write a one-paragraph statement outlining the ethical stand your organization will take with regard to program implementation.

WEBLINKS

1. **http://www.cc.nih.gov/ccc/protomechanics/chap_3.html#whatareinformca**
   National Institutes for Health (NIH)

   This is a page at the NIH website where you can get more information about informed consent and assent.

2. **http://www.hhs.gov/ocr/hipaa/index.html**
   United States Department of Health and Human Services (USDHHS)

   This is a page at the USDHHS website where you can get more information about the National Standards to Protect the Privacy of Personal Health Information.

3. **http://www.cdc.gov/communication/cdcynergy.htm**
   CDCynergy

   This is the Centers for Disease Control and Prevention's web page for the *CDCynergy* planning model. At this site you can read about Phase 6 of this model that deals with launching a program.

4. **http://www.thisdayinhistory.com/tdih/tdih.html**
   This Day in History

   This is a commercial web page. The site allows one to input a specific date to find out what historical events took place that day. It can be of use to planners when trying to plan the kick-off program "newsworthy" by linking it to a historical event.

Part III

Evaluating a Health Promotion Program

The chapters in this section of the book include an overview of the evaluation process, including how to plan an evaluation, analyze and interpret the data, and report the results. The chapters and topics presented in this section are:

CHAPTER 13

Evaluation
An Overview

Chapter Objectives

After reading this chapter and answering the questions at the end, you should be able to:

- Explain the difference between informal and formal evaluation.
- Compare and contrast the various types of evaluation.
- Identify some of the problems that may hinder an effective evaluation.
- List reasons why evaluation should be included in all programs.
- Explain the difference between internal and external evaluation.
- Describe several considerations in planning and conducting an evaluation.

Key Terms

baseline data	formal evaluation	process evaluation
evaluand	formative evaluation	outcome evaluation
evaluation	impact evaluation	stakeholders
evaluation consultant	informal evaluation	standards of acceptability
external evaluation	internal evaluation	summative evaluation

Whether they realize it or not, planners are constantly evaluating their health promotion efforts by asking questions such as: Did the program have an impact? How many people stopped smoking? Were the participants satisfied with the program? Should we change anything about the way the program was offered? What would happen if we just changed the time we offer the program? Should we expect a greater turnout than what we had tonight? Although all these questions are linked to evaluation, some will be of greater importance than others. The evaluation process that planners engage in can be classified into two categories of evaluation. The first is **informal evaluation.** Such evaluations:

> are characterized by an absence of breath and depth because they lack systematic procedures and formally collected evidence. As humans, we are limited in making judgments

by both the lack of opportunity to observe many different settings, clients, or students and by our own past experiences, which both informs and biases our judgments. Informal evaluation does not occur in a vacuum. Experience, instinct, generalization, and reasoning can all influence the outcome of informal evaluations, and any or all of these may be the basis for sound, or faulty judgments (Fitzpatrick, Sanders, & Worthen, 2004, p. 8–9).

There are times when informal evaluations are the only practical approach (Fitzpatrick et al., 2004). For example, planners may not have the resources or time to conduct a more formal evaluation. Informal evaluations are not inherently bad, but for many of the reasons outlined by Fitzpatrick and colleagues in the definition above they have the potential to be biased. Informal evaluations can be unbiased and useful when conducted by knowledgeable, experienced, and fair people (Fitzpatrick et al., 2004). If at all possible, we would only recommend informal evaluations when the stakes in evaluation outcomes are small. Examples might include changing the time of the program, adding an additional class session, consulting colleagues about a program concern, or making program changes based on participant feedback. Though informal evaluation processes are adequate in making minor changes in programs, when the stakes of program evaluation are high (i.e., conducting programs that have significant impact on the stakeholders), evaluation procedures need to become formal, explicit, and justifiable (CDC, 1999c). When these more major decisions are made, there is a need to use formal evaluation processes. **Formal evaluation** processes are characterized by "systematic well-planned procedures" (Williams & Suen, 1998, p. 308). They are processes that are designed to control a variety of extraneous variables that could produce evaluation outcomes that are not correct. Table 13.1 presents several different characteristics associated with formal and informal evaluation processes. Since informal evaluation has fewer restrictions on it than formal evaluation, and since informal evaluation skills are often learned on the job, the focus of the evaluation processes presented in this book are on formal evaluation.

Evaluation is critical for all health promotion programs. It is the only way to separate successful programs from those that are not; it is a driving force for planning new effective health promotion programs, improving existing programs, and demonstrating the results of resource investments (CDC, 1999c). For example, evaluation can help a planner determine whether participants were satisfied with a weight loss

Table 13.1 Characteristics of formal and informal evaluation

Characteristic	Formal	Informal
a. Degree of freedom	Planned activities	Spontaneous activities
b. Flexibility	Prescribed procedures or protocols	Flexible procedures or protocols
c. Information	Precision of information	Depth of information
d. Objectivity	Objective scores of measurement	Subjective impressions
e. Utility	Maximal comparability	Maximal informativeness
f. Bias	Potential narrowed scope	Subjective bias
g. Setting	Controlled settings	Natural settings
h. Inference	Strong inferences	Broad inferences

Source: Williams and Suen (1998). Permission granted by PNG Publications, publisher of *American Journal of Health Behavior.*

program, whether a smoking cessation workshop actually changed smoking behavior, or whether an exercise program should continue or not. Without adequate evaluation, accurate information is not gained, and decisions are based on speculation.

In order to generate useful and meaningful data about programs, the evaluation must be designed early in the process of program planning. As mentioned in Chapter 6, evaluation begins when the program goals and objectives are being developed. Evaluation will not only help determine whether program goals and objectives are met but it will also answer questions about the program as it is being implemented. If the evaluation is not designed until the program has ended, the information cannot be used to improve the program as it progresses. For example, low enrollment in a stress-management workshop might reflect an inadequate setting, inconvenient hours, or lack of publicity. All of these problems could be reduced or eliminated if evaluation was conducted in the planning stage.

The process of designing an evaluation should be a collaborative effort of program **stakeholders** (those individuals who have a vested interest in the program). Evaluation results must be relevant to the stakeholders in order to be used most effectively. For example, planners, administrators, program facilitators, and the representatives from the funding source all have specific questions they would like answered regarding the program's development and outcome. Planners may want to know if the program met the needs of the priority population; program administrators may want to know if the program is making any money; program facilitators may want to know if participants changed their behavior as a result of the program; and representatives from the funding source may be interested in knowing if the program was cost effective. If the evaluation is properly planned and implemented, it can provide answers to all of these questions and "the means to improve the quality of work for everyone involved" (Valente, 2002, p. 6).

Although evaluation is an important and necessary component of health promotion programs, planners need to understand that evaluation can be a political process. If evaluation is seen as a way to judge a program or determine its worth, it can be threatening. Judgment often "carries the possibilities of criticism, rejection, dismissal, and discontinuation" (Green & Lewis, 1986, p. 16). Thus those associated with a program may feel that negative results from an evaluation may reduce program funding and eliminate staff, parts of a program, or an entire program. Consequently, instead of using the term evaluation some use the terms *assessment, quality improvement,* or *quality control* to alleviate fears on the part of those who are being evaluated (Valente, 2002).

McDermott and Sarvela (1999) describe additional situations in which evaluations may be political. Results may be intentionally skewed by reporting only successes and not weaknesses to decision makers in order to prevent the elimination of a program. Even when results are reported fairly, political ramifications may occur—reviewing an unpopular but highly visible program, complying with governmental regulations, or complying with the evaluator's desire to publish the results. McDermott and Sarvela (1999) also indicate that an evaluation can be a political "hot potato." For example, if objective results lead to the recommendation that a drug abuse program serving poor, pregnant minority women be eliminated, what are the implications for the agency with regard to morale, racial harmony, and trust in governmental agencies?

Since evaluations may also have ethical considerations for the individuals involved, most colleges, universities, and school systems have boards to review the evaluation design. These groups are most often referred to as *institutional review boards (IRBs)* or *human subject review committees.* The purpose of these boards is to safeguard the rights, privacy, health, and well-being of the participants.

Basic Terminology

A number of definitions have been written for the word evaluation. In general terms, "evaluation is a process of reflection whereby the value of certain actions in relation to projects, programs, or policies are assessed" (Springett, 2003, p. 264). As it applies to health promotion, **evaluation** has been defined as "the comparison of an object of interest against a standard of acceptability" (Green & Lewis, 1986, p. 362). In this latter definition, the object of interest, also referred to as an **evaluand** (Scriven, 2000), could be the entire health promotion program or any part of that program. The **standards of acceptability** are the minimum levels of performance, effectiveness, or benefits used to judge the value (Green & Lewis, 1986) and are typically expressed in the "outcome" and "criterion" components of a program's objectives (see Chapter 6 for information about objectives). Box 13.1 lists a number of sources for standards of acceptability.

When determining the value of a program, planners can use several types of evaluation. The type of evaluation reflects whether the results are needed to improve a program before or during implementation, to assess the effectiveness and efficiency of a program, or to determine whether the program met the goals and objectives.

When describing evaluation activities usually one of two sets of evaluation terms is used. Some authors use the terms *process, impact,* and *outcome* to identify types of evaluation used to determine the value of a program. Other authors use the terms *formative* and *summative* to describe the evaluation that occurs during the program and after the program, respectively.

- **Process evaluation:** "Any combination of measurements obtained during the implementation of program activities to control, assure, or improve the quality of

Box 13.1 Standards of Acceptability

Standard of Acceptability	Examples
Mandate (policies, statutes, laws) of regulating agencies	Percent of children immunized for school; percent of priority population wearing safety belts
Priority population health status	Rates of morbidity and mortality compared to state and national norms
Values expressed in the local community	Type of school curriculum expected
Standards advocated by professional organizations	Passing scores, certification, or registration examinations
Norms established via research	Treadmill tests or percent body fat
Norms established by evaluation of previous programs	Smoking cessation rates or weight loss expectations
Comparison or control groups	Used in experimental or quasi-experimental studies

performance or delivery. Together with preprogram studies, makes up formative evaluation" (Green & Lewis, 1986, p. 364). Getting reactions from program participants about the times programs are offered or about program speakers are examples. Such measurements could be collected with a short questionnaire or focus group.

- **Impact evaluation:** Focuses on "the immediate observable effects of a program, leading to the intended outcomes of a program; intermediate outcomes" (Green & Lewis, 1986, p. 363). Measures of awareness, knowledge, attitudes, skills, and behaviors yield impact evaluation data.

- **Outcome evaluation:** Focuses on "an ultimate goal or product of a program or treatment, generally measured in the health field by morbidity or mortality statistics in a population, vital measures, symptoms, signs, or physiological indicators on individuals" (Green & Lewis, 1986, p. 364). Outcome evaluation is long-term in nature and takes more time and resources to conduct than impact evaluation.

- **Formative evaluation:** "Any combination of measurements obtained and judgments made before or during the implementation of materials, methods, activities or programs to control, assure or improve the quality of performance or delivery" (Green & Lewis, 1986, p. 362). Examples include, but are not limited to, a needs assessment or pilot testing a program.

- **Summative evaluation:** "Any combination of measurements and judgments that permit conclusions to be drawn about impact, outcome, or benefits of a program or method" (Green & Lewis, 1986, p. 366).

Even though the sets of terms are used to describe evaluation activities, there is some overlap among the terms (see Figure 13.1). Process evaluation occurs during the program and is a form of formative evaluation. Impact and outcome evaluation occur at the completion of the program and are considered forms of summative evaluation. Both sets of evaluation (process, impact, and outcome; formative and summative) take into account the need to conduct evaluation before and/or during the program, and at the end of the program. Plans for all types of evaluation should be in place before or during program implementation.

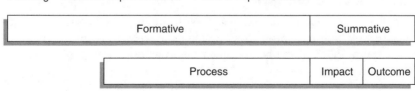

Figure 13.1 Comparison of evaluation terms

Purpose for Evaluation

Basically, programs are evaluated to gain information and make decisions. The types of evaluation are distinguished by how the information is going to be used. The information may be used by planners during the implementation of a program to make

improvements in services (process evaluation). It may be used to see if certain immediate outcomes—such as knowledge, attitude, skills, and behavior change—have occurred (impact evaluation). It may also be used at the end of a program to determine
whether long-term goals and objectives have been met (outcome evaluation). Capwell, Butterfoss, and Francisco (2000) identify six general reasons why stakeholders
may want programs evaluated:

1. *To determine achievement of objectives related to improved health status:* Probably the
   most common reason for program evaluation is to determine if objectives of the
   program have been met. Evaluation for this reason may also be used to determine
   which of several programs was most effective in reaching a given objective.

2. *To improve program implementation:* Planners should always be interested in improving a program. Program evaluation can help planners to understand why a
   particular intervention worked (Valente, 2002) or did not work, and thus, weak
   elements can be identified, removed, and replaced (Green & Lewis, 1986).

3. *To provide accountability to funders, community, and other stakeholders:* Many stakeholders are interested in the value of a program to a community, or if the program
   is worth its cost. Thus an evaluation may provide decision makers with the information to determine if the program funding should continue, discontinue, or expand.

4. *To increase community support for initiatives:* The results of an evaluation can increase
   the community awareness of a program. Positive evaluation information chan-
   neled through the media can help sell a program, which in turn may lead to additional funding.

5. *To contribute to the scientific base for community public health interventions:* Program
   evaluation can provide findings that can lead to new hypotheses about human
   behavior and community change, which in turn may lead to new and better programs.

6. *To inform policy decisions:* Program evaluation data can be used to impact policy
   within the community. For example, a number of communities have passed local
   ordinances based on the results of evaluative studies on secondhand smoke.

The Process for Evaluation

The process of evaluating a program begins with the initial program planning. Those
involved in developing new programs need to be aware of the importance of a well-
defined evaluation plan. The following list provides guidelines for planning and conducting an evaluation:

Planning
- Review the program goals and objectives.
- Meet with the stakeholders to determine what general questions should be
  answered.
- Determine whether the necessary resources are available to conduct the evalua-
  tion; budget for additional costs.
- Hire an evaluator, if needed.

- Develop the evaluation design.
- Decide which evaluation instrument(s) will be used and, if needed, who will develop the instrument.
- Determine whether the evaluation questions reflect the goals and objectives of the program.
- Determine whether the questions of various groups are considered, such as the program administrators, facilitators, planners, participants, and funding source.
- Determine when the evaluation will be conducted; develop a time line.

Data Collection
- Decide how the information will be collected: survey, records and documents, telephone interview, personal interview, observation (see Chapter 5).
- Determine who will collect the data.
- Plan and administer a pilot test.
- Review the results of the pilot test to refine the data collection instrument or the collection procedures.
- Determine who will be included in the evaluation—for example, all program participants, or a random sample of participants.
- Conduct the data collection.

Data Analysis
- Determine how the data will be analyzed.
- Determine who will analyze the data.
- Conduct the analysis, and allow for several interpretations of the data.

Reporting
- Write the evaluation report.
- Determine who will receive the results.
- Choose who will report the findings.
- Determine how (in what form) the results will be disseminated.
- Discuss how the findings of the process or formative evaluation will affect the program.
- Decide when the results of the impact, outcome, or summative evaluation will be made available.
- Disseminate the findings.

Application
- Determine how the results can be implemented.

Practical Problems or Barriers in Evaluation

Several authors (Solomon, 1987; Glasgow, Vogt, & Boles, 1999; Glasgow, 2002; NCI, 2002; Valente, 2002; Timmreck, 2003) have identified practical problems or barriers to effective evaluation. Some of the more common ones are presented below.

1. Planners either fail to build evaluation in the program planning process or do so too late (Solomon, 1987; Valente, 2002; Timmreck, 2003).

2. Resources (e.g., personnel, time, money) may not be available to conduct an appropriate evaluation (Solomon, 1987; NCI, 2002; Valente, 2002).

3. Organizational restrictions on hiring consultants and contractors (NCI, 2002).

4. Effects are often hard to detect because changes are sometimes small, come slowly, or do not last (Solomon, 1987; Glasgow, 2002; Valente, 2002).

5. Length of time allotted for the program and its evaluation (NCI, 2002).

6. Restrictions (i.e., policies, ethics, lack of trust in the evaluators) that limit the collection of data from those in the priority population (NCI, 2002).

7. It is sometimes difficult to distinguish between cause and effect (Solomon, 1987).

8. It is difficult to separate the effects of multistrategy interventions (Glasgow et al., 1999), or isolating program effects on the priority population from "real world" situations (NCI, 2002).

9. Conflicts can arise between professional standards and do-it-yourself attitudes (Solomon, 1987) with regard to appropriate evaluation design.

10. Sometimes people's motives get in the way (Solomon, 1987; Valente, 2002).

11. Stakeholders' perceptions of the evaluation's value (NCI, 2002).

12. Intervention strategies are sometimes not delivered as intended (i.e., type III error) (Glasgow, 2002), or are not culturally specific (NCI, 2002; Valente, 2002).

Examples of these problems in health promotion programs include not collecting initial information from participants because evaluation plans were not in place, failing to budget for the cost of the evaluation (e.g., printing questionnaires, additional staff, postage), or conducting the evaluation before a change can occur (e.g., changes in cholesterol level) or too long after program completion (e.g., long-term effects of a weight loss program). Those without evaluation expertise may conduct an evaluation without a sound design, such as not using appropriate sampling techniques or comparison groups. Program managers, who have a motivation to make their programs look cost effective, may minimize costs and exaggerate program benefits.

Awareness of these problems and development of strategies to deal with them may improve the accuracy of program evaluation. This chapter discusses many approaches that can help minimize these problems, such as including evaluation in the early stages of program planning, determining who will conduct the evaluation, carefully considering the evaluation design, increasing objectivity, and developing a plan to use the evaluation results.

Evaluation in the Program-Planning Stages

As discussed in Chapter 6, the evaluation design must reflect the goals and objectives of the program. The results of the evaluation will determine whether the goals and objectives were met. To be most effective, the evaluation must be planned in the early stages of program development and should be in place before the program begins. Results from evaluations conducted early in the program-planning process can assist in improving the program. Having a plan in place to conduct an evaluation before the end of a program will make collecting information regarding program outcomes much easier and more accurate.

Discussion on how evaluation plans can be included in program planning will focus on examples of formative and summative evaluations. The formative evaluation should provide feedback to the program administrator, with program monitoring beginning in the early stages. Collecting information and communicating it to the administrator quickly allows for the program to be modified and improved.

Data reflecting the initial status or interests of the participants **(baseline data)** or data from a needs assessment can be used for comparison to the early data collected from program participants. Additional information from the formative evaluation may indicate that the necessary staff have been hired, the program sites are available, brochures have been printed, participants are satisfied with the times the programs are offered, and classes are offered with the needs of the prospective participants in mind.

Early data regarding the program should be analyzed quickly to make any necessary adjustments to the program. This type of evaluation can improve both new and existing programs. Information from the formative evaluation can be useful in answering questions, such as whether the programs are provided at convenient locations for the community members, whether the necessary materials arrived on time, and whether people are attending the workshops at all the various times they are offered.

By developing the summative evaluation plan at the beginning of the program, planners can ensure that the results will be less biased. Early development of the summative evaluation plan ensures that the questions answered reflect the original objectives and goals of the program. This type of evaluation can provide answers to many questions, such as whether the group approach or the individual approach was more effective in reducing tobacco use among the participants in a smoking cessation program, whether the participants in a weight loss program lost weight and kept the weight off, and how many people in the priority population increased their knowledge, changed their attitudes, or reduced their risks.

Who Will Conduct the Evaluation?

At the beginning of the program, planners must determine who will conduct the evaluation. The program evaluator must be as objective as possible and should have nothing to gain from the results of the evaluation. The evaluator may be someone associated with the program or someone from outside.

If an individual trained in evaluation and personally involved with the program conducts the evaluation, it is called an **internal evaluation.** For example, a local health department may use one of its own employees to serve as the evaluator of its programs. An internal evaluator would have the advantage of 1) being more familiar with the organization and the program history, 2) knowing the decision making style of the organization, 3) being present to remind others of results now and in the future, and 4) being able to communicate technical results more frequently and clearly (Fitzpatrick et al., 2004). Conducting an internal evaluation is also less expensive than hiring additional personnel to conduct the evaluation. The major drawback, however, is the possibility of evaluator bias or conflict of interest. Someone closely involved with the program has an investment in the outcome of the evaluation and may not be completely objective. After all, a positive evaluation of the program may result in future funding that would secure the positions of the staff members.

An **external evaluation** is one conducted by someone who is not connected with the program. Often an external evaluator is referred to as an **evaluation consultant.** Having someone from the state health department conduct evaluations for the local health department would be an example of an external evaluator. External evaluators are somewhat isolated, lacking the knowledge and experience of the program that the internal evaluator possesses. Evaluation of this nature is also more expensive, since an additional person must be hired to carry out the work. However, an external evaluator: a) can provide a more objective outlook and a fresh perspective, b) can help to ensure an unbiased evaluation outcome, c) brings a global knowledge of evaluation having worked in a variety of settings, and d) "typically brings more breadth and depth of technical expertise" (Fitzpatrick et al., 2004, p. 23). Box 13.2 presents a list of characteristics that program planners can use when selecting an external evaluator. In addition, when selecting an external evaluator, planners should look for someone with formal training in evaluation methods and an affiliation with the American Evaluation Association (Anonymous reviewer, 2003).

Box 13.2 Characteristics of a Suitable Consultant

- Is not directly involved in the development or running of the program being evaluated
- Is impartial about evaluation results (i.e., has nothing to gain by skewing the results in one direction or another)
- Will not give in to any pressure by senior staff or program staff to produce particular findings
- Will give the staff the full findings (i.e., will not gloss over or fail to report certain findings for any reason)
- Has experience in the type of evaluation needed
- Communicates well with key personnel
- Considers programmatic realities (e.g., a small budget) when designing an evaluation
- Delivers reports and protocols on time
- Relates to the program
- Sees beyond the evaluation to other programmatic activities
- Explains both the benefits and risks of evaluation
- Educates program personnel about conducting evaluation, thus allowing future evaluations to be done in house
- Explains material clearly and patiently
- Respects all levels of personnel

Source: Thompson and McClintock (1998), p.13.

Whether an internal or external evaluator conducts the program evaluation, the main goal is to choose someone with credibility and objectivity. The evaluator must have a clear role in the evaluation design, accurately reporting the results regardless of the findings.

Evaluation Results

The question of who will receive the evaluation results is also an important consideration. The evaluation can be conducted from several vantage points, depending on whether the results will be presented to the program administrator, the funding source, the organization, or the public. These stakeholders may all have different sets of questions they would like answered. The evaluation results must be disseminated to groups interested in the program. Different aspects of the evaluation can be stressed, depending on the group's particular needs and interests. A program administrator may be interested in which approach was more successful, the funding source may want to know if all objectives were reached, and a community member may want to know if participants felt the program was beneficial.

The planning process of the evaluation should include a determination of how the results will be used. It is especially important in process and formative evaluation to implement the findings rapidly to improve the program. However, an action plan is needed in summative, impact, and outcome evaluation to ensure that the results are not filed away, but are used in the provision of future health promotion programs.

SUMMARY

Evaluation can be thought of as a way to make sound decisions regarding the worth or effectiveness of health promotion programs, to compare different types of programs, to eliminate weak program components, to meet requirements of funding sources, or to provide information about programs. The evaluation process takes place before, during, and after program implementation. If the evaluation is well designed and conducted, the findings can be extremely beneficial to the program stakeholders.

REVIEW QUESTIONS

1. What is the difference between informal and formal evaluation?
2. Give an example of a question that could be answered in a process evaluation, impact evaluation, and outcome evaluation.
3. What are some of the general reasons for evaluating a program?
4. Why can an evaluation be viewed as political?
5. What are some of the more common problems associated with or barriers to effective evaluation?
6. What different types of information could an evaluation provide for the various stakeholders (planners, the funding source, the administrators, and the participants)?
7. Why is it important to begin the evaluation process in the program-planning stages?
8. Explain how feedback from an evaluation can be used in program planning.
9. What are the components of the process of evaluation?

10. In what type of situation would an internal evaluation be more appropriate than an external evaluation?

11. What are the desirable characteristics of an external evaluator (evaluation consultant)?

ACTIVITIES

1. Describe how process, impact, and outcome evaluation could be used in a stress-management program for college students. Describe how formative and summative evaluation could be used.

2. Write a rationale to a funding source for hiring an external evaluator (evaluation consultant).

3. Review the evaluation component from a health promotion program in your community and/or discuss an evaluation plan with a planner or evaluator. Look for the planning process used, the rationale for the data collection method, and how the findings were reported.

4. Assume you are responsible for selecting an evaluator for a health promotion program you are planning. Would you select an internal or an external evaluator? Explain your rationale. If you select an external evaluator (evaluation consultant), where do you think you could find such a person?

WEBLINKS

1. **http://www.eval.org**
   American Evaluation Association (AEA)

   This is the website for the AEA. The AEA is an international professional association of evaluators devoted to the application and exploration of program evaluation, personnel evaluation, technology, and many other forms of evaluation.

2. **http://evaluationcanada.ca/site.cgi?=6=3**
   The Canadian Evaluation Society (CES)

   This is the website for the CES. The CES is a professional association of evaluators dedicated to the advancement of evaluation theory and practice. Information at this site is available in both English and French.

3. **http://www.wkkf.org/Programming/ResourceOverview.aspx?CID=281&ID=770**
   W.K. Kellogg Foundation (WKKF)

   This is a page from the WKKF webpage. At this site you will find the *WKKF Evaluation Handbook.* The handbook provides a framework for thinking about evaluation as a relevant and useful program tool. It was written primarily for project directors who have direct responsibility for the ongoing evaluation of W.K. Kellogg Foundation-funded projects.

4. **http://www.cdc.gov/eval/index.htm**
   Centers for Disease Control and Prevention (CDC)

   This is a page from the CDC website. This page is dedicated to the CDC Evaluation Working Group and its effort to promote program evaluation in public health. The site includes links to the CDC evaluation framework and additional resources that may help when applying the framework.

5. **http://www.nnfr.org/parented/links.html**
   National Network for Family Resiliency (NNFR)

   This is a page from the NNRR website. The page is called the "Electronic Resources for Evaluators" and provides many different links to resources that can be used in program evaluation. Example links include: Evaluation & Related Associations; Evaluation How-To; Assessment, Measurement, and Instruments; and Data and Statistics.

6. **http://hsc.usf.edu/CFH/cnheo**
   Coalition of National Health Education Organizations (CNHEO)

   This is the homepage for the CNHEO. The Coalition has as its primary mission the mobilization of the resources of the Health Education Profession in order to expand and improve health education, regardless of the setting. At this site you can print out a copy of the Code of Ethics for the Health Education Profession.

CHAPTER 14

Evaluation Approaches, Framework, and Designs

Chapter Objectives

After reading this chapter and answering the questions at the end, you should be able to:

- Describe the various evaluation approaches outlined.
- Identify the six steps and four standards of the framework for program evaluation.
- List some considerations in selecting an evaluation design.
- Compare and contrast quantitative and qualitative methods of evaluation.
- List the various qualitative methods that can be used in program evaluation.
- Differentiate among experimental, control, and comparison groups.
- Compare and contrast the major types of evaluation design.
- Identify the threats to internal and external validity and explain how evaluation design can increase control.

Key Terms

accreditation
blind
CIPP
COMlist
comparison group
control group
cost-benefit analysis
cost-effectiveness analysis
cost-feasibility analysis
cost-identification analysis
cost-utility analysis
deductive

double blind
economic evaluations
evaluation design
evaluation framework
experimental design
experimental group
external validity
generalizability
goal-free approach
inductive
internal validity
management-oriented approaches

measurement
nonexperimental design
objectives-oriented approaches
posttest
pretest
qualitative method
quantitative method
quasi-experimental design
systems analysis approaches
triple blind

This chapter presents several approaches to program evaluation, a framework for program evaluation, and a variety of evaluation designs. Washington (1987) indicates that each approach to evaluation represents a certain way of thinking, which in turn defines the evaluation questions that should be asked. For example, the evaluation questions may focus on the goals and objectives of the program, the effects of the intervention, the cost-benefit ratio of the program, and the behavior of the participants. The **evaluation framework** can be thought of as the "skeleton" of a plan that can be used to conduct an evaluation. It aids in focusing attention on important issues and puts in order the steps to be followed.

An **evaluation design** is used to organize the evaluation and to provide for planned, systematic data collection, analysis, and reporting. A well-planned evaluation design helps ensure that the conclusions drawn about the program will be as accurate as possible. The design is developed during the early stages of program planning and has program goals and objectives as its focus. Evaluators must give consideration to the audience and/or stakeholders who will read the results of the evaluation; the design must produce information that will answer their evaluation questions.

Evaluation Approaches

In setting up the program evaluation, evaluators have a variety of approaches from which to select; a single approach need not be selected. In fact, Popham (1988) suggests an eclectic approach. He believes that approaches can rarely be used in their pure form, so that choosing parts or categories may be more beneficial to the evaluator.

Several authors (House, 1980; McDermott & Sarvela, 1999; Fitzpatrick, Sanders, & Worthen, 2004) have written about various approaches to evaluation. A brief description of the approaches most often used in health promotion is presented here.

Systems Analysis Approaches

Systems analysis approaches of evaluation are based on efficiency—determining which are the most effective programs using inputs, processes, and outputs. They focus on the organization, determining whether appropriate resources are devoted to goal activities (and to nongoal activities, such as staff training or maintenance of the system). These approaches are centrally concerned with the measurement of general goals, but they do not focus on the achievement of a specific goal. This is due to the recognition that organizations function at different levels with various goals at each level.

Economic evaluations are typical strategies used in systems analysis approaches. **Economic evaluations** have been defined as the comparison of alternative courses of action in terms of both costs and outcomes (Blumenschein & Johannesson, 1996). Control over rising health care costs has forced many administrators and planners to be concerned about the cost of health promotion programs. Using cost analyses, decisions can be made regarding which programs are most effective within a certain budget. In order to be able to perform cost analyses, evaluators need to be able to measure both the costs and the outcomes associated with a program.

Some costs may be quite easy to determine, such as those for staff, books, and medical equipment. Other costs are more difficult to determine, such as those associated with years of productive life lost due to accidental death, loss of productivity due to absenteeism, and cost of pain and suffering.

Outcomes can be determined by a number of factors, including health care costs saved due to health promotion programs, years of life saved, number of smokers who quit, reduced absenteeism, and number of pounds lost.

Several different types of cost analysis can be used (McDermott & Sarvela, 1999; Levin & McEwan, 2001). **Cost-identification analysis** (or cost-feasibility analysis) is used to compare different interventions available for a program, often to determine which intervention would be the least expensive. With this type of analysis, evaluators identify the different items (i.e., personnel, facilities, curriculum, etc.) associated with a given intervention, determine a cost for each item, total the costs for that intervention, and then compare the total costs associated with each of several interventions. For example, if a health department was interested in providing a tobacco control program for a school district, it could conduct a cost-identification analysis on three different interventions: (1) teacher led, (2) peer education, and (3) voluntary agency provided. Costs for each of these interventions—such as staff time, staff benefits, curriculum materials, and volunteer training—would be identified, compared, and analyzed.

Cost-benefit analysis (CBA) looks at how resources can best be used. It will yield the dollar benefit received from the dollars invested in the program. **Cost-effectiveness analysis (CEA)** is used to quantify the effects of a program in monetary terms. It is more appropriate for health promotion programs than cost-benefit analysis, because a dollar value does not have to be placed on the outcomes of the program. Instead, a cost-effectiveness analysis will indicate how much it costs to produce a certain effect. For example, based on the cost of a program, the effect of years of life saved, number of smokers who stop smoking, or morbidity or mortality rates can be determined. A thorough explanation of both cost-benefit and cost-effectiveness analysis is presented in Appendix H in an article written by McKenzie (1986).

As noted in Appendix H, cost-benefit and cost-effectiveness analyses are not easy to carry out. You are referred to two sources (CDC, 1999a; Goetzel et al., 1998) presented in Chapter 3 that should be useful in understanding more fully the complexities of these cost analyses.

A fourth type of cost analysis that is used with health promotion programs is **cost-utility analysis (CUA).** This approach is different from the others in that the values of the outcomes of a program are determined by their subjective value to the stakeholders rather than their monetary cost. For example, an administrator may select a more expensive intervention for a program just because of the good public relations (i.e., the subjective value in the administrator's eye) for the organization. Or an administrator may survey those in the priority population to determine what outcomes they value from a program. Then, based on these data, the administrator selects the appropriate intervention.

Two advantages of the systems analysis approach are that the findings are objective and that the findings can convince decision makers that a program is effective in improving health status. A disadvantage, however, is that this is only one part of the data to be considered when making program decisions: information from program participants is not included. The fate of a program should not be based on a cost analysis alone.

Objective-Oriented Approaches

Probably the most commonly used approach to health promotion program evaluation is the objectives-oriented approach. **Objectives-oriented approaches** specify program goals and objectives and collect evidence to determine if the goals and objectives have been reached (Fitzpatrick et al., 2004). Success or failure is measured by the relationship between the outcome of the program and the stated goals and objectives. This type of approach is based on action, and the dependent variable is defined in terms of outcomes the program participant should be able to demonstrate at the end of the intervention.

In the objective-oriented approach, the program goals and objectives serve as the standards for evaluation. This type of evaluation was first used in education, to assess student behaviors. Competency testing is an example of objective-oriented evaluation, determining whether a student is able to pass an exam or advance to the next grade. This approach was later used in other fields, and more emphasis was placed on how objectives are to be measured. This approach is also found in business, where organizations use "management by objectives" (MBO) to determine how well they are meeting their objectives.

When using this approach, the general goal statement is the outcome of the program. The goal should be operationally defined—that is, it should consist of measurable objectives—and those objectives most critical in achieving the goal should be identified. An indicator of a performance episode refers to a measurable, observable outcome, based on normative criteria. Measurement should be standardized in order to compare outcomes from one program to another. (See Chapter 6 for a discussion of writing goals and objectives.)

A strength of the objective-oriented approach is its objectivity. The values of the evaluator do not interfere with the outcome of the evaluation. Another strength is that the goal is predetermined: The evaluation is based on whether the goal was met, not on whether it was appropriate. The goal can be expressed as measurable objectives, making it easier to determine whether the goal was met.

A possible limitation of this approach is how the goal is set, since the outcome of the evaluation is determined by the specification of the goal. The goal reflects the values or interests of the funding source, program staff, or consumers. Who sets the goal is an important factor, and consideration must be given to whose interests the goal represents. Fitzpatrick and colleagues (2004) have identified several other limitations of objectives-oriented approach raised by its critics. They point out that the approach:

(1) lacks a real evaluative component (facilitating measurement and assessment of objectives rather than resulting in explicit judgments of merit or worth), (2) lacks standards to judge the importance of observed discrepancies between objectives and performance levels, (3) neglects the value of the objectives themselves, (4) ignores important alternatives that should be considered in planning a program, (5) neglects the context in which the evaluation takes place, (6) ignores important outcomes other than those covered by the objectives (the unintended outcomes of the activity), (7) omits evidence of program value not reflected in its own objectives, and (8) promotes a linear, inflexible approach to evaluation. Collectively, these criticisms suggest that objectives-oriented evaluation can result in tunnel vision, which tends to limit evaluation's effectiveness and potential (pp. 82–83).

An example of these limitations would be a program that has its sole objective to change the behavior of its participants. If that is the only change that the evaluators are looking for, they could easily miss or overlook other positive changes such as changes in attitudes or knowledge.

Goal-Free Approach

The **goal-free approach** of evaluation was developed in response to the limitations of the objectives-oriented approaches. Scriven (1973), who developed the goal-free approach, believed that evaluation should not be based on goals in order to enable the evaluator to remain unbiased. The evaluator must search for all outcomes, including unintended positive or negative side effects. Thus the evaluator does not base the evaluation on reaching goals and remains unaware of the program goals.

Ideally, the evaluator suspends judgment concerning what the program is intended to accomplish and focuses on what actually happens. However, Popham (1988) sees this approach as oriented toward the output of the program and as a judgmental approach, since the evaluator is required to present a judgment regarding the program to the decision makers.

The techniques that the evaluator uses include examining preintervention test results, reading expert reviews, visiting program sites, reviewing the literature, examining similar programs, interviewing staff and clients, and examining materials. The techniques are generally qualitative methods, but quantitative methods can also be used.

The goal-free approach is not often used in health promotion program evaluation. It is difficult for evaluators to determine what to evaluate when goals and objectives are not to be used. One concern is that evaluators will substitute their own goals, since there is a lack of clear methodology as how to proceed. The goal-free evaluation approach may be most useful in combination with other approaches.

On the other hand, this approach has certain advantages. One is that it avoids classifying side effects and unanticipated effects as being of secondary interest, since these may be crucial to setting new priorities in a program. A classic example of this model was an evaluation of an educational program for coronary care patients. The results of the evaluation indicated no increase in knowledge, which was the program goal. However, an unanticipated side effect was reduction in patients' anxiety during exercise. Without the use of goal-free evaluation, this benefit of the program might not have been discovered.

The main differences between the objectives-oriented and goal-free approaches are presented in Table 14.1. The types of questions asked in each approach reflect the difference in focus of the evaluation.

Management-Oriented Approaches

Management-oriented approaches focus "on identifying and meeting the informational needs of managerial decision makers" (Fitzpatrick et al., 2004, p. 68). That is, good decision making is best made on good evaluative information. In this approach, the evaluators and managers work closely together to identify the decisions that must be made and the information needed to make them. The evaluators then collect the necessary data "about the advantages and disadvantages of each decision alternative to allow for fair judgment based on specified criteria. The success of the evaluation rests on the quality of the teamwork between evaluators and decision makers" (Fitzpatrick et al., 2004, p. 89).

The person who has been most associated with this approach to evaluation is Stufflebeam (1971; 2000; [Stufflebeam et al.,1971]). He views evaluation as a three-step process: delineating (focusing on information), obtaining (collecting, organizing,

Table 14.1 Comparison of the objectives-oriented and goal-free approaches

Objectives-Oriented Approach	Goal-Free Approach
Have the objectives been reached?	What is the outcome of the program?
Has the program met the needs of the priority population?	Who has been reached by the program?
How can the objectives be reached?	How is the program operating?
Are the needs of the program administrators and funding source being met?	What has been provided?

and analyzing information), and providing (synthesizing information so it will be useful) information for making decisions. Using this definition, Stufflebeam developed the CIPP evaluation model. The acronym **CIPP** stands for the four type decisions facing managers, **c**ontext, **i**nput, **p**rocess, and **p**roduct. Context evaluation describes the conditions in the environment, identifies unmet needs and unused opportunities, and determines why these occur. The purpose of input evaluation is to determine how to use resources to meet program goals. Process evaluation provides feedback to those responsible for program implementation. The purpose of product evaluation is to measure and interpret attainments during and after the program (Stufflebeam et al., 1971). It is the decision maker, not the evaluator, who uses this information to determine the worth of the program.

The main advantage to this type of approach is the increased likelihood that the information will actually be used by the decision makers. The information most relevant to them will be obtained by this type of evaluation. The advantage for the evaluator is that the evaluation is focused, with criteria already determined. A limitation of the decision-making approach is that the amount of input from administrators may reduce the objectivity of the evaluation.

Those interested in learning more about CIPP and management-oriented approaches can do so by going to the website of the The Evaluation Center at Western Michigan University noted in the *Weblinks* at the end of this chapter.

Consumer-Oriented Approaches

Consumer-oriented approaches focus on "developing evaluative information on 'products,' broadly defined, and accountability, for use by consumers in choosing among competing products" (Fitzpatrick et al., 2004, p. 68). This approach gets its "label" of consumer-oriented, in part, from the fact that it's an evaluation approach that helps "protect" the consumer by evaluating "products" used by the consumer. The consumer-oriented approach, which is summative in nature, primarily uses checklists and criteria to allow the evaluator to collect data that can be used to rate the "product." This is the approach used by: *Consumer Reports* when evaluating various consumer products, principals when evaluating their teachers, and instructors when they are evaluating the skill of their students to perform cardio-respiratory resuscitation (CPR). It is an approach that has been used extensively in evaluating educational materials and personnel.

A checklist has been defined as "a list of factors, properties, aspects, components, criteria, tasks, or dimensions, the presence or amount of which is to be separately considered, in order to perform a certain task" (Scriven, 2000, ¶2). The types and value of checklists vary greatly, but common to all is "that of being a mnemonic device. This function alone makes them useful in evaluation, since the nature of evaluation calls for a systematic approach to determining the merit, worth, etc., of what are often complex entities" (Scriven, 2000, ¶2).

Scriven (2000) has identified a hierarchy of checklists ranging from the least formal, a *laundry list* to a *sequential checklist* to *criteria of merit* (COM) *checklist* (or *COMlist*). A laundry list is not much more than a list of important items to consider when collecting evaluative data about a "product." For example, planners may use a laundry list when making sure they have completed all the tasks and arrangements for a stress management course. A sequential checklist is one in which the order of the items (or checkpoints) on the list must be followed in order to get valid results. This is the case when an instructor checks a student's skills in being able to perform CPR. That is, the student must first determine that a person is not breathing and that he/she does not have a pulse before starting CPR.

The highest level of checklist in the hierarchy is a COMlist. A **COMlist** is a checklist comprised of the criteria that essentially define the merit of the "product." For example, what are the criteria that define an excellent health promotion program, or an outstanding program facilitator, or exemplary instructional materials for a program? The criteria of merit (COM) are identified by being able to answer the question: "What properties are parts of the concept (the meaning) of 'a good X'?" (Scriven, 2000, ¶22). Thus if we were to apply this to program planning, we would ask the question "What are the criteria that define an excellent health promotion program?" Or, "What are the qualities of an outstanding facilitator?" Or, "What must be included for an instructional material to be considered exemplary?"

Checklists are often used in health promotion to plan, implement and evaluate programs. Several have already been presented in this book (see Chapter 10 for the "Checklist for Selecting Health Promotion Vendors" and the "Suitability Assessment of Materials," and Chapter 12 for "Checklist of Items to Consider when Developing an Emergency Care Plan"). Other checklists and more information about the use of checklists can be found at the website of the Evaluation Center at Western Michigan University noted in the *Weblinks* at the end of this chapter.

Expertise-Oriented Approaches

Expertise-oriented approaches, which are probably the oldest of the approaches to evaluation, rely "primarily on the direct application of professional expertise to judge the quality of whatever endeavor is evaluated" (Fitzpatrick et al., 2004, p. 68). Most of these approaches can be placed in one of three categories, formal professional review systems, or informal professional reviews, and individual reviews. Formal professional reviews are characterized by having:

(1) structure or organization established to conduct a periodic review; (2) published standards (and possibly instruments) for use in such reviews; (3) a prespecified schedule (for example, every five years) for when reviews will be conducted; (4) opinions of several experts combining to reach the overall judgments of value; and (5) an impact on the status of that which is reviewed, depending on the outcome (Fitzpatrick et al., 2004, p. 114).

The most common formal professional review system is that of accreditation. **Accreditation** is a process by which a recognized professional body evaluates the work of an organization (i.e., school, universities, and hospitals) to determine if such work meets prespecified standards. If they do, then the organization is approved or accredited. Examples of accreditation processes with which readers may be familiar are those of the National Council for the Accreditation of Teacher Education (NCATE) which accredits teacher education programs, including health education programs, and the Joint Commission on Accreditation of Healthcare Organizations (JCAHO) which accredits various healthcare facilities.

Another formal professional review system that is very similar to accreditation but organized a bit differently is approval review. An example of an approval review is that of the American Diabetes Association (ADA). The ADA reviews diabetes self-management education (DSME) programs. DSME programs that meet the standards of the ADA are referred to as Recognized Diabetes Education Programs (RDEP) (Task Force, 2002).

The second category of expert-oriented reviews is informal professional reviews. These reviews may have many of the qualities of formal professional reviews but lack one or more of the characteristics of formal professional reviews noted earlier. There are a number of informal professional reviews that are associated either directly or indirectly with health promotion. A local health department may regularly conduct internal reviews of it various units. One year the nursing unit may be reviewed, the next year the health education unit, the next year the environmental unit, and so on. The peer reviews of manuscripts for possible publication in a professional journal is another example of an informal professional review. Typically, those who make up the review team in these reviews are referred to collectively as review panels, jury of experts, blue-ribbon panels, or ad hoc review panels.

The third category of expert-oriented reviews is individual reviews. With such a review, an individual professional is selected for his/her expertise to judge the value of the item being reviewed (Fitzpatrick et al., 2004). The use of an external evaluator to review a program, such as when the lead health educator from the state department of health is asked to evaluate the health education unit of a local health department, provides an example of this type of review. Typically, this type of review is conducted to increase awareness and appreciation of a program in order to lead to improved standards and better performance (House, 1980).

Participant-Oriented Approaches

In all of the approaches presented so far in this chapter, the primary focus of each has been on something other than serving the needs of the priority population. It is not that those who use the previous approaches are unconcerned about the priority population, but the evaluation process does not begin with the priority population (Fitzpatrick et al., 2004). The **participant-oriented approaches** are different. They focus on a process "in which involvement of participants (stakeholders in that which is evaluated) are central in determining the values, criteria, needs, data, and conclusions for the evaluation" (Fitzpatrick et al., 2004, p. 68). In addition, their characteristics of less structure and fewer constraints, informal communication and reporting, and less attention to goals and objectives may be a drawback for those who want more formal, objective-type evaluation.

Fitzpatrick and colleagues (2004) have identified the following common elements of participant-oriented approaches:

1. *They depend on inductive reasoning.* Understanding an issue or event or process comes from grassroots observation and discovery. Understanding emerges; it is not the end product of some preordinate inquiry plan projected before the evaluation is conducted.

2. *They use multiplicity of data.* Understanding comes from the assimilation of data from a number of sources. Subjective and objective, qualitative and quantitative representations of the phenomena being evaluated are used.

3. *They do not follow a standard plan.* The evaluation process evolves as participants gain experience in the activity. Often the important outcome of the evaluation is a rich understanding of one specific entity with all the idiosyncratic contextual influences, process variations, and life histories. It is important in and of itself for what it tells about the phenomena that occurred.

4. *They record multiple rather than single realities.* People see things and interpret them in different ways. No one knows everything that happens in a school, or in the tiniest program. And no one perspective is accepted as *the* truth. Because only an individual can truly know what she has experienced, all perspectives are accepted as correct, and a central task of the evaluator is to capture these realities and portray them without sacrificing the program's complexity (pp. 133–134).

Examples of participant-oriented approaches include the responsive model (Stake, 1983), participatory evaluation, and empowerment evaluation. Responsive evaluation focuses on program activities rather than on goals or outcomes, looks at the priority population requirements for information, and considers the perspective of the participants in determining success or failure. The evaluator uses techniques such as observations and narratives about the program, validating the findings with participants and program staff. Much of this type of evaluation is informal, even the communication of the findings (Stake, 1983).

"Participatory approaches to evaluation attempt to involve in an evaluation all who have a stake in the outcomes, with a view to taking action and effecting change" (Springett, 2003, p. 264). The approach is one that grew out of the participatory research movement of the 1980s and 1990s (Fitzpatrick et al., 2004). As its title implies, those in the priority population are active participants in the evaluative process and have a joint responsibility for the evaluation. The participatory evaluation approach has been defined as evaluation that is carried out by having practice-based decision makers working in partnership with trained evaluators (Cousins & Earl, 1995). Table 14.2 provides a comparison of the differences between conventional evaluation and participatory evaluation. The application of participatory evaluation in health promotion is relatively new, but it has been used in some community health promotion programming. For those interested in learning more about participatory evaluation and its application to health promotion we refer you to Springett (2003).

Probably the most recently recognized approach to participant-oriented evaluation is empowerment evaluation. Though it was first discussed in the late 1980s, it became more visible in the mid-1990s. Empowerment evaluation is much like participatory evaluation but it includes the idea that evaluators not only facilitate the

Table 14.2 Differences between conventional evaluation
and participatory evaluation

	Conventional Evaluation	Participatory Evaluation
Who	External experts	Community, project staff facilitator
What	Predetermined indicators of success, primarily cost and health outcomes or gains	People identify their own indicators of success, which may include health outcomes and gains
How	Focus on "scientific objectivity," distancing evaluators from other participants; uniform, complex procedures; delayed, limited access to results	Self-evaluation; simple methods adapted to local culture; open, immediate sharing of results through local involvement in evaluation processes
When	Usually completion; sometimes also midterm	Merging of monitoring and evaluation; hence frequent small-scale evaluations
Why	Accountability, usually summative, to determine if funding continues	To empower local people to initiate, control, and take corrective action

Source: Springett, J. (2003). Issues in participatory evaluation. In M. Minkler & N. Wallerstein (Eds.), *Community-based participatory research for health* (pp. 263–288). San Francisco, CA: Jossey-Bass. p. 269.

participation of those from the priority population, "but also become advocates for societies' disenfranchised and voiceless minorities" (Fitzpatrick et al., 2004, p. 143). Thus as part of the evaluation process, evaluators also train those from the priority population to conduct their own evaluations and in turn the participants become more empowered. Participation then becomes more than just taking part; it is about engaging in a dialogue at all stages of the process of evaluation and shifting the power in favor of those in the priority population (Springett, 2003). Because of the newness of this approach to evaluation, only time will tell how useful it will become.

Framework for Program Evaluation

Once evaluators have selected the approach or approaches that will be used in the evaluation, they are ready to apply an evaluation framework. In 1999, the Centers for Disease Control and Prevention (CDC) (1999c) published an evaluation framework to be used with public health activities. Since the framework is applicable to all health promotion programs, an overview of it is provided here. The framework was developed by a working group that included evaluation experts, public health program managers and directors, state and local public health officials, teachers, researchers, U.S. Public Health Service agency representatives, and CDC staff.

The framework (see Figure 14.1) is comprised of six steps that must be completed in any evaluation, regardless of the setting. They are not a prescription; rather, they are starting points for tailoring the evaluation. The early steps provide the foundation, and all steps should be finalized before moving to the next step:

- *Step 1—Engaging stakeholders:* This step begins the evaluation cycle. Stakeholders must be engaged to insure that their perspectives are understood. The three primary groups of stakeholders are (1) those involved in the program operations,

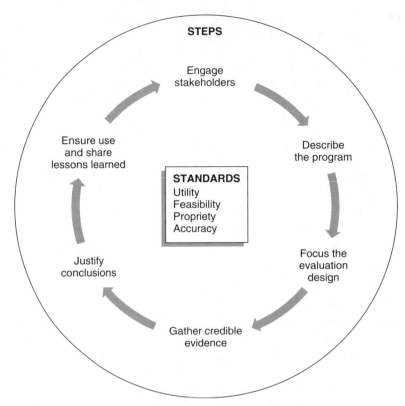

Figure 14.1 Framework for program evaluation

Source: Centers for Disease Control and Prevention (CDC) (1999c), p. 4.

(2) those served or affected by the program, and (3) the primary users of the evaluation results. The scope and level of stakeholder involvement will vary with each program being evaluated.

- *Step 2—Describing the program:* This step sets the frame of reference for all subsequent decisions in the evaluation process. At a minimum, the program should be described in enough detail that the mission, goals, and objectives are known. Also, the program's capacity to effect change, its stage of development, and how it fits into the larger organization and community should be known.

- *Step 3—Focusing the evaluation design:* This step entails making sure that the interests of the stakeholders are addressed while using time and resources efficiently. Among the items to consider at this step are articulating the purpose of the evaluation (i.e., gain insight, change practice, assess effects, affect participants), determining the users and uses of the evaluation results, formulating the questions to be asked, determining which specific design type will be used, and finalizing any agreements about the process.

- *Step 4—Gathering credible evidence:* This step includes many of the items mentioned in Chapter 5 of this text. At this step, evaluators need to decide on the measurement indicators, sources of evidence, quality and quantity of evidence, and logistics for collecting the evidence.

- *Step 5—Justifying conclusions:* This step includes the comparison of the evidence against the standards of acceptability; interpreting those comparisons; judging the worth, merit, or significance of the program; and creating recommendations for actions based upon the results of the evaluation.

- *Step 6—Ensuring use and sharing lessons learned:* This step focuses on the use and dissemination of the evaluation results. When carrying out this final step, concern must be given to each group of stakeholders.

In addition to the six steps of the framework, there are four standards of evaluation. These standards are noted in the box at the center of Figure 14.1. The standards provide practical guidelines for the evaluators to follow when having to decide among evaluation options. For example, these standards help evaluators avoid evaluations that may be "accurate and feasible but not useful or one that would be useful and accurate but is infeasible" (CDC, 1999c, p. 27). The four standards are:

- "Utility standards ensure that information needs of evaluation users are satisfied" (CDC, 1999c, p. 27).

- "Feasibility standards ensure that the evaluation is viable and pragmatic" (CDC, 1999c, p. 27).

- "Propriety standards ensure that the evaluation is ethical (i.e., conducted with regard for the rights and interests of those involved and effected)" (CDC, 1999c, p. 27).

- "Accuracy standards ensure that the evaluation produces findings that are considered correct" (CDC, 1999c, p. 29).

Selecting an Evaluation Design

As noted earlier in the chapter, evaluators must give careful consideration to the evaluation design, since the design is critical to the outcome of the program.

There are few perfect evaluation designs, because no situation is ideal, and there are always constraining factors, such as limited resources. The challenge is to devise an *optimal* evaluation—as opposed to an *ideal* evaluation (CDC, 1999c). Planners should give much thought to selecting the best design for each situation. The following questions may be helpful in the selection of a design:

- How much time do you have to conduct the evaluation?
- What financial resources are available?
- How many participants can be included in the evaluation?
- Are you more interested in qualitative or quantitative data?
- Do you have data analysis skills or access to computers and statistical consultants?
- In what ways can validity be increased?
- Is it important to be able to generalize your findings to other populations?
- Are the stakeholders concerned with validity and reliability?
- Do you have the ability to randomize participants into experimental and control groups?
- Do you have access to a comparison group?

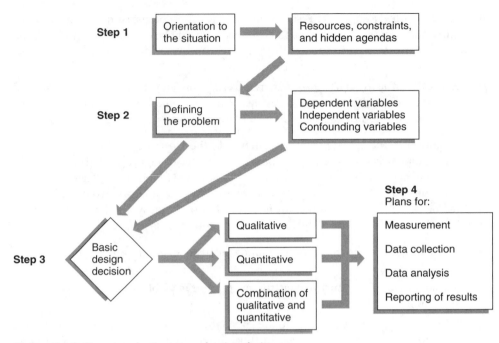

Figure 14.2 Steps in selecting an evaluation design

Source: From M.B. Dignan, *Measurement and Evaluation of Health Education,* third edition, 1995, p. 151. Courtesy of Charles C. Thomas Publisher, Ltd., Springfield, Illinois.

Dignan (1995) presents four steps in choosing an evaluation design. These four steps are outlined in Figure 14.2. The first step is to orient oneself to the situation. The evaluator must identify resources (time, personnel), constraints, and hidden agendas (unspoken goals). During this step, the evaluator must determine what is to be expected from the program and what can be observed.

The second step involves defining the problem—determining what is to be evaluated. During this step, definitions are needed for independent variables (what the sponsors think makes the difference), dependent variables (what will show the difference), and confounding variables (what the evaluator thinks could explain additional differences).

The third step involves making a decision about the design—that is, whether to use qualitative or quantitative methods of data collection or both. The **quantitative method** is **deductive** in nature (applying a generally accepted principle to an individual case), so that the evaluation produces numeric (hard) data, such as counts, ratings, scores, or classifications. Examples of quantitative data would be the number of participants in a stress-management program, the ratings on a participant satisfaction survey, and the pretest scores on a nutrition knowledge test. This method is suited to programs that are well defined and compares outcomes of programs with those of other groups or the general population. It is the method most often used in evaluation designs.

The **qualitative method** is an **inductive** method (individual cases are studied to formulate a general principle) and produces narrative (soft) data, such as descrip-

---

Box 14.1 Qualitative Methods Used in Evaluation

Case studies: In-depth examinations of a social unit, such as an individual, family, household, worksite, community, or any type of institution as a whole

Content analysis: A systematic review identifying specific characteristics of messages

Delphi techniques: See Chapter 4 for an in-depth discussion of the Delphi technique

Elite interviewing: Interviewing that focuses on a certain type ("elite") of respondent

Ethnographic studies: A variety of techniques (participant-observer, observation, interviewing, and other interactions with people) used to study an individual or group

Films, photographs, and videotape recording (film ethnography): Includes the data collection and study of visual images

Focus group interviewing: See Chapter 4 for an in-depth discussion of focus group interviewing

Historical analysis: A review of historical accounts that may include an interpretation of the impact on current events

In-depth interviewing: A less structured, deeper interview in which the interviewees share their view of the world

Kinesics: "The study of body communication" (p. 233)

Nominal group process: See Chapter 4 for an in-depth discussion of the nominal group process

Participant-observer studies: Those in which the observers (evaluators) also participate in what they are observing

Quality circle: "A group of people who meet at regular intervals to discuss problems and to identify possible solutions" (p. 236)

Unobtrusive techniques: "Data collection techniques that do not require the direct participation or cooperation of human subjects" (p. 236) and include such things as unobtrusive observation, review of archival data, and study of physical traces

Source: Adapted from McDermott and Sarvela (1999).

---

tions. This is a good method to use for programs that emphasize individual outcomes or in cases where other descriptive information from participants is needed. Box 14.1 provides a summary of the various qualitative methods presented by McDermott and Sarvela (1999).

Patton (1988) offers a checklist to determine whether qualitative data might be appropriate in a particular program evaluation. Collecting qualitative data may be a good strategy if there is a need to describe individual outcomes, to understand the dynamics and process of the programs, to obtain in-depth information on certain clients or sites, to focus on the diversity of program clients or sites; or to gather information to improve the program during formative evaluation.

Rather than choose one method, it may be advantageous to combine quantitative and qualitative methods. Steckler, McLeroy, and colleagues (1992) have discussed integrating qualitative and quantitative methods, since, to a certain extent, the weaknesses of one method is compensated for by the strengths of the other. Figure 14.3 illustrates four ways that the qualitative and quantitative methods might be integrated. In Model 1, qualitative methods are used to help develop quantitative methods and instruments. For example, evaluators could use a focus group with stakeholders to determine what type of questions should be included on a data collection instrument.

Model 1
Qualitative methods are used to help develop
quantitative measures and instruments.

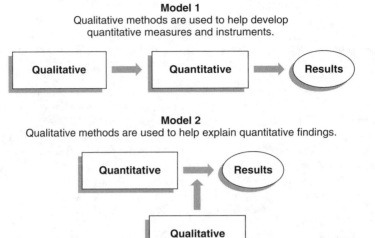

Model 2
Qualitative methods are used to help explain quantitative findings.

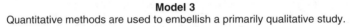

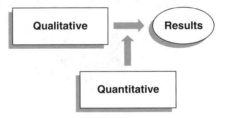

Model 3
Quantitative methods are used to embellish a primarily qualitative study.

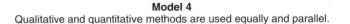

Model 4
Qualitative and quantitative methods are used equally and parallel.

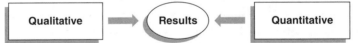

Figure 14.3 Four possible ways that qualitative and quantitative methods might be integrated

Source: A. Steckler, K.R. McLeroy, R.M. Goodman, S.T. Bird, & L. McCormick, "Toward Integrating Qualitative and Quantitative Methods: An Introduction," *Health Education Quarterly,* 19 (1), p. 5. Copyright © 1992 by Sage Publications, Inc. Reprinted by Permission of Sage Publications, Inc.

With Model 2, qualitative results are used to help interpret and explain findings from a quantitative evaluation. For example, evaluators could collect quantitative data from a large sample of people and more in-depth qualitative data from a few in the sample. Supplementing the hard data with anecdotal information further describes the findings. Model 3 is just the reverse of Model 2. In this model, quantitative results are used to help interpret predominately qualitative findings. For example, after observing a group of people for a period of time, evaluators may want to conduct a survey of the group. In the last model, Model 4, qualitative and quantitative are used equally and parallel to cross-validate the findings.

The fourth step in selecting an evaluation design includes choosing how to measure the dependent variable, deciding how to collect the data (these components were discussed in Chapter 5) and how the data will be analyzed, and determining how the results will be reported. (These components are discussed in Chapter 15.)

Experimental, Control, and Comparison Groups

As in research studies, when evaluating a health promotion program, the group of individuals who receive the intervention is known as the **experimental group.** The evaluation is designed to determine what effects the program has on these individuals. To make sure that the effects are caused by the program and not by some other factor, a **control group** should be used. The control group should be as similar to the experimental group as possible, but the members of this group do not receive the program (intervention or treatment) that is to be evaluated.

Without the use of a properly selected control group, the apparent effect of the program could actually be due to a variety of factors (confounding variables), such as differences in participants' educational background, environment, or experience. By using a control group, the evaluator can show that the results or outcomes are due to the program and not to confounding variables. In an ideal situation, participants should be randomly selected, then randomly assigned to one of two groups, and finally it should be randomly determined which group would become the experimental group and which the control group. Theoretically, this would evenly distribute the characteristics (independent variables) of the participants. This technique increases the credibility of the evaluation by controlling for extraneous events and factors.

It is not always possible or ethical to assign participants to a control group, especially if doing so would mean that they would be denied a necessary program or service. For example, a health promotion program could be designed for individuals with hypertension. Individuals diagnosed with hypertension could be referred by a physician into a health promotion class focused on reducing the risk factors associated with this disease. Denying some individuals access to the program in order to form a control group would clearly be unethical.

One way to deal with this problem is to provide the control group with an alternative program or to offer the regular program to the group at a later time (if a delay is not potentially harmful). Another alternative is to compare two programs: Offer an innovative program to some participants and continue the conventional program for others. Wagner and Guild (1989) see the advantage of this strategy as providing service to all participants (which fulfills a moral obligation) and still providing a comparison to assess the effectiveness of the innovative program.

Since the main purpose of social programs is to help clients, the client's viewpoint should be the primary one. It is important to keep this in mind when considering ethical issues in the use of control groups. Conner (1980) identifies four underlying premises for the use of control groups in social program evaluation:

1. All individuals have a right to status quo services.
2. All individuals involved in the evaluation are informed about the purpose of the study and the use of a control group.

3. Individuals have a right to new services, and random selection gives everyone a chance to participate.

4. Individuals should not be subjected to ineffective or harmful programs.

The ethical issues that must be considered involve the potential denial of a service and allocation of scarce resources. When randomization is not feasible, planners should consider an equitable process of providing services for individuals while maintaining control over the evaluation design.

When participants cannot be randomly assigned to an experimental or control group, a nonequivalent group may be selected. This is known as a **comparison group.** It is important to find a group that is as similar as possible to the experimental group, such as two classrooms of students with similar characteristics or a group of residents in two comparable cities. Factors to consider include participants' age, gender, education, location, socioeconomic status, and experience, as well as any other variable that might have an impact on program results.

Evaluation Designs

Measurements used in evaluation designs can be collected at three different times: after the program; both before and after the program; and several times before, during, and after the program. **Measurement** is defined by Green and Lewis (1986) as the method or procedure of assigning numbers to objects, events, and people. How such information is obtained has been discussed in Chapter 5.

Figure 14.4 presents evaluation designs commonly used in health promotion. In the figure, the letter O refers to measurement (or data collection), such as surveys, tests, interviews, observations, or other methods of gaining information. The O is also referred to as the dependent variable. When multiple measurements are taken, the subscript number behind each O indicates the order in which the measurements are made. Measurement before the program begins is known as the **pretest,** and measurement after the completion of the program is known as the **posttest.** The letter X represents the program (intervention, or independent variable); the relative positions of the two letters in the table indicate when measurements are made in relation to when the program is provided. The figure also shows which groups receive the program and when participants are randomly assigned to groups [(R)].

Windsor and colleagues (1994) differentiate among three types of evaluation designs: experimental, quasi-experimental, and nonexperimental. **Experimental design** offers the greatest control over the various factors that may influence the results (confounding variables). It involves random assignment to experimental and control groups with measurement of both groups. This evaluation design produces the most interpretable and defensible evidence of effectiveness. **Quasi-experimental design** results in interpretable and supportive evidence of program effectiveness, but usually cannot control for all factors that affect the validity of the results. There is no random assignment to the groups, and comparisons are made on experimental and comparison groups. **Nonexperimental design,** without the use of a comparison or control group, has little control over the factors that affect the validity of the results.

The most powerful design is the experimental design, in which participants are randomly assigned to the experimental and control groups. The difference between

Figure 14.4 Evaluation designs

I. Experimental design

1. Pretest-posttest design

—Experimental group	(R)	O_1	X	O_2			
—Control group	(R)	O_1		O_2			

2. Posttest-only design

—Experimental group	(R)		X	O			
—Control group	(R)			O			

3. Time series design

—Experimental group	(R)	O_1	O_2	O_3	X	O_4	O_5	O_6
—Control group	(R)	O_1	O_2	O_3		O_4	O_5	O_6

II. Quasi-experimental design

1. Pretest-posttest design

—Experimental group	O_1	X	O_2	
—Comparison group	O_1		O_2	

2. Time series design

—Experimental group	O_1	O_2	O_3	X	O_4	O_5	O_6
—Comparison group	O_1	O_2	O_3		O_4	O_5	O_6

III. Nonexperimental design

1. Pretest-posttest design

—Experimental group	O_1	X	O_2

2. Time series design

—Experimental group	O_1	O_2	O_3	X	O_4	O_5	O_6

Key: (R) = Random assignment
      O = Measurement/Observation
      X = Program/Intervention

designs I.1 and I.2 in Figure 14.4 is the use of a pretest to measure the participants before the program begins. Use of a pretest would help assure that the groups are similar and provide baseline measurement. Random assignment should equally distribute any of the variables (such as age, gender, and race) between the different groups. Potential disadvantages of the experimental design are that it requires a relatively large group of participants and that the intervention may be delayed for those in the control group.

A design more commonly found in evaluations of health promotion programs is the quasi-experimental pretest-posttest design using a comparison group (II.1 in Figure 14.4). This design is often used when a control group cannot be formed by random assignment. In such a case, a comparison group (a nonequivalent control group) is identified, and both groups are measured before and after the program. For example, a program on fire safety for two fifth-grade classrooms could be evaluated by using pre- and post-knowledge tests. Two other fifth-grade classrooms not receiving the program could serve as the comparison group. Similar pretest scores between the comparison and experimental groups would indicate that the groups were equal at the beginning of the program. However, without random assignment, it would be impossible to be sure that other variables (a unit on fire safety in a 4-H group, distribution of smoke detectors, information from parents) did not influence the results.

Sometimes participants cannot be assigned to a control group and no comparison group can be identified. In such cases, a nonexperimental pretest-posttest design (III.1 in Figure 14.4) can be used, but the results are of limited significance, since changes could be due to the program or to some other event. An example of this type of non-experimental design would be the incidence of safety belt use after a community program on that topic. An increase in use might mean that the program successfully motivated individuals to use safety belts; however, it could also reveal the impact of increased enforcement of the mandatory safety belt law, of a traffic fatality in the community, or a safety article in the local newspaper.

A time series evaluation design (I.3, II.2, III.2 in Figure 14.4) can be used to examine differences in program effects over time. Random assignment to groups (I.3) offers the most control over factors influencing the validity of the results. The use of a comparison group (II.2) offers some control; without a control group or comparison group (III.2), it is possible to determine changes in the participants over time, but one cannot be sure that the changes were due only to the program.

In the time series design, several measurements are taken over time both before and after the program is implemented. This process helps to identify other factors that may account for a change between the pretest and posttest measurements and is especially appropriate for measuring delayed effects of a program. A time series design could be used in a weight loss program to indicate the amount of weight loss over time and the ability to maintain a desired weight.

When more than one experimental group is part of the evaluation, they can be included in the designs we have discussed. These designs could be used to evaluate several types of programs—for example, to compare the effect of lectures, workshop, and self-study. Measurements could be collected from all groups at the same points in time, and programs could occur simultaneously.

Another design that may be used is the staggered treatment design (Figure 14.5), which is used to determine the effects of a program over time by including several measurements after the end of the program. It also indicates the effects of testing, since not all groups in this design receive a pretest. The staggered treatment design can also be used in quasi-experimental and nonexperimental designs, although with the limitations of not using a control group or comparison group.

Internal Validity

The **internal validity** of evaluation is the degree to which the program caused the change that was measured. Many factors can threaten internal validity, either singly or in combination, making it difficult to determine if the outcome was brought about by the program or some other cause. Cook and Campbell (1979) have identified some of the threats to internal validity, summarized as follows:

Figure 14.5 Staggered treatment design

Experimental group 1	(R)	X	O_1		O_2		O_3		O_4
Experimental group 2	(R)		O_1	X	O_2		O_3		O_4
Experimental group 3	(R)				O_1	X	O_2		O_3
Experimental group 4	(R)							X	O_1

Key: (R) = Random assignment
      O = Measurement/Observation
      X = Program

- *History* occurs when an event happens between the pretest and posttest that is not part of the health promotion program. An example of history as a threat to internal validity is having a national antismoking campaign coincide with a local smoking cessation program.

- *Maturation* occurs when the participants in the program show pretest-to-posttest differences due to growing older, wiser, or stronger. For example, in tests of muscular strength in an exercise program for junior high students, an increase in strength could be the result of muscular development and not the effect of the program.

- *Testing* occurs when the participants become familiar with the test format due to repeated testing. This is why it is helpful to use a different form of the same test for pretest and posttest comparisons.

- *Instrumentation* occurs when there is a change in the measuring between pretest and posttest, such as the observers becoming more familiar with or skilled in the use of the testing format over time.

- *Statistical regression* is when extremely high or low scores (which are not necessarily accurate) on the pretest are closer to the mean or average scores on the posttest.

- *Selection* reflects differences in the experimental and comparison groups, generally due to lack of randomization. Selection can also interact with other threats to validity, such as history, maturation, or instrumentation, which may appear to be program effects.

- *Mortality* refers to participants who drop out of the program between the pretest and posttest. For example, if most of the participants who drop out of a weight loss program are those with the least (or the most) weight to lose, the group composition is different at the posttest.

- *Diffusion or imitation of treatments* results when participants in the control group interact and learn from the experimental group. Students randomly assigned to an innovative drug prevention program in their school (experimental group) may discuss the program with students who are not in the program (control group), biasing the results.

- *Compensatory equalization of treatments* occurs when the program or services are not available to the control group and there is an unwillingness to tolerate the inequality. For instance, the control group from the previous example (students not enrolled in the innovative drug prevention program) may complain, since they are not able to participate.

- *Compensatory rivalry* is when the control group is seen as the underdog and is motivated to work harder.

- *Resentful demoralization of respondents receiving less desirable treatments* occurs among participants receiving the less desirable treatments compared to other groups, and the resentment may affect the outcome. For example, an evaluation to compare two different smoking cessation programs may assign one group (control) to the regular smoking cessation program and another group (experimental) to the regular program plus an exercise class. If the participants in the control group become aware that they are not receiving the additional exercise class, they may resent the omission, and this may be reflected in their smoking behavior and attitude toward the regular program.

The major way in which threats to internal validity can be controlled is through randomization. By random selection of participants, random assignment to groups, and random assignment of types of intervention or no intervention to groups, any differences between pretest and posttest can be interpreted as a result of the program. When random assignment to groups is not possible and quasi-experimental designs are used, the evaluator must make all threats to internal validity explicit and then rule them out one by one.

External Validity

The other type of validity that should be considered is **external validity,** or the extent to which the program can be expected to produce similar effects in other populations. This is also known as **generalizability.** The more a program is tailored to a particular population, the greater the threat to external validity, and the less likely it is that the program can be generalized to another group.

As with internal validity, several factors can threaten external validity. They are sometimes known as *reactive effects,* since they cause individuals to react in a certain way. The following are several types of threats to external validity:

- *Social desirability* occurs when individuals give a particular response to try to please or impress the evaluator. An example would be children who tell the teacher they brush their teeth every day, regardless of their actual behavior.

- *Expectancy effect* is when attitudes projected onto individuals cause them to act in a certain way. For example, in a drug abuse treatment program, the facilitator may feel that a certain individual will not benefit from the treatment; projecting this attitude may cause the individual to behave in self-defeating ways.

- *Hawthorne effect* refers to a behavior change because of the special status of those being tested. This effect was first identified in an evaluation of lighting conditions at an electric plant; workers increased their productivity when the level of lighting was raised as well as when it was lowered. The change in behavior seemed to be due to the attention given to them during the evaluation process.

- *Placebo effect* causes a change in behavior due to the participants' belief in the treatment.

Cook and Campbell (1979) discuss the threats to external validity in terms of statistical interaction effects. These include interaction of selection and treatment (the findings from a program requiring a large time commitment may not be generalizable to individuals who do not have much free time); interaction of setting and treatment (evaluation results from a program conducted on campus may not be generalizable to the worksite); and interaction of history and treatment (results from a program conducted on a historically significant day may not be generalizable to other days).

Conducting the program several times in a variety of settings, with a variety of participants, can reduce the threats to external validity. Threats to external validity can also be counteracted by making a greater effort to treat all subjects identically. In a **blind** study, the participants do not know what group (control or type of experimental group) they are in. In a **double blind** study, the type of group participants are in is not known by either the participants or the planners. In a **triple blind** study, this information is not available to the participants, planners, or evaluators.

It is important to select an evaluation design that provides both internal and external validity. This may be difficult, since lowering the threat to one type of validity may increase the threat to the other. For example, tighter evaluation controls make it more difficult to generalize the results to other situations. There must be enough control over the evaluation to allow evaluators to interpret the findings while sufficient flexibility in the program is maintained to permit the results to be generalized to similar settings.

SUMMARY

This chapter focused on evaluation approaches, an evaluation framework, and evaluation designs. Seven major approaches to evaluation were presented. No one approach is useful in all situations; therefore, evaluators should select an approach or parts of approaches to structure the evaluation based on the needs of the stakeholders involved with each program. The Framework for Program Evaluation in Public Health (CDC, 1999c) presents a process that is adaptable to all health promotion programs, yet is not prescriptive in nature.

The steps for selecting an evaluation design were also presented with a discussion about quantitative and qualitative methods. Evaluation design should be considered early in the planning process. Evaluators need to identify what measurements will be taken as well as when and how. In doing so, a design should be selected that controls for both internal and external validity.

REVIEW QUESTIONS

1. List the seven major approaches to evaluation presented in this chapter. What are the strengths and limitations of each of these approaches?

2. Of the seven major approaches to evaluation, which one is used most often with health promotion programs? Why?

3. What is the difference between cost-benefit analysis and cost-effectiveness analysis? Which is more appropriate for use in health promotion programs?

4. What are the six steps and four standards of the framework for program evaluation presented in this chapter? Why are the standards important?

5. What is the difference between quantitative and qualitative evaluation? When would one method be more appropriate than the other? How could they be combined in an evaluation design?

6. Name at least five different qualitative methods of evaluation and describe each.

7. What are the advantages of using a control group? What types of evaluation design do not use control groups? What is the difference between a control group and a comparison group?

8. What is the difference between experimental, quasi-experimental, and non-experimental designs? What are the strengths and weaknesses of each?

9. What is the difference between internal validity and external validity?

10. What are some considerations in the selection of an evaluation design presented in this chapter? What considerations can you add to this list?

ACTIVITIES

1. Identify which approach or approaches you would use in developing an evaluation for a program you are planning. Provide a rationale for your decision.

2. Look at an evaluation of a health promotion program that has been conducted in your community. Identify the evaluation approach that it most closely follows. Discuss your view with the program evaluator.

3. Talk with a program administrator or other decision makers about their view of evaluation; discuss the advantages and disadvantages of the major approaches from their perspective. For example, who should make the decision about how the evaluation results are used? What are the questions they would like answered? Conduct the same activity using program participants instead of administrators. How does the view of the participants differ from the view of administrators?

4. Develop an evaluation design for a program you are planning. Explain why you chose this design, and list the strengths and weaknesses of the design.

5. If you were hired to evaluate a safety belt program in a community, what evaluation design would you use and why? Assume you have all the resources you need to conduct the evaluation.

6. Explain what evaluation design you would use in evaluating the difference between two teaching techniques. Why would you choose this design?

WEBLINKS

1. **http://www.wmich.edu/evalctr/checklistl**
   The Evaluation Center at Western Michigan University (WMU)

   This is a page from the Evaluation Center at WMU website. This site provides evaluation specialists and users with refereed checklists. The site's purpose is to improve the quality and consistency of evaluations and enhance evaluation capacity through the promotion and use of high-quality checklists targeted to specific evaluation tasks and approaches. Visitors to this site can download a number of checklists and information on how to create them.

2. **http://www.cdc.gov/epo/mmwr/preview/mmwrhtml/rr4811a1.htm**
   Centers for Disease Control and Prevention

   This is a page from the CDC website that presents the entire issue of the *Morbidity and Mortality Weekly Report* [*MMWR* September 17, 1999 / 48(RR11);1-40] that presented the entire document *Framework for Program Evaluation in Public Health*. Visitors to this site can download the entire document.

3. **http://www.ucp-utica.org/uwlinks/outcomes.html**
   United Cerebral Palsy Association (UCPA), Greater Utica (N.Y.)

   This is a page from the UCPA of the Greater Utica area website. This page provides links to a variety of sites that provide information about outcome measurement and program evaluation.

4. **http://oerl.sri.com/**
   Online Evaluation Resource Library (OERL)

   This is the website for the OERL. This library, funded by the National Science Foundation (NSF), was developed for professionals seeking to design, conduct, document, or review project evaluations. OERL's resources include instruments, plans, and reports from evaluations that have proven to be sound and representative of current evaluation practices.

5. **http://www.ericae.net/main.htm**
   Educational Resources Information Center (ERIC)

   This is a page from the ERIC Clearinghouse on Assessment and Evaluation website. The site offers a variety of resources and seeks to provide balanced information concerning educational assessment, and resources to encourage responsible test use.

6. **http://national.unitedway.org/outcomes/**
   United Way of America (UWA)

   This is a page from UWA's website. This page is titled *Outcome Measurement Resource Network*. The *Resource Network* offers information, downloadable documents, and links to resources related to the identification and measurement of program- and community-level outcomes.

CHAPTER 15

Data Analysis and Reporting

Chapter Objectives

After reading this chapter and answering the questions at the end, you should be able to:

- Define data management.
- List examples of univariate, bivariate, and multivariate analysis and explain how they could be used in evaluation.
- Differentiate between descriptive and inferential statistics.
- Explain the difference between the null hypothesis and the alternative hypothesis in significance testing.
- Define *level of significance, Type I error,* and *Type II error.*
- Define *independent variable* and *dependent variable.*
- Describe how statistical results can be interpreted.
- Describe the format for the evaluation report, guidelines for presenting data, and ways to enhance the report.
- Discuss ways to increase the utilization of the evaluation findings.

Key Terms

alpha level
alternative hypothesis
analysis of variance (ANOVA)
bivariate data analysis
chi-square
correlation
data management
dependent variable
descriptive statistics
independent variable

inferential statistics
level of significance
mean
measures of central tendency
measures of spread or
  variation
median
missing data
mode
multiple regression

multivariate data analysis
null hypothesis
practical significance
program significance
range
statistical significance
Type I error
Type II error
univariate data analysis
variable

Like all other aspects of evaluation, the types of data analysis to be used in the evaluation should be determined in the program-planning stage. Basically, the analysis determines whether the outcome was different from what was expected. The evaluator then draws conclusions and prepares reports and/or presentations. The types of analysis to be used and how the information is presented are determined by the evaluation questions and the needs of the stakeholders.

This chapter describes different types of analyses commonly used in evaluating health promotion programs. To present them in detail or to include all possible techniques is beyond the scope of this text. If you need more information, refer to statistics textbooks, research methods and statistics courses, or statistical consultants.

Evaluations that suffer from major methodological problems are not likely to inspire confidence. A common problem is inadequate documentation of methods, results, and data analysis. The evaluation itself should be well designed; the report should contain a complete description of the program, objective interpretation of facts, information about the evaluation design and statistical analysis, and a discussion of features of the study that may have influenced the findings. In order to add accurate findings to the knowledge base of the profession, appropriate evaluation standards should be adopted to serve as guidelines for reporting and reviewing evaluation research (Moskowitz, 1989).

Data Management

Once the data have been collected (see Chapter 5 for data collection methods), they must be organized in such a manner that they can be analyzed in order to interpret the findings. To do this, the data, no matter if they are quantitative or qualitative, must be coded, cleaned, and organized into a usable format. These steps are collectively referred to as **data management.** By coded, we mean that the data are assigned labels so that they can be read and understood by a computer. To code data, a coding system must be established. The coding system outlines the process "through which raw data become translated for various forms of analysis (such as frequency counts, descriptive statistics, crosstabulations and other statistical procedures)" (McDermott & Sarvela, 1999, p. 77). For example, if the answer to a question on an instrument is yes, "yes" answers may be coded as the number "1" when entered into the computer, while "no" answers may be coded as a number "2." In addition to creating the coding scheme for raw data, a coding system also establishes rules for dealing with coding problems such as when respondents circle both "yes" and "no" for their answer to a question, or when neither "yes" nor "no" is circled but rather the space between the "yes" and "no" is circled.

Once the coded data have been entered into a computer system, they must be cleaned. "Data cleaning entails checking that the values are valid and consistent; i.e., all values correspond to valid question responses" (Valente, 2002, p. 136). For example, if the possible range of answers for a particular question is 1 to 3 and the frequency distribution identifies some 4s, those instruments with the 4s on them must be identified and checked to determine if the person completing the instrument made an error or if there was an error made by the person doing the data entry. If it was a data entry error, it should be corrected. If the person completing the data collection instrument made an error, it would be treated as no response to that question or as **missing data** (Cottrell & McKenzie, in press). Once the cleaning of the data has been completed, the appropriate data analysis can begin.

Data Analysis

The goal of data analysis is to reduce, organize, synthesize, and summarize information in order to make sense of it and to be able to make inferences about the priority population (Fitzpatrick et al., 2004; McDermott & Sarvela, 1999). Regardless of the type of data analysis to be used, the analysis begins with the identification of the variables of interest. A **variable** is a characteristic or attribute that can be measured or observed (Creswell, 2002). In program evaluation, the variables are divided into dependent and independent variables. **Independent variables** are ones that are either controlled by the evaluator or are not influenced by any other variable, whereas the **dependent variables** are the outcome variables being studied. "Independent variables influence dependent variables" (Valente, 2002, p. 165). Examples of independent variables include exposure to an intervention, gender, race, age, education, and income, while dependent variables may include, awareness, knowledge, attitudes, skills, and behaviors.

Statistics are used to analyze the variables. **Descriptive statistics** are used to organize, summarize, and describe characteristics of a group, while **inferential statistics** are concerned with relationships and causality in order to make generalizations (or inferences) about a population based upon findings from a sample. Statistical analyses also allow evaluators to measure the association and relationships between and among variables. When one variable is analyzed, it is called **univariate data analysis.** Analysis of two variables is called **bivariate** and analysis of more than two variables is referred to as **multivariate data analysis.**

The choice of a type of analysis is based on the evaluation questions, the type of data collected, and the audience who will receive the results (Newcomer, 1994). For some types of evaluation, descriptive data are all that is needed, and techniques are chosen to determine frequencies, counts or other univariate procedures. Other evaluation questions focus on testing a hypothesis about relationships between variables; in such cases, more elaborate statistical techniques are needed. Box 15.1 contains examples of the types of evaluation questions that can be answered by using different types of data analyses.

The level of measurement (i.e., nominal, ordinal, interval, or ratio, discussed in Chapter 5) is an important factor in selecting the type of data analysis. For the most part, analytical techniques have been developed for use with selected levels of measurement. In other words, not all analytical techniques can be used with all levels of measurement. For example, multiple regression analysis is a technique that has been reserved for use with interval and ratio data. Newcomer (1994) has created a very useful summary (see Table 15.1) to assist evaluators in selecting appropriate statistical techniques.

The issue of who will be the recipients of the final evaluation report should also be considered when selecting the type of analysis. Evaluators want to be able to present the evaluation results in a form that can be understood by the stakeholders. With regard to this issue, it is probably best to err on the side of too simple an analysis rather than one that is too complex.

> ## Box 15.1 Examples of Evaluation Questions Answered Using Univariate, Bivariate, and Multivariate Data Analysis
>
> | Univariate Analysis | Bivariate Analysis | Multivariate Analysis |
> |---|---|---|
> | What was the average score on the cholesterol knowledge test? | Is there a difference in smoking behavior between the individuals in the experimental and control groups after the healthy lifestyle program? | Can the risk of heart disease be predicted using smoking, exercise, diet, and heredity? |
> | How many participants at the worksite attended the healthy lifestyle presentation? | Is peer education or classroom instruction more effective in increasing knowledge about the effects of drug abuse? | Can mortality risk among motorcycle drivers be predicted from helmet use, time of day, weather conditions, and speed? |
> | What percentage of the participants in the corporate fitness program met their target goal? | Do students' attitudes about bicycle helmets differ in rural and urban settings? | |

Finally, regardless of the type of analysis selected for an evaluation, the method should be chosen early in the evaluation process and should be in place before the data are collected.

Univariate Data Analyses

Univariate data analysis examines one variable at a time. It is common for univariate analysis to be descriptive in nature. As noted earlier, descriptive statistics are used to describe, classify, and summarize data. Summary counts (frequencies) are totals, and they are the easiest type of data to collect and report. Summary counts could be used in formative evaluation—for example, to count the number of participants in blood pressure screening programs at various sites. The information would assist the planners in publicizing sites with low attendance or adding additional personnel to busy sites. Other examples of frequencies, or summary counts, are, for instance, the number of participants in a workshop, those who scored over 80% on a knowledge posttest, or the number of individuals wearing a safety belt.

Measures of central tendency are other forms of univariate data analyses. The **mean** is the arithmetic average of all the scores. The **median** is the midpoint of all the scores, dividing scores ranked by size into equal halves. The **mode** is the score that occurs most frequently. These are all useful in describing the results, and reporting all three measures of central tendency will be especially helpful if extreme scores are found.

Measures of spread or variation refers to how spread out the scores are. **Range** is the difference between the highest and lowest scores. For example, if the high score is 100 and the low score is 60, the range is 40. Measures of spread or variation—such as range, standard deviation, or variance—can be used to determine whether scores from groups are similar or spread apart.

Table 15.1 Selecting statistical techniques

Purpose of the Analysis	How the Variables Are Measured	Appropriate Technique	Appropriate Test for Statistical Significance	Appropriate Measure of Magnitude
To compare a sample distribution to a population distribution	Nominal/ordinal	Frequency counts	Chi-square	NA
	Interval	Means/medians, Standard deviations/interquartile range	Chi-square	NA
To analyze a relationship between two variables	Nominal/ordinal	Contingency tables	Chi-square	Percentage difference
	Interval	Contingency tables/test of differences of means	Chi-square or t	Difference in means
To reduce data through identifying factors that explain variation in a set of measures	Nominal/ordinal	NA	NA	NA
	Interval	Factor analysis	t	Pearson's correlations
To sort units into similar clusters or groupings	Nominal/ordinal	NA	NA	NA
	Interval	Cluster or discriminant analysis	t	Equivalent of R-square
To predict or estimate program impact	Nominal/ordinal	Loglinear regression	t and F	R-square, beta weights
	Interval	Regression	t and F	beta weights
To describe or predict a trend in a series of data collected over time	Nominal/ordinal	Regression	t and F	R-square, beta weights
	Interval	Regression	t and F	Same as above

Note: NA = not applicable

Bivariate Data Analyses

Bivariate data analyses are used to study two variables simultaneously. Such analyses "are usually used to determine the presence of relationships or differences between groups" (McDermott & Sarvela, 1999, p. 300). When using bivariate analyses, it is common to state evaluation questions in the form of hypotheses. The **null hypothesis** holds that there is no observed difference between the groups. The **alternative hypothesis** says that there is a difference between the groups. For example, a null hypothesis might state that there is no difference between the two groups, say men and women, in knowledge about cancer risk factors, while the alternative hypothesis states that there is a difference.

Statistical tests are used to determine if the relationships or differences between groups are statistically significant. **Statistical significance** "refers to whether the observed differences between the two or more groups are real or not, or whether they are chance occurrences" (McDermott & Sarvela, 1999, p. 300). In other words, statistical tests are used to determine whether the null hypothesis can be rejected (meaning a relationship between the groups probably does exist) or whether it should be retained (indicating that any apparent relationship between groups is due to chance).

There is the possibility that the null hypotheseis can be rejected when it is, in fact, true; this is known as **Type I error.** There is also the possibility of failing to reject the null hypothesis when it is, in fact, not true; this a **Type II error.** The probability of making a Type I error is reflected in the alpha level. The **alpha level,** or **level of significance,** is established before the statistical tests are run and is generally set at .05 or .01. This indicates that the decision to reject the null hypothesis is incorrect 5% (or 1%) of the time; that is, there is a 5% probability (or 1% probability) that the outcome occurred by chance alone.

When a smaller alpha level is used (.01 or .001), the possibility of making a Type I error is reduced; at the same time, however, the possibility of a Type II error increases. An example of a Type I error is the adoption of a new program due to higher scores on a knowledge test, when, in reality, increases in knowledge occurred by chance and the new program is not more effective than the existing program. An example of a Type II error is not adopting the new program when it is, in reality, more effective.

Bivariate analyses that are commonly used in program evaluation include chi-square, *t*-tests, analysis of variance, and correlations. **Chi-square** is a statistical test "that measures the association between two nominal and/or ordinal variables" (Valente, 2002, p. 170). An example of this type of analysis would be measuring the association of grade levels (i.e., third and fifth grades) with the attitudes of children toward the use of bicycle helmets (i.e., strongly agree, agree, disagree, and strongly disagree).

While chi-square is used to study nominal and/or ordinal variables, *t*-tests and **analysis of variance (ANOVA)** are statistical tests used to study group differences when the dependent variables are interval or ratio data (e.g., scores on a test). There are several situations in which a *t*-test could be used. The most common use of a *t*-test is to determine whether a variable changed significantly in one group at two different points in time, say between baseline before the intervention (referred to as a pre-test) and at follow-up after the intervention (referred to as a post-test). This type of *t*-test is called a dependent *t*-test. A second common use of a *t*-test is to study the differences between two groups at a single point in time. An example of such a situation is the comparison of nutrition knowledge test scores after two groups have been exposed to different nutrition education interventions. This type of *t*-test is called an independent *t*-test.

ANOVA is a statistical test that could be used to study differences between two groups just like a *t*-test, but is more commonly used to study differences between more than two groups. For example, an ANOVA could be used to determine if there was a difference in the test scores of three groups (i.e., different age groups like 15–24, 24–45, and 46–65 year olds) on a physical activity knowledge test following exposure to a single health promotion intervention.

While the bivariate analyses discussed so far are used to determine if differences exist between groups, **correlations** are used to study the strength and direction of relationships between two variables (McDermott & Sarvela, 1999). Correlations are expressed as values between +1 (a positive correlation) and −1 (a negative correlation), with a 0 indicating no relationship between the variables. "The higher the value of the correlation coefficient is (regardless of direction) the stronger the relationship between the two variables" (McDermott & Sarvela, 1999, p. 304).

Correlation between variables only indicates a relationship; this technique does not establish cause and effect. An example of the use of correlation would be to determine the relationship between safety belt use and age of the driver. If older people were found to wear their safety belts more often than younger people, that would constitute a positive correlation between age and belt use. If younger people wore their safety belts more often, it would be a negative correlation. If age made no difference in who wore the belts more often, the correlation would be 0.

Multivariate Data Analyses

Multivariate data analyses are used to study three or more variables simultaneously. Typically, such analyses are used in more advanced evaluation designs, and thus will not be discussed in detail here because of the scope of this text. Examples of multivariate analyses include multiple regression, discriminant analysis, and factor analysis. Of these, the one most commonly used in health promotion evaluation is **multiple regression.** "There are many different types of multiple regression, including stepwise regression, logistic regression, and general linear regression" (McDermott & Sarvela, 1999, p. 305). Though the procedures and applications for various types of regression differ, they are "useful in exploring relationships among variables or in exploring the independent effects of many variables on one dependent variable" (Fitzpatrick et al., 2004, p.359). An example of the later would be trying to predict the risk of heart disease (the dependent variable) using the independent variables of smoking, exercise, diet, and family history.

Applications of Data Analyses

Many evaluation concepts have been presented—so many, in fact, that you might find it difficult to keep them all clear in your mind or to apply them. Therefore a few examples here will help you see how to move from a program goal to an intervention to an evaluation design to data analysis. To illustrate these concepts, a couple of statistics have been selected that are commonly used with health promotion programs: chi-square and *t*-tests.

Case #1

Program goal: Reduce the prevalence of smoking in the priority population
Priority population: The seventy smoking employees of Company XYZ
Intervention (independent variable): Two different smoking cessation programs
Variable of interest (dependent variable): Smoking cessation after one year
Evaluation design:

$$R \quad A \quad X_1 \quad O_1$$
$$R \quad B \quad X_2 \quad O_1$$

where:

$$R = \text{random assignment}$$
$$A = \text{group A}$$
$$B = \text{group B}$$
$$X_1 = \text{method 1}$$
$$X_2 = \text{method 2}$$
$$O_1 = \text{self-reported smoking behavior}$$

Data collected: Nominal data; quit yes or no

	Smoking Employees	
	Group A Method 1	Group B Method 2
Quit	24%	33%
Did not quit	76%	67%

Data analysis: A chi-square test of statistical significance can be used to test the null hypothesis that there is no difference in the success of the two groups.

Case #2

Program goal: Increase the AIDS knowledge of the priority population
Priority population: The 1,200 new freshmen at ABC University
Intervention (independent variable): A two-hour lecture-discussion program given during the freshmen orientation program
Variable of interest (dependent variable): AIDS knowledge
Evaluation design:

$$O_1 \quad X \quad O_2$$

where:

$$O_1 = \text{pretest scores}$$
$$X = \text{two-hour program at freshman orientation}$$
$$O_2 = \text{posttest scores}$$

Data collection: Ratio data; scores on 100-point-scale test

	Test Results	
	Pretest	Posttest
Number of students	1,200	1,200
Mean score	69.0	78.5

Data analysis: A dependent *t*-test of statistical significance can be used to test the null hypothesis that there is no difference between the pre- and post-test means on the knowledge test.

Case #3

Program goal: To improve the testicular self-examination skills of the priority population

Priority population: All boys enrolled in the eighth grade at Jones Junior High School

Intervention (independent variable): Two-week unit on testicular cancer

Variable of interest (dependent variable): Score on testicular self-exam skills test

Evaluation design:

$$A \quad O_1 \quad X \quad O_2$$
$$B \quad O_1 \qquad O_2$$

where:

$$A = \text{eighth-grade boys at Jones Junior High School}$$
$$B = \text{eighth-grade boys at Hastings Junior High School}$$
$$O_1 = \text{pretest scores}$$
$$X = \text{two-week unit on testicular cancer}$$
$$O_2 = \text{posttest scores}$$

Data collected: Ratio data; scores on 100-point skills test

Test Results

	Jones Junior High ($n = 142$)	Hastings Junior High ($n = 131$)
Pre	62	63
Post	79	65

Data analysis: An independent *t*-test of statistical significance can be used to (1) test the null hypothesis that there is no difference in the pretest scores of the two groups, since the groups were not randomly assigned, and (2) test the null hypothesis that there is no differences in the posttest scores of the two groups.

Interpreting the Data

With the data analyses completed, attention must turn to interpreting the data. By interpretation we mean, attaching meaning to the analyzed data and drawing conclusions (Fitzpatrick et al., 2004). "Interpretation should be characterized by careful, fair, open methods of inquiry. Anyone who claims that the 'numbers speak for themselves' is either naive or a shyster" (Fitzpatrick et al., 2004, p. 364).

To insure that the interpretation is fair and as objective as possible, it is recommended that the interpretation not be the sole responsibility of the evaluator or, for that matter, any other single person. At the beginning of Chapter 13 when we began our discussion of evaluation, we spoke of the importance of making sure that the evaluation process is a collaborative process that includes representation from all of the stakeholders. That principle applies not only to the planning of the evaluation, but also to the interpretation of the data. Several authors (Fitzpatrick et al., 2004; Patton, 1986; Solomon, 1987; Weiss, 1984) have recommended bringing the stakeholders and evaluator together in one or more meetings to systematically review the findings. Such meetings take advantage of the diverse perspectives of the stakeholders, as well as allow for a discussion of the implications of various interpretative conclusions.

There is no single method used to interpret data. In fact, there are a number of different methods that could be used. Fitzpatrick and colleagues (2004) have identified eight methods that have served well in the recent past. They include:

1. Determining whether objectives have been achieved;
2. Determining whether laws, democratic ideals, regulations, or ethical principles have been violated;
3. Determining whether assessed needs have been reduced;
4. Determining the value of accomplishments;
5. Asking critical reference groups to review the data and to provide their judgments of successes and failures, strengths, and weaknesses;
6. Comparing results with those reported by similar entities or endeavors;
7. Comparing assessed performance levels on critical variables to expectations of performance or standards;
8. Interpreting results in light of evaluation procedures that generated them (p. 364).

Finally, the interpretation of the results must distinguish between **program significance** (**practical significance**) and statistical significance. Programmatic significance measures the meaningfulness of a program regardless of statistical significance. Statistical significance is determined by statistical testing. It is possible—especially when a large number of people are included in the data collection—to have statistically significant results that indicate gains in performance but are not meaningful in terms of program goals. For example, say the mean scores on a knowledge test of two groups are 70 and 69 (out of 100 points). If the groups are large enough, it would be possible that the difference in the scores (i.e., 1 point) could be statistically significant. But in practical terms, does the group with a mean score of 70 have more knowledge that will translate more informed consumers? Probably not! Thus spending extra dollars on the program that generated the mean score of 70 versus the less expensive program that generated a mean score of 69 would really not be cost-effective. Statistical significance is similar to reliability in that they are both measures of precision. It is important to consider whether statistical significance justifies the development, implementation, and costs of a program (Fink & Kosecoff, 1978).

Evaluation Reporting

The results and interpretation of the data analyses, as well as a description of the evaluation process, are incorporated into the final report to be presented to the stakeholders. The report itself generally follows the format of a research report, including an introduction, methodology, results, conclusions, and discussion.

Some may see the creation of an evaluation report as a waste of time or a nonessential step in the larger process of evaluation, however an evaluation report is essential for several reasons (Wurzbach, 2002). An evaluation report can provide:

- the discipline to help you critically analyze the results of the evaluation and think about any changes you should make as a result

- a tangible product for your agency

- evidence that your program or materials have been carefully developed—to be used as a sales tool with gatekeepers (e.g., television station public service directors)

- a record of your activities for use in planning future programs

- assistance to others who may be interested in developing similar programs or materials

- a foundation for evaluation activities in the future (e.g., it is easier to design a new questionnaire based upon one you have previously used than to start anew) (p. 590)

The number and type of reports needed are determined at the beginning of the evaluation based on the needs of the stakeholders. For a formative evaluation, reports are needed early and may be provided on a weekly or monthly basis. The formative evaluations may be formal or informal, ranging from scheduled presentations to informal telephone calls. They must be submitted on time in order to provide immediate feedback so that program modifications can be made. Generally, a report is submitted at the end of an evaluation and may be written and/or oral.

Evaluators must be able to communicate to all audiences when presenting the results of the evaluation. The reaction of each audience—participants, media, administrators, funding source—must be anticipated in order to prepare the necessary information. In some cases, technical information must be included; in other cases, anecdotal information may be appropriate. The evaluator must fit the report to the audience as well as prepare for a negative response if the results of the evaluation are not favorable. This involves looking critically at the results and developing responses to anticipated reactions.

The format for communicating the evaluation results may include several methods, such as a technical report, journal article, news release, meeting, presentation, press conference, letter, or workshop. Generally, more than one method is selected in order to meet the needs of all stakeholders. For example, following an innovative worksite health promotion program, the evaluator might prepare a news release for the community, a letter to all staff who participated, a technical report for the funding source, and an executive summary for the administrators.

Designing the Written Report

As previously mentioned, the evaluation report follows a similar format to that used in a research report. The evaluation report generally includes the following sections:

- *Abstract or executive summary:* This is a summary of the total evaluation including goals and objectives, methods, results, conclusions, and recommendations. It is a concise presentation of the evaluation since it may be the only portion of the report that some of the stakeholders may read. Most abstracts/executive summaries range in length from 150 to 600 words.

Box 15.2 What to Include in the Evaluation Report

Abstract/executive summary	Overview of the program and evaluation
	General results, conclusions, and recommendations
Introduction	Purpose of the evaluation
	Program and participant description (including staff, materials, activities, procedures, etc.)
	Goals and objectives
	Evaluation questions
Methods/procedures	Design of the evaluation
	Priority population
	Instrumentation, including information on validity and reliability
	Sampling procedures
	Data collection procedures
	Pilot study results
	Limitations
	Data analyses procedures
Results	Description of findings from data analyses
	Answers to evaluation questions
	Addresses any special concerns
	Explanation of findings
	Charts and graphs of findings
Conclusions/recommendations	Interpretation of results
	Conclusions about program effectiveness
	Program recommendations
	Determining if additional information is needed

- *Introduction:* This section of the report includes a complete description of the program and the evaluation. Goals and objectives of the program are listed, as are the evaluation questions to be answered.

- *Methods/procedures:* The methods/procedures section of the report includes information on the evaluation design, the priority groups, the instruments used, and how the data were collected and analyzed.

- *Results:* This section is the main part of the report. It includes the findings from the evaluation, summarizing and simplifying the data and presenting them in a clear, concise format. Data are presented for every evaluation question.

- *Conclusions/recommendations:* This section uses the findings (presented in the previous section) to answer the evaluation questions. The results are interpreted to determine significance and explanations. Judgments and recommendations are included in this section; they may have been made by the evaluator and/or the administrator, depending on the evaluation model used.

Box 15.2 summarizes what is included in the evaluation report.

Presenting Data

The data that have been collected and analyzed are presented in the evaluation report. The presentation of the data should be simple and straightforward. Graphic displays and tables may be used to illustrate certain findings; in fact, they are often a central part of the report. They also often make it easier for the readers of a written report or the audience for an oral report to understand the findings of an evaluation. When presenting the data in graphic form it is often helpful to include a frame of reference— such as a comparison with national, state, local, or other data—and explain any limitations of the data. If graphic displays are used in a report, it is recommended (USDHHS, CDC, no date) that such displays are appropriate for the results:

1. Use horizontal bar charts to focus attention on how one category differs from another.
2. Use vertical bar charts to focus attention on a change in a variable over time.
3. Use cluster bar charts to contrast one variable among multiple subgroups.
4. Use line graphs to plot data for several periods and show a trend over time.
5. Use pie charts to show the distribution of a set of events or a total quantity.

If many tables are included, the main ones can be placed in the text of the report and the rest relegated to an appendix. Box 15.3 lists guidelines to follow when presenting data in the evaluation report and/or presentation.

How and When to Present the Report

Evaluators must consider carefully the logistics of presenting the evaluation findings. They should discuss this with the decision makers involved in the evaluation. An evaluator may be in the position of presenting negative results, encountering distrust among staff members, or submitting a report that will never be read. Following are several suggestions for enhancing the evaluation report:

- Give key decision makers advance information on the findings; this increases the likelihood that the information will actually be used and prevents the decision makers from learning about the results from the media or another source.

- Maintain anonymity of individuals, institutions, and organizations; use sensitivity to avoid judging or labeling people in negative ways; maintain confidentiality of the final report according to the wishes of the administrators; maintain objectivity throughout the report (Windsor et al., 1994).

- Choose ways to report the evaluation findings so as to meet the needs of the stakeholders, and include information that is relevant to each group.

Increasing Utilization of the Results

Far too often an evaluation will be conducted and a report submitted to the decision makers, but the recommendations will not be implemented. This occurs for a variety of reasons. Decision makers may not use findings because they are conducting the evaluation only to fulfill the requirements of the funding source, to serve their own self-interest, or to gain recognition for a successful program. Even decision makers who plan to use the evaluation results in their health promotion program may find

---

Box 15.3 Guidelines for Presenting Data

1. Use graphic methods of presenting numerical data whenever possible.
2. Build the results and discussion section of the evaluation report—and perhaps other sections as well—around tables and figures. Prepare the tables and graphs first; then write text to explain them.
3. Make each table and figure self-explanatory. Use a clear, complete title, a key, label, footnotes, and so forth.
4. Discuss in the text the major information to be found in each table and figure.
5. Play with, and consider using, as many graphs as you have the time and ingenuity to prepare. Not only do they communicate clearly to your audiences, they also help you to see what is happening.
6. Since graphs tend to convey fewer details than numerical tables, consider providing both tables and graphs for the same data, where appropriate.
7. If you have used a mixed evaluation design with both quantitative and qualitative data collection procedures, use the direct quotations and descriptions from the qualitative results to add depth and clarity to information reported graphically.
8. When presenting complicated graphs to a live audience, give some instruction about how to read the graph and a few sample interpretations of simpler versions, then present the real data.
9. When a complete draft of the report has been completed, ask yourself the following questions:
   a. Do the figure titles give a comprehensive description of the figures? Could someone leafing through the report understand the graphs?
   b. Are both axes of every graph clearly labeled with a name?
   c. Is the interval size marked on all axes of graphs?
   d. Is the number of cases on which each summary statistic has been based indicated in each table or on each graph?
   e. Are the tables and figures labeled and numbered throughout the report?
   f. If the report is a lengthy one, does it include a list of tables and figures at the front following the table of contents?

Source: L. L. Morris, C. T. Fitz-Gibbon, and M. E. Freeman, *How to Communicate Evaluation Findings* (pp. 75–76). Copyright © 1987 by Sage Publications, Inc. Reprinted by permission of Sage Publications, Inc.

---

that they are unable to state the evaluation question or that the final report contains language and concepts that are unfamiliar to them. Weiss (1984) sees the need to improve the quality both of evaluation and of modes of disseminating the findings. Weiss developed the following guidelines to increase the chances that evaluation results will actually be used:

1. Plan the study with program stakeholders in mind and involve them in the planning process.
2. Continue to gather information about the program after the planning stage; a change in the program should result in a change in the evaluation.

3. Focus the evaluation on conditions about the program that the decision makers can change.

4. Write reports in a clear, simple manner and submit them on time. Use graphs and charts within the text, and include complicated statistical information in an appendix.

5. Base the decision on whether to make recommendations on how specific and clear the data are, how much is known about the program, and whether differences between programs are obvious. A joint interpretation between evaluator and stakeholders may be best.

6. Disseminate the results to all stakeholders, using a variety of methods.

7. Integrate evaluation findings with other research and evaluation about the program area.

8. Provide high-quality research.

SUMMARY

Evaluation questions developed in the early program-planning stages can be answered once the data have been analyzed. Descriptive statistics can be used to summarize or describe the data, and inferential statistics can be used to generate or test hypotheses. These statistics are generated by applying the appropriate univariate, bivariate, and/or multivariate analysis. Evaluators then interpret the data and present the results to the stakeholders via a formal or informal report.

REVIEW QUESTIONS

1. What are some common problems with evaluations, and how can these problems be reduced or overcome?

2. What is meant by the term data management?

3. What is the difference between descriptive and inferential statistics?

4. What are some types of univariate data analyses used in evaluation? When would these be used?

5. How are bivariate and multivariate data analyses used in evaluation?

6. Explain the concepts of hypothesis testing, level of significance, Type I error, and Type II error.

7. What is the role of evaluators and decision makers in interpreting the results and making recommendations?

8. What is the difference between statistical significance and program significance?

9. What information is included in the written evaluation report? How is the information modified for various audiences?

10. What are some guidelines for presenting data in an evaluation report?

11. How can the evaluation report be enhanced?

12. How can the evaluator increase the likelihood of utilization of the evaluation findings?

ACTIVITIES

1. Obtain an actual report from a program evaluation. Look for the type of statistical tests used, the level of significance, the independent and dependent variables, the interpretation of the findings, recommendations, and format for the report.

2. Discuss evaluation with a decision maker from a health agency. Find out what types of evaluation have been conducted, who has conducted them, what the findings have been, whether the findings were implemented, and how the information was reported.

3. Compare an evaluation report with a research report. What are the similarities and differences? How could you improve the report?

4. Using data that you have generated or data presented by your instructor, create one table and one graph.

WEBLINKS

1. **http://www.astho.org/**
   Association of State and Territorial Health Officials (ASTHO)

   This is the website for the ASTHO. The ASTHO is the national nonprofit organization representing the state and territorial public health agencies of the United States, the U.S. Territories, and the District of Columbia. ASTHO's members are the chief health officials of these jurisdictions. At this site you can link to all the state and territorial public health agencies where you can find various examples of the presentation of health data using charts, graphs, and tables.

2. **http://www.cancercontrol.cancer.gov/index.html**
   National Cancer Institute (NCI)

   This is a web page from the NCI website. This is the page that provides information on cancer control and population sciences. This site includes evaluation reports on a number of cancer education programs including the well known 5ADay program.

3. **http://www.adb.org/Evaluation/reports/asp**
   Asian Development Bank (ADB)

   This is a web page from the ADB website. The ADB, established 1966, is a multilateral development finance institution dedicated to reducing poverty in Asia and the Pacific. At this web page you can find a number of the final evaluation reports created by the ADB. These reports provide good examples of how final evaluation reports are formatted. Some of the reports deal with health-related topics.

4. **http://www.cdc.gov/train.htm**
   Centers for Disease Control and Prevention (CDC)

   This is a web page from the CDC website that lists training and employment opportunities. Several of the training opportunities relate to statistical data analysis and reporting.

5. **http://www.cdc.gov/nchs/**
   National Center for Health Statistics (NCHS)

   This is the website for the NCHS. It is a rich source of information about America's health and provides many examples of the presentation of health data.

6. **http://www.nhtsa.dot.gov/stsi/**
   State Traffic Safety Information (STSI)

   This is a web page from the National Center for Statistical Analysis of the National Highway Traffic Safety Administration website. STSI is a by-State profile of traffic safety data and information including: crash statistics, economic costs, legislation status, funding programs, and more. It provides a lot of examples of the presentation of health data using charts, graphs, and tables.

Appendixes

Examples of a News Release and Copy for a Newspaper Column

NEWS RELEASE

Delaware City-County Health Department

For Immediate Release   **Contact: Susan Sutherland**
                                              Phone: (740) 368–1700

Food Safety: A Health Department Priority at Fair

Health Inspectors are busy this week checking every food concession stand at the fair for food safety. Health Department staff are looking for proper food temperatures, concession stand cleanliness, a safe water supply, and proper control of insects.

"The Health Department provides this service to ensure that our community and guests to our county are protected from food borne illnesses such a E. coli and Salmonella," said Susan Sutherland, Food Protection Program Manager. Sutherland and her staff will be reminding all food handlers to wash their hands before they touch foods, thoroughly cook food and test for temperature by using a reliable food thermometer. "It's as simple as keeping hot foods hot and cold foods cold," advised Sutherland.

Should you have any questions about food safety, please contact Ms. Sutherland at the Health Department.

The Delaware City-County Health Department promotes good health and improved quality of life in Delaware County. For more information contact the Delaware City-County Health Department at (740)368–1700 or (740)548–7055. You may e-mail Susan Sutherland at ssutherland@iwaynet.net or you may visit the Health Department's home page at www.health.co.delaware.oh.us

–end–

Source: Reprinted by permission of Delaware City-County Health Department.

Delaware Gazette Bi-monthly Column
Roger Wren, Health Educator
February 24, 2000

WHICH AILMENT: COLD OR FLU?

Delaware City-County Health Department

Much to the displeasure of a great many people, winter is still alive and well. Colds and influenza are still around too, and it looks like they will be for awhile. When you catch one of these bugs, how do you know one from the other?

People associate sneezing, stuffy nose, and sore throat with both ailments, but they are more common with the cold than with the flu. People can have the flu and have none of these symptoms.

Chest congestion and coughing are common in both illnesses, but can be more severe with the flu. Being less severe, a cold's symptoms are usually limited to sneezing, runny nose, sore throat, coughing, and chest congestion, with the occasional complications of sinus infection and earache.

The flu has much more to offer! Sudden onset of high fever, headaches, muscle aches, and fatigue are in store with influenza. Fever is characteristic of the flu and usually ranges between 102 and 104 degrees Fahrenheit and lasts three to four days. Headaches are prominent, and fatigue, usually not much of a problem with a cold, hits early and hard and tends to last from two to three weeks.

Although sinus infections and earaches are annoying complications of a cold, flu can give you a nasty dose of bronchitis or even pneumonia as an encore. Suffice it to say that the flu is usually much more severe than your common cold.

The only thing preferable about the flu over a cold is that there are preventative measures and treatment for influenza but not for a cold. You have to ride out a cold, getting only temporary relief of the symptoms. An annual flu vaccination is a good start from a prevention standpoint, but if you are unfortunate enough to get the flu anyway, your doctor may be able to prescribe antiviral drugs. Both illnesses are caused by a virus, so anti*biotic* drugs will not work.

This year, the influenza season started late and is expected to last a little longer than usual. The yearly flu vaccine lasts roughly four months, so people who got theirs early, in September or early October, may be at risk of contracting the flu, since the immunity may wear off. However, the Centers for Disease Control and the Ohio Department of Health are not recommending that people get an additional flu shot.

Remember, with or without the flu shot, there are still steps you can take to increase your chances of staying well! You can still affect your good health by doing the things that tend toward wellness—keep eating right, get enough rest, exercise, and wash your hands often to prevent the spread of germs. By staying fit, you can keep your immune system working effectively so it will fight off those scourges of winter—colds and flu.

The Delaware City-County Health Department promotes good health and improved quality of life in Delaware County. For more information, contact the Health Department at (740)368–1700 or (740) 548–7055. You can also e-mail the health education staff at **<healthed@rrcol.com>** *or go to* **<www.health.co.delaware.oh.us>** *and visit the Health Department's home page.*

—30—

Examples of PSAs for Radio and Television

30-SECOND PUBLIC SERVICE ANNOUNCEMENT

Delaware City-County Health Department

For Immediate Release   **Contact: Roger Wren**
                                              (740) 368–1700 or (740) 548–7055

Concern for the environment begins at home. Proper waste disposal has increasingly become a critical environmental concern, both globally and locally.

Recycling is an important part of the solution to this dilemma since it saves valuable land-fill space and conserves natural resources.

Let's keep our home—Delaware County—an environmentally conscientious community.

Recycle. Because it's important.

Keep Delaware County beautiful.

Source: Reprinted by permission of Delaware City-County Health Department.

CABLE TELEVISION—PUBLIC SERVICE ANNOUNCEMENT

Delaware City-County Health Department

For Immediate Release

Contact: Melissa Sever
Delaware Health Dept.
(740) 368–1700

Cable Television

Most car seats aren't
installed safely!
Free car seat check up
at Nourse Chevrolet
1101 Columbus Pike
Saturday, Feb. 20th from 9 to 12 A.M.
Delaware Health Department
(740) 368–1700

Source: Reprinted by permission of Delaware City-County Health Department.

Examples of Smoking Policies

SAMPLE POLICY I

Totally Smoke-Free

A. SCOPE

All (company's name) employees, on-site contractors, and visitors.

B. PURPOSE

At (company name), our employees are one of our most valuable resources and in recognition of that we promote the health, safety, and well-being of each individual through progressive health and benefit programs.

C. POLICY

Since our obligation includes concerns for all employees in all areas with known hazards; and since tobacco smoke is the major cause of heart and lung and respiratory diseases and causes or aggravates allergic reactions, all of which lead to impaired performance and increased health care cost, therefore, because of the aforementioned, smoking is prohibited in Company building(s) (or on property), company vehicles, and in those areas of other buildings used, operated or occupied by (company's name).

D. EFFECTIVE DATE

This company smoking policy will take effect on (date).

E. ADMINISTRATION AND PROCEDURES

1. Cigarette machines will not be permitted on company property.
2. Prior to implementation of this policy and continuing thereafter, smoking treatment programs will be offered to employees and their dependents. Please contact (department/person).

(continues)

(continued)

3. (appropriate individuals) will be responsible for ensuring compliance with this policy.
4. All prospective employees will be informed of the guidelines and of the company's commitment to a smoke-free work environment.
5. Any questions regarding the policy should be referred to (department/person).
6. Noncompliance with this policy will result in disciplinary actions.

F. EDUCATIONAL RESOURCES
1. The Human Resource Department will provide written materials for safety meetings emphasizing current medical concerns about smoking.
2. Any questions regarding the policy should be referred to the Human Resource Department.

SAMPLE POLICY II

Designated Smoking Room

A. SCOPE

All (company's name) employees, on-site contractors, and visitors.

B. PURPOSE

At (company name), our employees are one of our most valuable resources and in recognition of that we promote the health, safety, and well-being of each individual through progressive health and benefit programs.

C. POLICY

Since our obligation includes concerns for all employees in all areas with known hazards; and since tobacco smoke is the major cause of heart and lung and respiratory diseases and causes or aggravates allergic reactions, all of which lead to impaired performance and increased health care cost, therefore, because of the aforementioned, smoking will be limited to a designated room with outside ventilation. Smoking is permitted only in the following designated room: _____

D. EFFECTIVE DATE

This company smoking policy will take effect on (date).

E. ADMINISTRATION AND PROCEDURES
   1. Cigarette machines will not be permitted on company property.
   2. Prior to implementation of this policy and continuing thereafter, smoking treatment programs will be offered to employees and their dependents. Please contact (department/person).
   3. (appropriate individuals) will be responsible for ensuring compliance with this policy.
   4. All prospective employees will be informed of the guidelines and of the company's commitment to a smoke-free work environment.
   5. Any questions regarding the policy should be referred to (department/person).
   6. Noncompliance with this policy will result in disciplinary actions.

F. EDUCATIONAL RESOURCES
   1. The Human Resource Department will provide written materials for safety meetings emphasizing current medical concerns about smoking.
   2. Any questions regarding the policy should be referred to the Human Resource Department.

Source: Coalition for a Smoke-Free Valley. (1995). *Working it out.* Allentown, PA: Author. pp. 7–9.

Health Behavior Contract

Being of sound mind and in need of health behavior change, I (insert name of person wanting to make the change) do hereby commit myself to the following health behavior change for the next eight weeks. This contract with (insert the name of the other person who is entering into this contract) shall be in effect from (insert starting date) to (insert ending date). For completing this contract, I will be rewarded/reinforced with (insert reward or reinforcer). This reward/reinforcer will be received when I (insert desired behavior). If I do not successfully fulfill this contract, I will (insert what will happen if person is not successful).

A. The behavior I plan to change is:

_____

_____

B. The reason I want to change this behavior is because:

_____

_____

C. I have set the following objectives for myself (Reminder: objectives must be measurable so that you will know if you have reached them. For example, choose practicing relaxation techniques once a day, 5 times per week as an objective rather than indicating stress reduction as a goal).

1. _____

2. _____

3. _____

D. To meet these objectives, I will (provide a description of your daily/weekly activity):

_____

_____

(continues)

(*continued*)

E. To carry out my plan, I am going to solicit the help of (names of friends, family, room-
mate, or significant others and how they will help):

_____

_____

F. I expect to receive the following benefits from this activity:

_____

_____

Your signature: _____   Date: _____

Facilitator's signature: _____   Date: _____

Example of an Informed Consent Form for a Cholesterol Screening Program

I hereby grant permission to the Institute for Health Promotion personnel to perform a cholesterol screening on me. I am engaging in this screening voluntarily. I have been told that this screening is an analysis of total blood cholesterol and that my blood will be taken from a fingerstick blood sample by a trained employee. I understand that the results of this screening are considered to be preliminary in nature and in no way conclusive. Results of a blood cholesterol screening like this can be affected by a number of factors including, but not limited to, smoking, stress level, amount of exercise, hormone levels, foods eaten, heredity, and pregnancy. I also understand that my physician can perform a more complete blood lipid (fat) analysis for me, if I so desire.

Further, I have been told that all information related to this screening is considered confidential.

I have read the above statement and understand what it means. I have also had an opportunity to ask questions about the screening, and all my questions have been answered to my satisfaction.

_____ _____ _____
Participant's Signature   Date   Signature of Witness

To ensure it meets with all related local and state laws, this form, or any others like it, should be submitted to legal counsel before use.

Sample Medical Clearance Form

I hereby certify that (name of participant) has been examined and cleared by me to participate, with the noted restrictions, in the programs indicated below. This person should not be placed into any of the other programs until he/she has been cleared by me to do so.

❏ Vigorous exercise programs. This type of program would include all-out effort for the development of cardiovascular endurance, muscular strength, and flexibility.

Physician's comments: _____

_____

_____

❏ Moderate exercise program. This type of program is for those participants who would be unable to participate in the vigorous exercise program because of physical limitations. These programs should be modified as per my instructions.

Physician's comments: _____

_____

_____

❏ Mild exercise program. This type of program is for those participants who would be unable to participate in the moderate exercise program because of physical limitations. These programs should be modified as per my instructions.

Physician's comments: _____

_____

_____

_____   _____
Physician's Signature   Date

Code of Ethics for the Health Education Profession

Unabridged Version

Preamble

The Health Education profession is dedicated to excellence in the practice of promoting individual, family, organizational, and community health. Guided by common ideals, Health Educators are responsible for upholding the integrity and ethics of the profession as they face the daily challenges of making decisions. By acknowledging the value of diversity in society and embracing a cross-cultural approach, Health Educators support the worth, dignity, potential, and uniqueness of all people.

The Code of Ethics provides a framework of shared values within which Health Education is practiced. The Code of Ethics is grounded in fundamental ethical principles that underlie all health care services: respect for autonomy, promotion of social justice, active promotion of good, and avoidance of harm. The responsibility of each health educator is to aspire to the highest possible standards of conduct and to encourage the ethical behavior of all those with whom they work.

Regardless of job title, professional affiliation, work setting, or population served, Health Educators abide by these guidelines when making professional decisions.

Article I: Responsibility to the Public

A Health Educator's ultimate responsibility is to educate people for the purpose of promoting, maintaining, and improving individual, family, and community health. When a conflict of issues arises among individuals, groups, organizations, agencies, or institutions, health educators must consider all issues and give priority to those that promote wellness and quality of living through principles of self-determination and freedom of choice for the individual.

Section 1 Health Educators support the right of individuals to make informed decisions regarding health, as long as such decisions pose no threat to the health of others.

Section 2 Health Educators encourage actions and social policies that support and facilitate the best balance of benefits over harm for all affected parties.

Section 3 Health Educators accurately communicate the potential benefits and consequences of the services and programs with which they are associated.

Section 4 Health Educators accept the responsibility to act on issues that can adversely affect the health of individuals, families, and communities.

Section 5 Health Educators are truthful about their qualifications and the limitations of their expertise and provide services consistent with their competencies.

Section 6 Health Educators protect the privacy and dignity of individuals.

Source: The Coalition of National Health Education Organizations, Ethics Task Force, November 9, 1999 <www.med.usf.ed/~kmbrown/CNHEO.htm>. Reprinted by permission.

Section 7 Health Educators actively involve individuals, groups, and communities in the entire educational process so that all aspects of the process are clearly understood by those who may be affected.

Section 8 Health Educators respect and acknowledge the rights of others to hold diverse values, attitudes, and opinions.

Section 9 Health Educators provide services equitably to all people.

Article II: Responsibility to the Profession

Health Educators are responsible for their professional behavior, for the reputation of their profession, and for promoting ethical conduct among their colleagues.

Section 1 Health Educators maintain, improve, and expand their professional competence through continued study and education; membership, participation, and leadership in professional organizations; and involvement in issues related to the health of the public.

Section 2 Health Educators model and encourage nondiscriminatory standards of behavior in their interactions with others.

Section 3 Health Educators encourage and accept responsible critical discourse to protect and enhance the profession.

Section 4 Health Educators contribute to the development of the profession by sharing the processes and outcomes of their work.

Section 5 Health Educators are aware of possible professional conflicts of interest, exercise integrity in conflict situations, and do not manipulate or violate the rights of others.

Section 6 Health Educators give appropriate recognition to others for their professional contributions and achievements.

Article III: Responsibility to Employers

Health Educators recognize the boundaries of their professional competence and are accountable for their professional activities and actions.

Section 1 Health Educators accurately represent their qualifications and the qualifications of others whom they recommend.

Section 2 Health Educators use appropriate standards, theories, and guidelines as criteria when carrying out their professional responsibilities.

Section 3 Health Educators accurately represent potential service and program outcomes to employers.

Section 4 Health Educators anticipate and disclose competing commitments, conflicts of interest, and endorsement of products.

Section 5 Health Educators openly communicate to employers, expectations of job-related assignments that conflict with their professional ethics.

Section 6 Health Educators maintain competence in their areas of professional practice.

Article IV: Responsibility in the Delivery of Health Education

Health Educators promote integrity in the delivery of health education. They respect the rights, dignity, confidentiality, and worth of all people by adapting strategies and methods to meet the needs of diverse populations and communities.

Section 1 Health Educators are sensitive to social and cultural diversity and are in accord with the law, when planning and implementing programs.

Section 2 Health Educators are informed of the latest advances in theory, research, and practice, and use strategies and methods that are grounded in and contribute to development of professional standards, theories, guidelines, statistics, and experience.

Section 3 Health Educators are committed to rigorous evaluation of both program effectiveness and the methods used to achieve results.

Section 4 Health Educators empower individuals to adopt healthy lifestyles through informed choice rather than by coercion or intimidation.

Section 5 Health Educators communicate the potential outcomes of proposed services, strategies, and pending decisions to all individuals who will be affected.

Article V: Responsibility in Research and Evaluation

Health Educators contribute to the health of the population and to the profession through research and evaluation activities. When planning and conducting research or evaluation, health educators do so in accordance with federal and state laws and regulations, organizational and institutional policies, and professional standards.

Section 1 Health Educators support principles and practices of research and evaluation that do no harm to individuals, groups, society, or the environment.

Section 2 Health Educators ensure that participation in research is voluntary and is based upon the informed consent of the participants.

Section 3 Health Educators respect the privacy, rights, and dignity of research participants, and honor commitments made to those participants.

Section 4 Health Educators treat all information obtained from participants as confidential unless otherwise required by law.

Section 5 Health Educators take credit, including authorship, only for work they have actually performed and give credit to the contributions of others.

Section 6 Health Educators who serve as research or evaluation consultants discuss their results only with those to whom they are providing service, unless maintaining such confidentiality would jeopardize the health or safety of others.

Section 7 Health Educators report the results of their research and evaluation objectively, accurately, and in a timely fashion.

Article VI: Responsibility in Professional Preparation

Those involved in the preparation and training of Health Educators have an obligation to accord learners the same respect and treatment given other groups by providing quality education that benefits the profession and the public.

Section 1 Health Educators select students for professional preparation programs based upon equal opportunity for all, and the individual's academic performance, abilities, and potential contribution to the profession and the public's health.

Section 2 Health Educators strive to make the educational environment and culture conducive to the health of all involved, and free from sexual harassment and all forms of discrimination.

Section 3 Health Educators involved in professional preparation and professional development engage in careful preparation; present material that is accurate, up-to-date, and timely; provide reasonable and timely feedback; state clear and reasonable expectations; and conduct fair assessments and evaluations of learners.

Section 4 Health Educators provide objective and accurate counseling to learners about career opportunities, development, and advancement, and assist learners to secure professional employment.

Section 5 Health Educators provide adequate supervision and meaningful opportunities for the professional development of learners.

Abridged Version

Preamble

The Health Education profession is dedicated to excellence in the practice of promoting individual, family, organizational, and community health. The Code of Ethics provides a framework of shared values within which Health Education is practiced. The responsibility of each Health Educator is to aspire to the highest possible standards of conduct and to encourage the ethical behavior of all those with whom they work.

Article I: Responsibility to the Public

A Health Educator's ultimate responsibility is to educate people for the purpose of promoting, maintaining, and improving individual, family, and community health. When a conflict of issues arises among individuals, groups, organizations, agencies, or institutions, health educators must consider all issues and give priority to those that promote wellness and quality of living through principles of self-determination and freedom of choice for the individual.

Article II: Responsibility to the Profession

Health Educators are responsible for their professional behavior, for the reputation of their profession, and for promoting ethical conduct among their colleagues.

Article III: Responsibility to Employers

Health Educators recognize the boundaries of their professional competence and are accountable for their professional activities and actions.

Article IV: Responsibility in the Delivery of Health Education

Health Educators promote integrity in the delivery of health education. They respect the rights, dignity, confidentiality, and worth of all people by adapting strategies and methods to meet the needs of diverse populations and communities.

Article V: Responsibility in Research and Evaluation

Health Educators contribute to the health of the population and to the profession through research and evaluation activities. When planning and conducting research or evaluation, health educators do so in accordance with federal and state laws and regulations, organizational and institutional policies, and professional standards.

Article VI: Responsibility in Professional Preparation

Those involved in the preparation and training of Health Educators have an obligation to accord learners the same respect and treatment given other groups by providing quality education that benefits the profession and the public.

Cost-Benefit and Cost-Effectiveness as a Part of the Evaluation of Health Promotion Programs

Abstract

Economic evaluation should be a component of program evaluation. To encourage and help with this process, definitions of common economic terms, a review of the literature, steps for conducting an economic evaluation, and the use of economic evaluation, with health promotion program is presented.

Introduction

The idea of promoting good health practices is not new in the United States. However, it is only in recent years that the concept of health promotion has grown in popularity and that the number of health promotion programs has flourished. The growth has occurred because of the "... increasing evidence of an association between patterns of lifestyle and health status of individuals and population groups, and associations between environmental and workplace hazards and the health and well-being of communities and workers" (Work Group on Health Promotion/Disease Prevention, 1987).

Though the number of health promotion programs continues to increase, the evaluation of said programs lags behind. There are several reasons for this. First, many of the first generation health promotion programs were developed without regard to an appropriate plan of evaluation. Thus data were not and could not be collected. Second, the very nature of health promotion programs, that of being "in the field" and being geared toward the long-term outcome of "impovered health," makes them difficult to evaluate. Concerns such as evaluation expertise, confidentiality of participants, and resources of time, money, and personnel have proven to be stumbling blocks in collecting the needed data.

If health promotion programs are to prosper and grow, empirical evidence of their worth should be provided. This can be done only through appropriate evaluation of the programs; evaluation that pays considerable attention to problems of design and measurement, and that can be reproducible. Green (1979) stated that "Evaluation of a health promotion plan certifies its appropriateness and its effectiveness and ensures that the practitioner is accountable to the patient (consumer), the community, and the hospital administrator." Though Green's comments were directed toward hospital health promotion programs these same ideas can be transferred to any health promotion setting because all program planners need to be accountable to the consumer (Work Group on Health Promotion/Disease Prevention, 1987).

The question now is not whether or not health promotion programs should be evaluated

Source: J. F. McKenzie "Cost-Benefit and Cost-Effectiveness as a Part of the Evaluation of Health Promotion Programs," *The Eta Sigma Gamman, 18*(2) (1986): 10–16. Reprinted by permission from *Journal of Eta Sigma Gamma: The Health Educator,* formerly *The Eta Sigma Gamman.*

but how should it be done? Green (1979) has defined three different levels of evaluation—process, impact, and outcome. Process evaluation deals with the professional practice of those presenting the health promotion program. Impact evaluation is concerned with the immediate difference that the health promotion program has on the knowledge, attitude, behavior, and environment. Outcome evaluation focuses on long-term concerns such as morbidity, morality, and years of survival following the health promotion program. There are many strategies for evaluating health promotion programs within each of these levels, and they have been thoroughly covered in the works of Windsor, Baranowski, Clark, and Cutter (1984) and Green and Lewis (1986). However, there is one evaluation strategy that these authors have addressed that merits further discussion because of the importance being placed on it in today's practice: the economic evaluation of health promotion programs. In the business world the economic evaluation of a program is often referred to as the "bottom line."

In writing about corporate health promotion programs, Fielding (1982, p. 85) has stated:

> Although current evidence suggests a very favorable return on investment for disease prevention and health promotion programs, much more information is needed to quantify costs and benefits and to suggest which models work best in different corporate settings. Therefore, it is imperative that all efforts include long-term evaluation of effects of programs on both direct and indirect costs.

The remaining portion of this paper will focus on the economic evaluation of health promotion programs. This refers to the cost-benefit and cost-effectiveness analysis (CBA and CEA, respectively) of the programs.

Definitions of CBA and CEA

Simply stated, CBA and CEA are formal analytical techniques used for comparing the negative and positive consequences of alternative uses of resources. They are not formulas for making decisions, but rather they are tools to help individuals make decisions (Warner & Luce, 1982).

More specifically, Green and Lewis (1986, p. 361) have defined cost-benefit as "a measure of the cost of an intervention relative to the benefits it yields, usually expressed as a ratio of dollars saved or gained for every dollar spent on the program," and cost-effectiveness as "a measure of the cost of an intervention relative to its impact, usually expressed in dollars per unit of effect." Common CEA measures may include years of life saved, days of morbidity and disability avoided, number of smokers who quit, and number of pounds lost.

When first reading these definitions, they appear to be very much alike. The basic technical distinction between CBA and CEA lies in the process of valuing the desirable consequences of health promotion programs (Warner & Luce, 1982). CBA requires that all desirable consequences be expressed in monetary (dollar) terms. For many of the consequences this is a manageable task, but there are some desirable consequences that researchers have found most difficult to quantify in dollars—the value of human life may be the most notable. Several researchers (Rice, 1966; Cooper and Rice, 1976; Acton, 1976) have offered means of dealing with the problem.

More recently the difference between CBA and CEA seems to be fading. Warner and Luce have pointed out that as they have reviewed the literature on CBA and CEA, the two techniques are becoming more alike in the way analysts are applying the concepts. They have indicated that "recent sophisticated health care CEAs are incorporating some dollar-valued benefits into the cost side of the equation (as negative costs), and increasing recognition of the meaning of CBA in health care is bringing it closer to CEA. The human capital approach to measuring indirect benefits in CBA values livelihood, not life itself; thus a CBA is really a net dollar benefit for some nonmonetized health outcomes. The newer more sophisticated CEA seems to be a significant step forward in that it combines the best of both CBA and CEA" (Warner & Luce, 1982, p. 213).

The Popularity of CBA and CEA

The evaluation techniques of CEA and CBA are by no means new concepts, for they can be traced back hundreds of years. However, there has been a tremendous growth in their use and interest in the health professions in the past fifteen years. Much of this growth has paralleled the increase of health care costs during the same period of time. Many feel that this burgeoning interest of CEA and CBA in the health professions has resulted from health professionals seeking to identify and convey the meaning of cost-beneficial and cost-effective health care interventions. It is now quite common to find CBA and CEA citations on most all health care topics.

Review of Literature

As Warner and Hutton (1980) have pointed out, the contributions to the health care CBA and CEA literature have grown exponentially in recent years. Over the years the majority of the literature has dealt with medical interventions. Since this paper is focused on nonmedical interventions—health promotion activities—the medical intervention CBA and CEA literature is not reviewed here. However, it is well presented in Warner and Luce (1982).

The references to the nonmedical CBA and CEA literature are much more limited. The nonmedical literature falls into three major areas—public health measures (i.e., water fluoridation, food inspection, etc.), identification of health risks via screenings (for hypertension, cancer and other diseases), and personal health lifestyle (i.e., exercise, smoking, nutrition, stress, etc.). Public health measures have generally not been considered a part of health promotion activities. And even though screenings have been a portion of a number of health promotion programs, it is the category of personal health lifestyle on which most health promotion programs are planned. It is this literature that is reviewed below.

A number of reviews of the CBA and CEA of health promotion type activities have been found in the literature (Fielding, 1982; Rogers, Eaton, & Bruhn, 1981; Scheffler & Paringer, 1980; and Warner, 1979). These reviews report on basically two types of studies. One group includes studies that have calculated a CBA or CEA on a specific health problem in terms of what the costs and benefits would be for the entire United States if a health promotion pro-

gram were implemented. One such paper is presented by Kristein (1977). In his paper, Kristein examines several different health concerns such as hypertension, cancer of the colon, heavy cigarette smoking, alcohol abuse, and breast cancer. A summary of his heavy cigarette smoking calculations provides a good example of this approach. He calculated that the costs of heavy cigarette smoking were approximately $20.3 billion (in 1975 dollars). This includes the cost of hospital care, medical care, absenteeism, and premature deaths. If a smoking cessation program were implemented for the 22 million heavy smokers in the United States (a 1975 estimate) at $125 per person and there was a 25% success rate, Kristein estimated a cost-benefit ratio of 1.8 to 1.0. This means that for every dollar put into such a program a $1.80 could be saved. This type of CBA is useful in showing that smoking cessation programs can provide financial benefits, but the exactness of the figures must be put into perspective because of the lack of detail in the analysis.

The other major group of studies that appear in the reviews are those which report on the results of a CBA or CEA calculated on a specific health promotion activity offered by a specific organization. For example, Fielding (1982) has reviewed the results of a number of employee health promotion programs. His findings show that a number of different techniques have been used to calculate CBAs and CEAs, that calculations are based on a number of assumptions and thus the results are difficult to compare. In another paper, Fielding (1984) offers the following example:

> Campbell's analysis of the savings attributable to their colorectal cancer screening programs hinges on assumptions regarding the number of cases of colorectal cancer that would have occurred in the absence of screening, and the direct and indirect costs associated with each case. It also assumes that all cases prevented were due to on-site screening rather than screening that occurred in another setting (e.g., doctor's office or HMO) at the encouragement of an outside health professional. While these estimates of savings due to health promotion measures are useful in showing the value companies themselves have

placed in the savings, it is difficult to know if their assertions can be applied to other companies. (p. 259)

Further indication of the inconsistency in the way CBA and CEA for health promotion activities have been calculated was noted by Rogers et al. (1981, p. 333)—". . . carefully designed cost analyses have not been conducted so that various approaches can be compared as to the expense, as well as to short-term impact and long-term outcome." There is clearly a need for authors to describe in detail all the steps they follow in calculating their CBA or CEA so that other evaluators can use the same steps and thus be able to compare results.

The health promotion literature includes more reports of CBAs and CEAs on identification of health risks than in personal health lifestyle change, with the more reports dealing with hypertension screening programs than any other (Alderman, Madhavan, & Davis, 1983; Erfurt & Foote, 1984; Foote & Erfurt, 1977; Ruchlin & Alderman, 1980; and Ruchlin, Melcher, & Alderman, 1984). Only two recent reports on personal health lifestyle change could be found. One dealt with weight loss (Seidman, Sevelius, & Ewald, 1984) and the other with smoking cessation (Weiss, Jurs, Lesage, & Iverson, 1984). Scheffler and Paringer (1980) have pointed out the need for empirical evidence of the economic soundness of other lifestyle change programs such as physical exercise and dietary changes.

Finally, there are many more reports using CEA than CBA in the health promotion literature. Only two reports of CBA (Alderman et al., 1983; and Weiss et al., 1984) could be found. All others were CEAs. The reasons for this will become clear from subsequent discussion.

Calculating CBAs and CEAs

As suggested in preceding portions of this paper, the calculation of CBAs and CEAs for health promotion activities is no easy task. In most cases they will be difficult and in some cases impossible to calculate. However, if evaluations of health promotion activities are going to be complete, they should be attempted.

Though there are certain processes that must be included in calculating CBAs and CEAs, the exact steps one could use may vary.

The important point to remember is that whatever steps are used, they should be reported accurately and in detail so others can replicate and compare results. The steps presented below are a combination of techniques suggested by a governmental agency and several different individuals (OTA, 1978; OTA, 1980; Rogers et al., 1981; Shepard & Thompson, 1979; and Warner & Luce, 1982).

Step 1: Defining the Problem   The initial step in calculating a CBA or CEA is defining the problem to be analyzed. The problem should be stated as clearly and explicitly as possible. Seemingly small differences in the definition of the problem could have a large impact on the calculated costs, benefits and effects. The statement of the problem should also clearly specify for whom the analysis is going to be calculated. For example, a cost-analysis of a health promotion program would differ greatly if it were being calculated from the employer's point of view as opposed to the costs, benefits, and effects experienced by the employee.

Commonly defined problems for which health promotion programs are usually designed deal with either a specific health concern or an economic issue. An example of a problem that deals with a health concern might be to reduce the risk of cardiovascular disease in white collar employees, while a problem revolving around an economic issue may be to reduce the amount of money the company spends on health insurance claims per year. Both of these problems would be appropriate for calculating a CBA or CEA; however, for the purposes of this paper, the cardiovascular disease problem will be used as an example through the remaining steps in the process.

Step 2: Specifying the Objectives   Closely related to defining the problem is setting one or more objectives against which programmatic alternatives are to be evaluated. If the defined problem is not readily measurable, further specification may help qualify it. For example, the problem of reducing cardiovascular disease in white collar employees is too broad to be readily quantified.

A possible specification of an appropriate objective would be to reduce the risk of cardiovascular disease in this employee group by getting 50% of the high-risk employees in an appropriate exercise program. It is known that the high-risk group includes individuals who have hypertension and are overweight. These individuals cost a company more money in medical care, accidents, etc. than individuals without them. Exercise has been shown to help both of these health concerns.

Step 3: Identifying Alternatives   To determine if a specific approach to a problem is cost-effective or cost-beneficial, it needs to be compared to other approaches that could also be used to achieve the stated objectives. Again using the problem of cardiovascular disease as an example, an alternative approach may be to reduce disease via a nutrition and weight control program as opposed to the exercise program.

When identifying alternatives for health promotion programs, it should be noted that the alternatives do not need to attack the problem using similar approaches. For example, if the problem is to reduce health costs due to cigarette smoking within an organization, one cost analysis may be completed on an educational smoking cessation approach. Another analysis of costs could be calculated on the alternative which mandates, via a company policy, that there be no smoking in the workplace.

It is helpful to keep the following concerns in mind when identifying appropriate alternatives: (1) select only alternatives that are believed to be potentially quite cost-effective, (2) select alternatives that offer variety in their approach, and (3) select alternatives that would be appropriate for comparison—do not select an alternative that is obviously an inappropriate approach for solving the problem (i.e., getting *every* employee to adopt a specific exercise program).

Step 4: Describing Production Relationships
The first three steps of this process set the conceptual framework for calculating a CBA or CEA. When one describes the production relationships, he/she is creating the technical framework for the quantitative assessment and comparison of costs and benefits of the alternatives. This may be the most important step in the CBA and CEA processes. To set up the technical framework, the evaluator must identify the resources necessary to carry out the alter-

native, explain how the resources are combined, and then predict the outcome(s). As Warner and Luce (1982) have pointed out, this can be completed in several different ways ranging from a simple flow chart to a sophisticated, multi-equation computer simulation.

In the cardiovascular disease problem, the resources would include personnel time—of both the high-risk employees participating in this program and the program leaders, educational materials (i.e., booklets, films, handouts, etc.), supplies (i.e., exercise clothing, laundry expenses, etc.), pre- and post-program exercise testings, pre-program medical examinations, fee for facility use, and any other preparticipant program expenses. The outcomes of the program may include 50% of the participants getting involved in a life-long exercise program, 50% reducing their weight, and 75% getting their blood pressure under control. These in turn may result in fewer health insurance claims because of reduced illness, less absenteeism, and fewer accidents, thus increasing productivity. In the long run it is hoped these programs will decrease both morbidity and premature mortality.

As one can see from this example, this step can become quite involved. One may need to examine previous programs—conducted either in house or in another setting—or obtain the services of a technical consultant to try to adequately identify all resources and outcomes. However, the evaluator of the health promotion programs should be aware that even this additional work may not ensure the identification of all health outcomes. It is because of this inability to identify specific health outcomes that the use of CBA with health promotion programs has been limited. If the health benefits of a program cannot be identified, then one cannot put a dollar value on them and thus the cost of the benefit cannot be analyzed. For example, what are the health benefits of a nutrition education program? Unless these benefits can be identified,* CBA would be an inappropriate cost analysis technique to use with health promotion programs.

---

*See the related literature section of this paper for examples of where evaluators have been able to apply CBA to health promotion programs.

On the other hand, CEA can be applied very well to some health promotion programs. For the outcomes of concern are not benefits but effects, and with a CEA the evaluator is not required to put a dollar value on the effects. Thus when analyzing the nutrition education program, one can identify effects such as the reduction of calorie intake or the reduction of serum fat levels without trying to identify the health benefit of such. It should be noted that these effects are immediate (i.e., reduction in calories) or intermediate (i.e., decrease in serum fat levels) outcomes only and not long-term (i.e., decreased premature mortality) like some financiers of health promotion programs want to see.

Whether one is using CBA or CEA, the more completely the production relationships have been described, the easier it will be to complete steps 5 and 6 in the process—analyzing costs, benefits, and effectiveness.

Step 5: Analyzing the Costs   Costs should be defined as those resources that one must give up to gain some benefit or effect (Warner & Luce, 1982). This would include not only those direct controllable costs but also overhead uncontrollable costs.

The cost of some resources may be obvious. Using the cardiovascular disease example, it may be very easy to determine the cost of the educational materials because they can be purchased at a cost of Y per set. The cost of the group leader may be obvious, too, but how about the cost ∪. the four volunteers who are helping conduct the program? Since the program could not be run without the four volunteers, this is a cost to the program. In this situation the economic concept of "opportunity cost" would be used. "The opportunity cost is its value in another use" (Warner & Luce, 1982, p. 77). So if these volunteers were not helping in this program, how much would they be worth in another setting? It may be found that they would be worth $7.50 per hour working in a similar capacity at a local health agency. Therefore their cost could be determined with this figure.

Since one of the major reasons for calculating CBA and CEA is to be able to compare alternatives, it is important that costs (and for that matter benefits and effects) of the different alternatives are calculated in a similar manner. For example, if one is comparing different cardiovascular exercise programs and both programs include the help of volunteers, the same opportunity costs should be used in determining the total cost of volunteers.

Step 6: Analyzing Benefits and Effectiveness
There are usually numerous desired outcomes (benefits) that result from health promotion programs. Some are obvious while others are much more difficult to identify. For this reason, it may help the evaluator to try to categorize the different outcomes. Warner and Luce (1982) have identified the following classification scheme for outcomes associated with health care activities: (1) Personal health benefits—improvements in health such as increased life expectancy, decreased morbidity, and reduced disability; (2) Health care resource benefits—the saving of unused resources resulting from the implementation of an activity (for example, an exercise program could reduce the resources put into cardiac surgery); (3) Other economic benefits—desired outcomes that are not identified as either health or health care benefits, such as work productivity; (4) Other social benefits—desired outcomes that have positive social effects like increased access to health services or compassion; and (5) Intermediate outcomes—benefits that occur prior to a final outcome. Because it is sometimes difficult to measure final outcomes, one often must use the intermediate outcome. For example, the long-term impact of an exercise program on one's health would be difficult to determine, but one could measure the intermediate outcome of weight loss.

It should be noted that not all outcomes are benefits. The best example of this appears in screening programs when false positive outcomes appear. If such outcomes do exist, they need to be treated as costs.

The measurement of benefits and effectiveness is very much like the measurement of costs in that some aspects are straightforward while others are very difficult. For example, not all social benefits can be quantified, such as compassion. There is no standard unit of compassion on which one could attach a dollar value.

It is at this point in the calculations of CBA and CEA that the differences in the two analyses can be seen. The CEA ends with the measurement of effectiveness. No dollar value is placed on the outcomes. Thus, the number of lives saved, trips to the health clinic, or persons involved in the exercise program are all that are needed. However, in order to calculate a CBA, monetary units must be attached to each outcome. This is not too difficult when market prices are available. But they are not always available, and the one area that has caused considerable discussion is trying to put a monetary label on the "value of life." Techniques that have been used include (1) human capital—value of being productively employed in the labor market plus direct benefit of health care resource savings, (2) willingness to pay—value that individuals place on reducing risks of death and illness, (3) court awards in civil cases—value of productive life and emotional costs, and (4) life insurance holdings—value of one's life insurance.

Step 7: Discounting   A necessary step in calculating an accurate CBA or CEA is that of discounting. Since the costs and benefits of some programs do not occur entirely in the present, for comparison purposes all future costs and monetary values of future benefits should be discounted to their present value. In other words, a dollar today is worth more to an individual than the promise of having the dollar tomorrow and more still than having the dollar the day after tomorrow. "The discount rate attempts to adjust for what a dollar invested today would earn in interest" (Collen & Goodman, 1985). ". . . Discounting is particularly important in the case of preventive activities since so many of the benefits occur well into the future. In addition, discounting helps to explain how 'postponing' illness costs can have the effect of 'containing them'" (Warner, 1979).

To carry out the discounting process, one must first decide on a discount rate. The discount rate expresses the degree to which tomorrow's dollar loses value relative to today's dollar. Since there is little consensus on what discount rate should be used and because the particular discount rate chosen can have a substantial impact on the outcome of the analysis [In relative terms, low discount rates tend to favor projects whose benefits occur in the distant future (OTA, 1980)], CBAs and CEAs are usually calculated using several different rates, usually ranging from 3–10%. This process of using several different rates is called sensitivity analysis.

For example, if one wanted to spend $1,000 today on an exercise program expecting to save $2,000 in medical costs in five years, there would be a need to discount the benefit ($2,000) to its estimated present value. For the sake of the example the discount rate will be set at 5%. The present discounted value today of the net benefit would be $567 ($1,567–1,000) and not $1,000 ($2,000–$1,000).

Both time (in years) and the discount rate have an impact on the discounted value. Tables 1 and 2 are presented to illustrate the effect of each. Table 1 shows how an expected $2,000 benefit decreases in value over time when the discount rate stays constant (5% in this example).

Table 2 illustrates how again a $2,000 benefit decreases in value as the discount rate increases and the time stays constant (5 years in this example).

It is obvious from these tables that given a large enough discount rate and/or a substantial number of years, the net benefit could be a negative number. Such a number would indicate that the costs would outweigh the benefits and the cost-benefits ratio would be less than one point zero (1.0) to 1.0. In other words, it would cost more than one dollar to get a dollar worth of benefit.

For those interested in other examples of the discounting process, see Collen and Goodman (1985) and Warner and Luce (1982).

Step 8: Analyzing Uncertainties   As has been demonstrated throughout this discussion of calculating a CBA or CEA, there will be times when the evaluator will be uncertain of some data that need to be included. In such cases there are several alternatives available to the evaluator. As with discounting, the evaluator could use a sensitivity analysis. For example, if the evaluator were figuring a CEA on a smoking cessation program and was not sure of the cost of an instructor for the program, he/she could make several different estimates of the cost. Each of these estimates could then be "plugged into" the analysis to give the evaluator a range for the CEA.

Another approach to dealing with uncertainties would be to elicit the help of a group of

TABLE 1 Effect of time on discounted value

Discount Rate	Time (in years)	Present Value of Cost	Present Value of Benefit	Present Value of Net Benefit
.05	0	$1,000	$2,000	$1,000
.05	1	$1,000	$1,905	$905
.05	2	$1,000	$1,814	$814
.05	5	$1,000	$1,567	$567
.05	10	$1,000	$1,228	$228
.05	20	$1,000	$754	$–246

experts in the field. Such a technique is called consensus development. With this technique a group of experts is brought together to listen to a presentation of uncertain areas. Following the presentation, the group is then isolated to discuss the presentation and to reach a consensus as to what should be used in place of the uncertain data.

Step 9: Interpreting the Results   Because of all the concerns noted in calculating a CBA or CEA, one needs to be careful in interpreting the results of an analysis. There are many assumptions and uncertainties that both the evaluator and/or the interpreter of the results could overlook. Thus, one needs to proceed with caution when reading the analysis reports.

Assuming all steps have been carried out properly and appropriate CBA and CEA data have been calculated, the decision maker must not forget that the economic evaluation is only one piece of the data needed to make decisions about programs. Most programs have important ethical, legal, and/or societal issues that must be identified and discussed before final program decisions can be made.

Using CBAs and CEAs with Health Promotion Programs   The need for incorporating an economic component in the evaluation of a health promotion program should be obvious. The question that remains is, what specific technique would be most appropriate? In most situations the answer would be CEA. The reasons for using CEA as opposed to CBA with health promotion programs are: (1) the inability to determine and then measure all the effects of a program, and (2) the inability to put a monetary value on the measured effect. These inabilities of not being able to identify the effects and then in turn being able to determine the value (in dollars) of these effects are critical steps in the CBA process. Without them an evaluator could not calculate an accurate CBA. It would probably be a rare situation in which a CBA would be an appropriate technique to use in an evaluation of a health promotion program. Even if an evaluator were able to determine these values, there are some (Fielding, 1979; Kristein, 1983) who believe the cost-benefit ratio would not favor the health promotion programs. These individuals have indicated that there are several cost issues that evaluators

TABLE 2 Effect of discount rate on discounted value

Discount Rate	Time (in years)	Present Value of Cost	Present Value of Benefit	Present Value of Net Benefit
0	5	$1,000	$2,000	$1,000
3	5	$1,000	$1,725	$725
5	5	$1,000	$1,567	$567
7	5	$1,000	$1,426	$426
10	5	$1,000	$1,242	$242
15	5	$1,000	$994	$–6

to date have not considered when calculating a CBA. One of these issues revolves around the additional costs of human longevity. When an individual lives longer, he/she is more likely to have incurred additional medical costs and an employee will have to pay pensions for a longer period of time.

Conclusion

Many of the early health promotion programs planned in this country were implemented on the premise that it was more economically sound to spend health care dollars on prevention activities than on curing disease. At the present time, there is little empirical data to prove such economic evaluation—even though CBA and CEA have been used in many other areas of the health care system. As one looks to the future, it seems reasonable that if health promotion program planners are going to convince policy makers that such programs are an effective means of improving health status, then economic evaluation must be a part of the total evaluation process.

References

Acton, J. (1976). Measuring the monetary value of lifesaving programs. *Law and Contemporary Problems, 40,* 46.

Alderman, M. H., Madhavan, S., & Davis, T. (1983). Reduction of cardiovascular disease events by worksite hypertension treatment. *Hypertension, 5* (supplement V). V138–V143.

Collen, M., & Goodman, C. (1985). Cost-effectiveness and cost-benefit analysis. In Institute of Medicine, *Assessing Medical Technologies* (pp. 136–144, 160–164). Washington, D.C.: National Medical Press.

Cooper, B., & Rice, D. (1976). The economic cost of illness revisited. *Social Security Bulletin, 39,* 21.

Erfurt, J.C., & Foote, A. (1984). Cost-effectiveness of work-site blood pressure control programs. *Journal of Occupational Medicine, 26,* 892–900.

Fielding, J. E. (1982). Effectiveness of employee health improvement programs. *Journal of Occupational Medicine, 24,* 907–916.

Fielding, J. E. (1984). Health promotion and disease prevention at the worksite. In L. Breslow (Ed.), *Annual Review in Public Health* (pp. 237–265). Palo Alto, California: Annual Reviews, Inc.

Fielding, J. E. (1979). Preventive medicine and the bottom line. *Journal of Occupational Medicine, 21,* 79–88.

Foote, A., & Erfurt, J. C. (1977). Controlling hypertension: A cost-effective model. *Preventive Medicine, 6,* 319–343.

Green, L. W. (1979). How to evaluate health promotion. *Hospitals, 53,* 106–108.

Green, L. W., & Lewis, F. M. (1986). *Measurement and evaluation in health education and health promotion.* Palo Alto, California: Mayfield Publishing Company

Kristein, M. M. (1977). Economic issues in prevention. *Preventive Medicine, 6,* 252–264.

Kristein, M. M. (1983). How much can business expect to profit from smoking cessation? *Preventive Medicine, 12,* 358–381.

Office of Technology Assessment, U.S. Congress. (1978). *Assessing the efficacy and safety of medical technologies.* Washington, D.C.: U.S. Government Printing Office.

Office of Technology Assessment, U.S. Congress (1980). *The implications of cost-effectiveness analysis of medical technology/background paper #1: Methodological issues and literature review.* Washington, D.C.: U.S. Government Printing Office.

Rogers, P. J., Eaton, E. K., & Bruhn, J. G. (1981). Is health promotion cost effective? *Preventive Medicine, 10,* 324–339.

Rice, D. (1966). *Estimating the cost of illness.* U.S. Department of Health, Education and Welfare, PHS, Health Economic Series No. 6.

Ruchlin, H. S., & Alderman, M. H. (1980). Cost of hypertension control at the workplace. *Journal of Occupational Medicine, 22,* 795–800.

Ruchlin, H. S., Melcher, L. A., & Alderman, M. H. (1984). A comparative economic analysis of work-related hypertension care programs. *Journal of Occupational Medicine, 26,* 45–49.

Scheffler, R. M., & Paringer, L. (1980). A review of the economic evidence on prevention. *Medical Care, 18,* 473–484.

Schwartz, R. M., & Rollins, P. L. (1985). Measuring the cost benefit of wellness strategies. *Business and Health, 2,* 10, 24–26.

Seidman, L. S., Sevelius, G. G., & Ewald, P. (1984). A cost-effective weight loss program at the worksite. *Journal of Occupational Medicine, 26,* 725–730.

Shepard, D. S., & Thompson, M. S. (1979). First principles of cost-effectiveness analysis in health. *Public Health Reports, 94,* 535–543.

Warner, K. E., & Hutton, R. C. (1980). Cost-benefit and cost-effective analysis in health care. *Medical Care, 18,* 1069–1084.

Warner, K. E., & Luce, B. R. (1982). *Cost-benefit and cost-effectiveness in health care: Principles, practice, and potential.* Ann Arbor, Michigan: Health Administration Press.

Warner, K. E. (1979). The economic implications of preventive health care. *Social Science and Medicine, 13C,* 227–237.

Weiss, S. J., Jurs, S., Lesage, J. P., & Iverson, D. C. (1984). A cost-benefit analysis of a smoking cessation program. *Evaluation and Program Planning, 7,* 337–346.

Windsor, R. A., Baranowski, T., Clark, N., & Cutter, G. (1984). *Evaluation of health promotion and education programs.* Palo Alto, California: Mayfield Publishing Company.

Work Group on Health Promotion/Disease Prevention. (1987). Criteria for the development of health promotion and education programs. *American Journal of Public Health, 77,* 89–92.

References

Ad Hoc Work Group of the American Public Health Association. (1987). Criteria for the development of health promotion and education programs. *American Journal of Public Health, 77*(1), 89–92.

Agency for Health Care Policy and Research (AHCPR). (1996). *Smoking cessation: Clinical practice guideline no. 18.* (AHCPR Publication No. 96-0692). Rockville, MD: Author.

Ajzen, I. (1988). *Attitudes, personality, and behavior.* Chicago: Dorsey Press.

Albrecht, T. L. (1997). Defining social marketing: Twenty five years later. *Social Marketing Quarterly, 3*, 21–23.

Albrecht, T. L., & Bryant, C. (1996). Advances in segmentation modeling for health communication and social marketing campaigns. *Journal of Health Communication, 1*, 65–80.

Aldana, S. G. (2001). Financial impact of health promotion programs: A comprehensive review of the literature. *American Journal of Health Promotion, 15*(5), 296–320.

Alexander, G. (1999). Health risk appraisal. In G. C. Hyner, K. W. Peterson, J. W. Travis, J. E. Dewey, J. J. Foerster, & E. M. Framer (Eds.), *SPM handbook of health assessment tools* (pp. 5–8). Pittsburgh, PA: The Society of Prospective Medicine.

Alinsky, S. D. (1971). *Rules for radicals: A pragmatic primer for realistic radicals.* New York: Random House.

Altschuld, J. W., & Witkin, B. R. (2000). *From needs assessment to action: Transforming needs into solution strategies.* Thousand Oaks, CA: Sage Publications, Inc.

American Association for Health Education (AAHE), National Commission for Health Education Credentialing, Inc. (NCHEC), & Society for Public Health Education (SOPHE). (1999). *A competency-based framework for graduate-level health educators.* Reston, VA: Authors.

American Association of School Administrators (AASA). (1990). *Healthy kids for the year 2000: An action plan for schools.* Arlington, VA: Author.

American College Health Association (ACHA). (2002). *Healthy Campus 2010: Making it Happen.* Baltimore, MD: Author.

American Indian Health Care Association (AIHCA). (no date). *Promoting health traditions workbook—A Guide to the healthy people 2000 campaign.* St. Paul, MN: Author.

American Public Health Association. (1991). *Healthy communities 2000: Model standards—Guidelines for community attainment of the year 2000 national health objectives* (3rd ed.). Washington, DC: Author.

Anderson, D. R., & O'Donnell, M. P. (1994). Toward a health promotion research agenda: "State of the science" reviews. *American Journal of Health Promotion, 8*(6), 462–465.

Anderson, P., & Fenichel, E. (1989). *Serving culturally diverse families of infants and toddlers with disabilities.* Washington, DC: National Center for Clinical Infant Programs.

Andreasen, A. (1995). *Marketing sound change: Changing behavior to promote health, social development, and the environment.* San Francisco: Jossey-Bass.

Anspaugh, D. J., Dignan, M. B., Anspaugh, S. L. (2000). *Developing health promotion programs.* Boston, MA: McGraw-Hill.

Anspaugh, D. J., Hunter, S., & Savage, P. (1996). Enhancing employee participation in corporate health promotion programs. *American Journal of Health Behavior, 20*(3), 112–120.

Archer, S. E., & Fleshman, R. P. (1985). *Community health nursing.* Monterey, CA: Wadsworth Health Sciences.

Archer, S. E., Kelly, C. D., & Bisch, S. A. (1984). *Implementing change in communities: A collaborative process.* St. Louis: C. V. Mosby.

Arkin, E. B. (1990). Opportunities for improving the nation's health through collaboration with the mass media. *Public Health Reports, 105*(3), 219–223.

Association for the Advancement of Health Education (AAHE). (1994). *Cultural awareness and sensitivity: Guidelines for health educators.* Reston, VA: Author.

Auld, E. (1997). Practical tips for influencing public policy. *Health Education & Behavior, 24*(3), 272–274.

Babbie, E. (1992). *The practice of social research* (6th ed.). Belmont, CA: Wadsworth Publishing Company.

Backer, T. E., & Rogers, E. M. (1998). Diffusion of innovations theory and worksite AIDS programs. *Journal of Health Communication, 1,* 17–28.

Bakker, A. B. (1999). Persuasive communication about AIDS prevention: Need for cognition determines the impact of message format. *AIDS Education and Prevention, 11,* 150–162.

Bandura, A. (1977a). Self-efficacy: Toward a unifying theory of behavioral change. *Psychological Review, 84*(2), 191–215.

Bandura, A. (1977b). *Social learning theory.* Englewood Cliffs, NJ: Prentice-Hall.

Bandura, A. (1986). *Social foundations of thought and action.* Englewood Cliffs, NJ: Prentice-Hall.

Bandura, A. (2001). Social cognitive theory: An agentic perspective. *Annual review of psychology, 52,* 1–26.

Baranowski, T., (1985). Methodologic issues in self-report of health behavior. *Journal of School Health, 55*(5), 179–182.

Baranowski, T., Perry, C. L., & Parcel, G. S. (2002). How individuals, environments, and health behavior interact. In K. Glanz, B. K. Rimer, & F. M. Lewis (Eds.), *Health behavior and health education: Theory, research, and practice* (3rd ed., pp. 165–184). San Francisco, CA: Jossey-Bass.

Barnes, M. D., Neiger, B. L., & Thackeray, R. (2003). Health communication. In R. J. Bensley & J Brookins-Fisher (Eds.), *Community health education methods* (2nd ed., pp. 51–82). Boston, MA: Jones and Bartlett Publishers.

Bartholomew, L. K., Parcel, G. S., Kok, G., & Gottlieb, N. H. (2001). *Intervention mapping: Designing theory- and evidenced-based health promotion programs.* Mountain View, CA: Mayfield Publishing Company.

Bartlett, E. E., Windsor, R. A., Lowe, J. B., & Nelson, G. (1986). Guidelines for conducting smoking cessation programs. *Health Education, 17*(1), 31–37.

Bartol, K. M., & Martin, D. C. (1991). *Management.* New York, NY: McGraw-Hill Inc.

Bates, I. J., & Winder, A. E. (1984). *Introduction to health education.* Palo Alto, CA: Mayfield.

Becker, M. H. (Ed.). (1974). The health belief model and personal health behavior. *Health Education Monographs, 2* (entire issue).

Becker, M. H., Drachman, R. H., & Kirscht, J. P. (1974). A new approach to explaining sick-role behavior in low income populations. *American Journal of Public Health, 64*(March), 205–216.

Becker, M. H., & Green, L. W. (1975). A family approach to compliance with medical treatment, a selective review of the literature. *International Journal of Health Education, 18*(3), 2–11.

Beckwith, H. (1997). *Selling the invisible: A field guide to modern marketing* (p. 31). New York: Warner Books.

Behrens, R. (1983). *Work-site health promotion: Some questions and answers to help you get started.* Washington, DC: Office of Disease Prevention and Health Promotion.

Bellicha, T., & McGrath, J. (1990). Mass media approaches to reducing cardiovascular disease risk. *Public Health Reports, 105*(3), 245–252.

Bensley, L. B. (1989). A review of the use of mass media and marketing in health education: A look at theory and practice. *Eta Sigma Gamman, 21*(1), 18–23.

Bensley, L. B. (1991). Schoolsite health promotion: Ways of sustaining interest. *Journal of Health Education, 22*(2), 86–89.

Berkman, L. F., & Syme, S. L. (1979). Social networks, host resistance and mortality: A nine-year follow-up of Alameda County residents. *American Journal of Epidemiology, 109*(2), 186–204.

Berwick, D. M. (2003). Disseminating innovations in health care. *Journal of the American Medical Association, 15,* 1969–1975.

Blackburn, H. (1983). Research and demonstration projects in community cardiovascular disease prevention. *Journal of Public Health Policy, 4*(4), 398–421.

Bloomquist, K. (1981). Physical fitness programs in industry: Applications of social learning theory. *Occupational Health Nursing, 29*(7), 30–33.

Blumenschein, K., & Johannesson, M. (1996). Economic evaluation in healthcare. *Pharmacoeconomics, 10,* 114–122.

Borg, W. R., & Gall, M. D. (1989). *Educational research: An introduction* (5th ed.). New York: Longman.

Borras, J. M., Fernandez, E., Schiaffino, A., Borrell, C., & LaVecchia, C. (2000). Pattern of smoking initiation in Catalonia, Spain, from 1948 to 1992. *American Journal of Public Health, 9,* 1459–1462.

Bourque, L. B., & Fielder, E. P. (1995). *How to conduct self-administered and mail surveys.* Thousand Oaks, CA: Sage.

Bowling, A. (1997). *Measuring health: A review of quality of life measurement scales* (2nd ed.). Philadelphia, PA: Open University Press.

Bowling, A. (2002). *Research methods in health: Investigating health and health services* (2nd ed.). Buckingham, UK: Open University Press.

Brager, G., Specht, H., & Torczyner, J. L. (1987). *Community organizing.* New York: Columbia University Press.

Braithwaite, R. L., Murphy, F., Lythcott, N., & Blumenthal, D. S. (1989). Community organization and development for health promotion within an urban black community: A conceptual model. *Health Education, 20*(5), 56–60.

Breckon, D. J. (1997). *Managing health promotion programs: Leadership skills for the 21st century.* Gaithersburg, MD: Aspen.

Breckon, D. J., Harvey, J. R., & Lancaster, R. B. (1998). *Community health education: Settings, roles, and skills for the 21st century* (4th ed.). Gaithersburg, MD: Aspen.

Breen, M. (1999). Researching grants on the Internet. *Community Health Center Management,* March/April, p. 29.

Breslow, L. (1999). From disease prevention to health promotion. *Journal of the American Medical Association, 281*(11), 1030–1033.

Brownson, R. C., Koffman, D. M., Novotny, T. E., Hughes, R. G., & Eriksen, M. P. (1995). Environmental and policy interventions to control tobacco use and prevent cardiovascular disease. *Health Education Quarterly, 22*(4), 478–498.

Bryant, C. (1998, June). *Social marketing: A tool for excellence.* Eighth annual conference on social marketing in public health, Clearwater Beach, FL.

Burdine, J. N., & McLeroy, K. R. (1992). Practitioners' use of theory: Examples from a workgroup. *Health Education Quarterly, 19*(3), 331–340.

Butterfoss, F. D., & Whitt, M. D. (2003). Building and sustaining coalitions. In R. J. Bensley & J. Brookins-Fisher (Eds.), *Community health education methods* (2nd ed., pp. 325–356). Boston, MA: Jones and Bartlett Publishers.

Buxton, T. (1999). Effective ways to improve health education materials. *Journal of Health Education, 30*(1), 47–50.

Campbell, M. K., Devellis, B. M., Strecher, V. J., Ammerman, A. S., Devillis, R. F., & Sandler, R. S. (1994). Improving dietary behavior: The effectiveness of tailored messages in primary care settings. *American Journal of Public Health, 84*(5), 783–787.

Campinha-Bacote, J. (1994). Cultural competence in psychiatric mental health nursing: A conceptual model. *Nursing Clinics of North America, 29,* 1–8.

Capwell, E. M., Butterfoss, F., & Francisco, V. T. (2000). Why evaluate? *Health Promotion Practice, 1*(1), 15–20.

Centers for Disease Control and Prevention (CDC), U.S. Department of Health and Human Services (USDHHS). (no date). *Planned approach to community health: Guide for local coordinator.* Atlanta, GA: Author.

Centers for Disease Control and Prevention (CDC), U.S. Department of Health and Human Services (USDHHS). (1999a). *An ounce of prevention... What are the returns?* (2nd ed.). Atlanta, GA: Author.

Centers for Disease Control and Prevention (CDC), U.S. Department of Health and Human Services (USDHHS). (1999b). *Best practices for comprehensive tobacco control programs.* Atlanta, GA: Author.

Centers for Disease Control and Prevention (CDC). (1999c). Framework for program evaluation in public health. *Morbidity and Mortality Weekly Report, 48* (RR-11), 1–40.

Centers for Disease Control and Prevention (CDC). (1999d). Ten great public health achievements—United States, 1900–1999. *Morbidity and Mortality Weekly Report, 48*(12), 241–243.

Centers for Disease Control and Prevention (CDC), U.S. Department of Health and Human Services (USDHHS). (2003). *CDCynergy 3.0: Your Guide to Effective Health Communication* (CD-ROM Version 3.0). Atlanta, GA: Author.

Centers for Disease Control and Prevention (2000). *Healthy plan-it: A tool for planning and managing public health programs. Sustainable Management Development Program.* Atlanta, GA: Author.

Centers for Disease Control and Prevention (2001). *Injury fact book: 2001–2002.* Atlanta, CA: National Center for Injury Prevention.

Centers for Disease Control and Prevention (2003a). *Assessing health risk behaviors among young people: Youth risk behavior system, At a Glance.* Atlanta, GA: National Center for Chronic Disease Prevention and Health Promotion.

Chaplin, J. P., & Krawiec, T. S. (1979). *Systems and theories of psychology* (4th ed.). New York: Holt, Rinehart & Winston.

Chapman, L. S. (1997). Securing support from top management. *The Art of Health Promotion, 1*(2), 1–7.

Chapman, L. S. (2003). Meta-evaluation of worksite health promotion economic return studies. *The Art of Health Promotion, 6*(6), 1–14.

Chapman, L. S. (2003a). Biometric screening in health promotion: Is it really as important as we think? *The Art of Health Promotion, 7*(2), 1–12.

Checkoway, B. (1989). Community participation for health promotion: Prescription for public policy. *Wellness Perspectives: Research, Theory and Practice, 6*(1), 18–26.

Chenoweth, D. H. (1987). *Planning health promotion at the worksite.* Indianapolis: Benchmark Press.

Cinelli, B., Rose-Colley, M., & Hayes, D. M. (1988). Health promotion efforts in Pennsylvania schools. *American Journal of Health Promotion, 2*(4), 36–44.

Clapp, J. D., Packard, T. R., & Stanger, L. A. (1993). Community organizing in alcohol and other drug prevention coalition building: The role of strategic decisions. *Journal of Health Education, 24*(3), 157–161.

Clark, N. M., Janz, N. K., Dodge, J. A., & Sharpe, P. A. (1992). Self-regulation of health behavior: The "take PRIDE" program. *Health Education Quarterly, 19*(3), 341–354.

Cleary, M. J., & Neiger, B. L. (1998). *The certified health education specialist: A self-study guide for professional competency* (3rd ed.). Allentown, PA: The National Commission for Health Education Credentialing.

Cohen, S., & Lichtenstein, E. (1990). Partner behaviors that support quitting smoking. *Journal of Consulting and Clinical Psychology, 58,* 304–309.

Colletti, G., & Brownell, K. (1982). *The physical and emotional benefits of social support: Application to obesity, smoking and alcoholism.* In M. Eisler et al. (Eds.), *Progress in behavior modification* (vol. 13). New York: Academic Press.

Conner, R. F. (1980). Ethical issues in the use of control groups. In R. Perloff & E. Perloff (Eds.), *New Directions for Program Evaluation* (pp. 63–75). San Francisco: Jossey-Bass.

Connor, D. M. (1968). *Strategies for development.* Ottawa: Development Press.

Cook, T. D., & Campbell, D. T. (1979). *Quasi-experimentation: Design and analysis issues for field settings.* Boston: Houghton Mifflin.

Cottrell, R. R., & McKenzie, J. F. (in press). *Health promotion & education research methods: Using the 5 chapter thesis/dissertation model.* Boston, MA: Jones & Bartlett.

Cottrell, R. R., Girvan, J. T., & McKenzie, J. F. (2002). *Principles and foundations of health promotion and foundations* (2nd ed.). San Francisco, CA: Benjamin Cummings.

Cousins, J. B., & Earl, L. M. (Eds.). (1995). *Participatory evaluation in education: Studies in evaluation use and organisational learning.* Washington, DC: Falmer.

Cowdery, J. E., Wang, M. Q., Eddy, J. M., & Trucks, J. K. (1995). A theory driven health promotion program in a university setting. *Journal of Health Education, 26*(4), 248–250.

Creswell, J. W. (2002). *Educational research: Planning, conducting and evaluating quantitative and qualitative research.* Merrill Prentice Hall: Upper Saddle River, NJ.

Crosby, R. A., Kegler, M. C., & DiClemente, R. J. (2002). Understanding and applying theory in health promotion practice and research. In R. J. DiClemente, R. A. Crosby, & M. C. Kegler (Eds.), *Emerging theories in health promotion practice and research: Strategies for improving public health.* (pp. 1–15). San Francisco, CA: Jossey-Bass.

Cummings, C., Gordon, J. R., & Marlatt, G. A. (1980). Relapse: Prevention and prediction. In W. R. Miller (Ed.), *Addictive behaviors* (pp. 291–322). Oxford, U.K.: Pergamon Press.

Cummings, K., Becker, M. H., & Maile, M. (1980). Bringing the models together in an empirical approach to combining variables used to explain health actions. *Journal of Behavioral Medicine, 3*(2), 123–145.

D'Onofrio, C. N. (1992). Theory and the empowerment of health education practitioners. *Health Education Quarterly, 19*(3), 385–403.

Dane, F. C. (1990). *Research Methods.* Pacific Grove, CA: Brooks/Cole Publishing Company.

Daniel, E. L., & Balog, J. E. (1997). Utilization of the world wide web in health education. *Journal of Health Education, 28*(5), 260–267.

Davis, J. (1990). Employee health newsletters: Analysis of characteristics. *AAOHN Journal, 38*(8), 360–367.

Davis, N. A., Lewis, M. J., Rimer, B. K., Harvey, C. M., & Koplan, J. P. (1997). Evaluation of a phone intervention to promote mammography in a managed care plan. *American Journal of Health Promotion, 11*(4), 247–249.

Davis, T. C., Mayeaux, E. J., Fredrickson, D., Bocchini, J. A., Jackson, R. H., & Murphy, P. W. (1994). Reading ability of parents compared with reading level of pediatric patient education materials. *Pediatrics, 93,* 460–468.

Deeds, S. G. (1992). *The health education specialist: Self-study for professional competence.* Los Alamitos, CA: Loose Canon.

DiBlase, D. (1985). Small businesses lead into wellness. *Business Insurance,* (December 2), 16.

DiClemente, R. J., Crosby, R. A., & Kegler, M. C. (Eds.). (2002). *Emerging theories in health promotion practice and research: Strategies for improving public health.* San Francisco, CA: Jossey-Bass.

Dignan, M. B. (1995). *Measurement and evaluation of health education* (3rd ed.). Springfield, IL: Charles C. Thomas.

Dignan, M. B., & Carr, P. A. (1992). *Program planning for health education and health promotion.* Philadelphia: Lea & Febiger.

Dishman, R. K., Sallis, J. F., & Orenstein, D. R. (1985). The determinants of physical activity and exercise. *Public Health Reports, 100*(2), 158–171.

Doak, C. C., Doak, L. G., & Root, J. H. (1996). *Teaching patients with low literacy skills* (2nd ed.). Philadelphia, PA: J. B. Lippincott Company.

Dollahite, J., Thomson, C., & McNew, R. (1996). Readability of printed sources of diet and health information. *Patient Education and Counseling, 27*(2), 123–134.

Dunbar, J. M., Marshall, G. D., & Howell, M. F. (1979). Behavioral strategies for improving compliance. In R. B. Haynes, D. W. Taylor, & D. L. Sackett (Eds.), *Compliance in health care* (pp. 174–190). Baltimore: Johns Hopkins University Press.

EBSCO (2003). *ERIC.* Retrieved October 17, 2003, from http://www.epnet.com/academic/eric.asp

Eddy, J. M., Donahue, R. E., Webster, R. D., & Bjornstad, E. D. (2002). Application of an ecological worksite health promotion: A review. *American Journal of Health Studies, 17*(4), 197–202.

Edington, D. W. (2001). Emerging research: A view from one research center. *American Journal of Health Promotion, 15*(5)341–349.

Edington, D. W., & Yen, L. (1992). Is it possible to simultaneously reduce risk factors and excess health care costs? *American Journal of Health Promotion, 6*(6), 403–406, 409.

Elliott, S. (Ed.). (1998). *Health and productivity management: Consortium benchmarking study, Best-practice report.* Houston, TX: American Productivity and Quality Center.

Emont, S. L., & Cummings, K. M. (1989). Adoption of smoking policies by automobile dealerships. *Public Health Reports, 104*(5), 509–514.

Emont, S. L., & Cummings, K. M. (1992). Using low-cost prize-drawing incentive to improve recruitment rate at a workshop smoking cessation clinic. *Journal of Occupational Medicine, 34*(8), 771–774.

Erfurt, J. C., Foote, A., Heirich, M. A., & Gregg, W. (1990). Improving participation in worksite wellness: Comparing health education classes, a menu approach, and follow-up counseling. *American Journal of Health Promotion, 4*(4), 270–278.

Erickson, A. C., McKenna, J. W., & Romano, R. M. (1990). Past lessons and new uses of the mass media in reducing tobacco consumption. *Public Health Reports, 105*(3), 239–244.

Faerber, M. (Ed.). (1999). *Gale directory of databases: Volume 1: Online databases.* Detroit, MI: Gale Group, Inc.

Feldman, R. H. L. (1983). Strategies for improving compliance with health promotion programs in industry. *Health Education, 14*(4), 21–25.

Fennell, R., & Beyrer, M. K. (1989). AIDS: Some ethical considerations for the health educator. *Journal of American College Health, 38*(November), 145–147.

Ferrence, R. (1996). Using diffusion theory in health promotion: The case of tobacco. *Canadian Journal of Public Health, Supp2,* 24–27.

Fink, A., & Kosecoff, J. (1978). *An evaluation primer.* Washington, DC: Capitol Publications.

Finkler, S. A. (1992). *Budgeting concepts for nurse managers* (2nd ed.). Philadelphia: W. B. Saunders.

Fishbein, M. (Ed.) (1967). *Readings in attitudes theory measurement.* New York, NY: Wiley.

Fishbein, M., & Ajzen, I. (1975). *Belief, attitude, intention and behavior: An introduction to theory and research.* Reading, MA: Addison-Wesley.

Fitzpatrick, J. L., Sanders, J. R., & Worthen, B. R. (2004). *Program evaluation: Alternative approaches and practical guidelines* (3rd ed.). Boston, MA: Pearson, Allyn & Bacon.

Forster, J., Jeffery, R., Sullivan, S., & Snell, M. (1985). A worksite weight control program using financial incentives collected through payroll deduction. *Journal of Occupational Medicine, 27*(11), 804–808.

Frankish, C. J., Lovato, C. Y., & Shannon, W. J. (1998). Models, theories, and principles of health promotion with multicultural populations. In R. M. Huff & M. V. Kline (Eds.), *Promoting health in multicultural populations* (pp. 41–72). Thousand Oaks, CA: Sage.

Franklin, B. A. (Ed.). (2000). *ACSM's Guidelines for exercise testing and prescription* (6th ed.). Philadelphia, PA: Lippincott Williams & Wilkins.

Frederiksen, L. (1984). Using incentives in worksite wellness. *Corporate Commentary, 1*(2), 51–57.

Freimuth, V. S., & Mettger, W. (1990). Is there a hard-to-reach audience? *Public Health Reports, 105*(3), 232–238.

Freire, P. (1973). *Education: The practice of freedom.* London: Writer's and Reader's Publishing.

Freire, P. (1974). *Pedagogy of the oppressed.* New York: Seabury Press.

French, S. A., Jeffery, R. W., & Oliphant, J. A. (1994). Facility access and self-reward as methods to promote physical activity among healthy sedentary adults. *American Journal of Health Promotion, 8*(4), 257–259, 262.

French, S. A., Jeffery, R. W., Story, M., Hannan, P., & Snyder, M. P. (1997). A pricing strategy to promote low-fat snack choices through vending machines. *American Journal of Public Health, 87*(5), 849–851.

Gilbert, G., & Sawyer, R. (2000). *Health education: Creating strategies for school and community health* (2nd ed.). Boston: Jones & Bartlett.

Gilmore, G. D., & Campbell, M. D. (1996). *Needs assessment strategies for health education and health promotion* (2nd ed.). Madison, WI: WCB Brown & Benchmark.

Glanz, K., & Rimer, B. K. (1995). *Theory at a glance: A guide for health promotion practice* [NIH Pub. No. 95–3896]. Washington, DC: National Cancer Institute.

Glanz, K., Lewis, F. M., & Rimer, B. K. (Eds.). (2002a). *Health behavior and health education: Theory, research, and practice.* San Francisco, CA: Jossey-Bass.

Glanz, K., Lewis, F. M., & Rimer, B. K., (2002b). Theory, research, and practice in health behavior and health education. In K. Glanz, B. K. Rimer, & F. M. Lewis (Eds.), *Health behavior and health education: Theory, research, and practice.* (3rd ed, pp. 22–39.) San Francisco, CA: Jossey-Bass.

Glasgow, R. E. (2002). Evaluation of theory-based interventions: The RE-AIM model. In K. Glanz, B. K. Rimer, & F. M. Lewis (Eds.), *Health behavior and health education: Theory research, and practice* (3rd. ed, pp. 530–544). San Francisco, CA: Jossey-Bass.

Glasgow, R. E., Vogt, T. M., & Boles, S. M. (1999). Evaluating the public health impact of health promotion interventions: The RE-AIM framework. *American Journal of Public Health, 89*(9), 1322–1327.

Godin, G., & Kok, G. (1996). The theory of planned behavior: A review of its applications to health-related behaviors. *American Journal of Health Promotion, 11*(2), 87–98.

Goetzel, R. Z., Anderson, D. R., Whitmer, R. W., Ozminkowski, R. J., Dunn, R. L., & Wasserman, J., The Health Enhancement Research Organization (HERO) Research Committee. (1998). The relationships between modifiable health risks and health care expenditures. *Journal of Occupational and Environmental Medicine, 40* (10), 843–854.

Golaszewski, T. (2001). Shining lights: Studies that have most influenced the understanding of health promotion's financial impact. *American Journal of Health Promotion, 15*(5), 332–340.

Golaszewski, T. J., Yen, L., Clearie, A., Lynch, W., & Vickery, D. (1989, September). Characteristics of employees reporting medical visits saved from use of the medical self-care text, Take care of yourself: The consumer's guide to medical care (pp. 152–161). In *Proceedings of the 25th Annual Meeting of the Society of Prospective Medicine.* Indianapolis, IN: Society of Prospective Medicine.

Goldman, K. D. (1994). Perceptions of innovations as predictors of implementation levels: The diffusion of nation-wide health education campaign. *Health Education and Behavior, 21*(4), 429–444.

Goldman, K. D. (1998). Promoting new ideas on the job: Practical theory-based strategies. *The Health Educator, 30*(1), 49–52.

Goldstein, M. G., DePue, J., Kazura, A., & Niaura, R. (1998). Models for provider-patient interaction: Applications to health behavior change. In S. A. Shumaker, E. B. Schron,

J. K. Ockene, & W. L. McBee (Eds.), *The handbook of health behavior change* (2nd ed., pp. 85–113). New York: Springer.

Goodman, R. M., & Steckler, A. (1989). A model for the institutionalization of health promotion programs. *Family and Community Health, 11*(4), 63–78.

Goodman, R. M., McLeroy, K. R., Steckler, A. B., & Hoyle, R. H. (1993). Development of level of institutionalization scales for health promotion programs. *Health Education Quarterly, 20*(2), 161–178.

Graber, M. A., Roller, C. M., & Kaeble, B. (1999). Readability levels of patient education material on the World Wide Web. *The Journal of Family Medicine, 48*(1), 58–61.

Granat, J. P. (1994). *Persuasive advertising for entrepreneurs and small business owners: How to create more effective sales messages.* Binghamton, NY: Haworth Press.

Green, L. W. (1974). Toward cost-benefit evaluations of health education: Some concepts, methods, and examples. *Health Education Monographs, 2* (Suppl. 1), 34–64.

Green, L. W. (1975). Evaluation of patient education programs. Criteria and measurement techniques. In *Rx: Education for the patient: Proceedings of the Continuing Education Institution, Southern Illinois University* (pp. 89–98). Carbondale, IL: Southern Illinois University Press.

Green, L. W. (1976). Methods available to evaluate the health education components of preventive health programs. In *Preventive Medicine, USA* (pp. 162–171). New York: Prodist.

Green, L. W. (1979). National policy on the promotion of health. *International Journal of Health Education, 22,* 161–168.

Green, L. W. (1980). Healthy People: The Surgeon General's report and the prospects. In W. J. McNervey (Ed.), *Working for a healthier America* (pp. 95–110). Cambridge, MA: Ballinger.

Green, L. W. (1981a). Emerging federal perspectives on health promotion. In J. P. Allegrante (Ed.), *Health Promotion Monographs* (28 pp.). New York: Teachers College, Columbia University.

Green, L. W. (1981b). The objectives for the nation in disease prevention and health promotion: A challenge to health education training. *Proceedings of the National Conference for Institutions Preparing Health Educators,* (DHHS Publication No. 81–50171) (pp. 61–73). Washington, DC: U.S. Office of Health Information and Health Promotion.

Green, L. W. (1982). Reconciling policy in health education and primary care. *International Journal of Health Education, 24* (Suppl. 3), 1–11.

Green, L. W. (1983a). New policies in education for health. *World Health* (April–May), 13–17.

Green, L. W. (1983b). *New policies for health education in primary health care* (Background document for the technical discussions of the 36th World Health Assembly, May 1983). Geneva: World Health Organization.

Green, L. W. (1984a). A triage and stepped approach to self-care education. *Medical Times, 111,* 75–80.

Green, L. W. (1984b). Health education models. In J. D. Matarazzo, S. M. Weiss, & J. A. Herd (Eds.), *Behavioral health: A handbook of health enhancement and disease prevention* (pp. 181–198). New York: Wiley.

Green, L. W. (1984c). La educacion para la salud en el medio urbano. In *Conferencia Inter-Americana de Educacion Para La Salud* (pp. 80–82). Mexico City: Sector Salud, SEP, and International Union for Health Education and World Health Organization.

Green, L. W. (1984d). Modifying and developing health behavior. *Annual Review of Public Health, 5,* 215–236.

Green, L. W. (1986a, October). *Applications and trials of the PRECEDE framework for planning and evaluation of health programs.* Paper presented at the meeting of the American Public Health Association, Las Vegas, NV.

Green, L. W. (1986b). Evaluation model: A framework for the design of rigorous evaluation of efforts in health promotion. *American Journal of Health Promotion, 1*(1), 77–79.

Green, L. W. (1986c). *New policies for health education in primary health care.* Geneva: World Health Organization.

Green, L. W. (1986d). Research agenda: Building a consensus on research questions. *American Journal of Health Promotion, 1*(2), 70–72.

Green, L. W. (1986e). The theory of participation: A qualitative analysis of its expression in national and international health policies. In W. B. Ward (Ed.), *Advances in Health Education and Promotion* (pp. 211–236). Greenwich, CT: JAI Press.

Green, L. W. (1987a). How physicians can improve patients' participation and maintenance in self-care. *Western Journal of Medicine, 147,* 346–349.

Green, L. W. (1987b). *Program planning and evaluation guide for Lung Associations.* New York: American Lung Association.

Green, L. W. (1989, March). *The health promotion program of the Henry J. Kaiser Family Foundation.* Paper presented at a public lecture at Mankato State University, Mankato, MN.

Green, L. W. (1990). The revival of community and the public obligation of academic health centers. In R. E. Bulger and S. J. Reiser (Eds.), *Integrity in institutions: Humane environments for teaching* (pp. 163–178). Iowa City: University of Iowa Press.

Green, L. W. (1999). Health education's contributions to public health in the twentieth century: A glimpse through health promotion's rear-view mirror. In J. E. Fielding, L. B. Lave, & B. Starfield (Eds.), *Annual review of public health* (pp. 67–88). Palo Alto, CA: Annual Reviews.

Green, L. W., & Allen, J. (1980). *Toward a healthy community: Organizing events for community health promotion* (PHS Publication No. 80–50113). Washington, DC: USDHHS, Office of Disease Prevention and Health Promotion.

Green, L. W., Glanz, K., Hochbaum, G. M., Kok, G., Kreuter, M. W., Lewis, F. M., Lorig, K., Morisky, D., Rimer, B. K., & Rosenstock, I. M. (1994). Can we build on, or must we replace, the theories and models of health education? *Health Education Research, 9*(3), 397–404.

Green, L. W., & Kreuter, M. W. (1991). *Health promotion planning: An educational and environmental approach* (2nd ed.). Mountain View, CA: Mayfield.

Green, L. W., & Kreuter, M. W. (1992). CDC's planned approach to community health as an application of PRECEDE and an inspiration for PROCEED. *Journal of Health Education, 23*(3), 140–147.

Green, L. W., & Kreuter, M. W. (1999). *Health promotion planning: An educational and ecological approach* (3rd ed.). Mountain View, CA: Mayfield.

Green, L. W., Kreuter, M. W., Deeds, S. G., & Partridge, K. B. (1980). *Health education planning: A diagnostic approach.* Palo Alto, CA: Mayfield.

Green, L. W., Levine, D. M., & Deeds, S. G. (1975). Clinical trials of health education for hypertensive outpatients: Design and baseline data. *Preventive Medicine, 4,* 417–425.

Green, L. W., & Lewis, F. M. (1986). *Measurement and evaluation in health education and health promotion.* Palo Alto, CA: Mayfield.

Green, L. W., & McAlister, A. L. (1984). Macrointervention to support health behavior: Some theoretical perspectives and practical reflections. *Health Education Quarterly, 11,* 323–339.

Green, L. W., Mullen, P. D., & Friedman, R. (1986). An epidemiological approach to targeting drug information. *Patient Education and Counseling, 8,* 255–268.

Green, L. W., Wang, V. L., Deeds, S. G., Fisher, A. A., Windsor, R., & Rogers, C. (1978). Guidelines for health education in maternal and child health programs. *International Journal of Health Education, 21* (suppl.), 1–33.

Green, L. W., Wilson, A. L., & Lovato, C. Y. (1986). What changes can health promotion achieve and how long do these changes last? The tradeoffs between expediency and durability. *Preventive Medicine, 15,* 508–521.

Green, L. W., Wilson, R. W., & Bauer, K. G. (1983). Data required to measure progress on the objectives for the nation in disease prevention and health promotion. *American Journal of Public Health, 73,* 18–24.

Greenberg, J. (1978). Health education as freeing. *Health Education, 9*(2), 20–21.

Grunbaum, J. A., Gingiss, P., Orpinas, P., Batey, L. S., & Parcel, G. S. (1995). A comprehensive approach to school health program needs assessment. *Journal of School Health, 65*(2), 54–59.

Guyer, M. (1999). Grants: Finding a funding source. *Grant Source* (pp. 1–3). Columbus, OH: Office of the Auditor, State of Ohio.

Hall, C. L. (1943). *Principles of behavior.* New York: Appleton-Century-Crofts.

Hallfors, D., & Godette, D. (2002). Will the principles of effectiveness improve prevention practice? Early findings from a diffusion study. *Health Education Research, 4,* 461–470.

Hancock, T., & Minkler, M. (1997). Community health assessment of healthy community assessment. In M. Minkler (Ed.), *Community organizing and community building for health* (pp. 139–156). New Brunswick, NJ: Rutgers University Press.

Hanlon, J. J. (1974). *Administration of public health.* St. Louis: C. V. Mosby.

Harris, J. H. (2001). Selecting the right vendor for your health promotion program. *Absolute Advantage, 1*(4), 4–5.

Harris, J. H., McKenzie, J. F., & Zuti, W. B. (1986). How to select the right vendor for your company's health promotion program. *Fitness in Business, 1*(October), pp. 53–56.

Hayden, J. (2000). *The health education specialist: A study guide for professional competence* (4th ed.). Allentown, PA: The National Commission for Health Education Credentialing, Inc.

Health Insurance Association of America. (1983). *Your guide to wellness at the worksite.* Pamphlet issued by the Public Relations Division of the Health Insurance Association of America, Washington, DC.

Healthy people: The Surgeon General's report on health promotion and disease prevention. (1979). (Publication No. 79–55071). Washington, DC: Department of Health, Education, and Welfare (Public Health Service).

Heiser, P. F., & Begay, M. E. (1997). The campaign to raise the tobacco tax in Massachusetts. *American Journal of Public Health, 87*(6), 968–973.

Hellerstedt, W. L., & Jeffery, R. W. (1997). The effects of a telephone-based intervention on weight loss. *American Journal of Health Promotion, 11*(3), 177–182.

Hertoz, J. K., Finnegan, J. R., Rooney, B., Viswanath, K., & Potter, J. (1993). *Health Communication, 5*(1), 21–40.

Hinkle, D. E., Oliver, J. D., & Hinkle, C. A. (1985). How large should the sample be? Part II-the one-sample case for survey research. *Educational and Psychological Measurement 45*(2), 271–280.

Hochbaum, G. M., Sorenson, J. R., & Lorig, K. (1992). Theory in health education practice. *Health Education Quarterly, 19*(3), 295–313.

Hopkins, K. D., Stanley, J. C., & Hopkins, B. R. (1990). *Educational and psychological measurement and evaluation* (7th ed.). Englewood Cliffs, NJ: Prentice-Hall.

Horman, S. (1989). The role of social support on health throughout the lifestyle. *Health Education, 20*(4), 18–21.

Horne, W. M. (1975). Effects of a physical activity program on middle-aged, sedentary corporation executives. *American Industrial Hygiene Journal,* (March), 241–245.

Hosokawa, M. C. (1984). Insurance incentives for health promotion. *Health Education, 15*(6), 9–12.

House, E. R. (1980). *Evaluating with validity.* Beverly Hills, CA: Sage.

Hoyert, D. L., Kochanek, K. D., & Murphy, S. L. (1999). *Deaths: Final data for 1997.* Hyattsville, MD: U.S. Department of Health and Human Services, Public Health Service, CDC, National Center for Health Statistics.

Huff, R. M., & Kline, M. V. (1999). Health promotion in the context of culture. In R. M. Huff & M. V. Kline (Eds.), *Promoting health in multicultural populations* (pp. 3–22). Thousand Oaks, CA: Sage.

Hunt, W. A., Barnett, L. W., & Branch, L. G. (1971). Relapse rates in addiction programs. *Journal of Clinical Psychology, 27*(4), 455–456.

Hurlburt, R. T. (2003). *Comprehending behavioral statistics* (3rd ed.). Belmont, CA: Wadsworth/Thomson Learning.

Hyner, G. C., Peterson, K. W., Travis, J. W., Dewey, J. E., Foerster, J. J., & Framer, E. M. (Eds.). (1999). *SPM handbook of health assessment tools.* Pittsburgh, PA: The Society of Prospective Medicine.

Institute of Medicine (IOM). (1988). *The future of public health.* Washington, DC: National Academy Press.

Israel, B. A., Checkoway, B., Schulz, A., & Zimmerman, M. (1994). Health education and community empowerment: Conceptualizing and measuring perceptions of individual, organizational, and community control. *Health Education Quarterly, 21*(2), 149–170.

Jacobsen, D., Eggen, P., & Kauchak, D. (1989). *Methods for teaching: A skills approach* (3rd ed.). Columbus, OH: Merrill, an imprint of Macmillan Publishing Company.

Jadad, A. R., & Gagliardi, A. (1998). Rating health information on the Internet. *Journal of the American Medical Association, 279,* 611–614.

Janz, N. K., & Becker, M. H. (1984). The health belief model: A decade later. *Health Education Quarterly, 11*(1), 1–47.

Janz, N. K., Champion, V. L., & Strecher, V. J. (2002). The health belief model. In K. Glanz, B. K. Rimer, & F. M. Lewis (Eds.), *Health behavior and health education: Theory, research, and practice* (3rd. ed., pp. 45–66). San Francisco, CA: Jossey-Bass.

Jason, L. A., Jayaraj, S., Blitz, C. C., Michaels, M. H., & Klett, L. E. (1990). Incentives and competition in a worksite smoking cessation intervention. *American Journal of Public Health, 80*(2), 205–206.

Jeffery, R. W., Forster, J. L., Baxter, J. E., French, S. A., & Kelder, S. H. (1993). An empirical evaluation of the effectiveness of tangible incentives in increasing participation and behavior change in a worksite health promotion program. *American Journal of Health Promotion, 8*(2), 98–100.

Jessor, R., & Jessor, S. L. (1977). *Problem behavior and psychosocial development: A longitudinal study of youth.* New York: Academic Press.

Johnson, G., Scholes, K., & Sexty, R. W. (1989). *Exploring strategic management.* Scarborough, Ontario: Prentice Hall.

Joint Committee on Terminology. (2001). Report of the 2000 Joint Committee on Health Education and Promotion Terminology. *American Journal of Health Education, 32*(2), 89–103.

Kaplan, B., & Cassel, J. (1977). Social support and health. *Medical Care, 15*(5), 47–58.

Kendall, R. (1984). Rewarding safety excellence. *Occupational Hazards,* (March), 45–50.

Kerlinger, F. N. (1986). *Foundations of behavioral research.* (3rd ed.). Austin, TX: Holt, Rinehart, & Winston.

Keyser, B. B., Morrow, M. J., Doyle, K., Ogletree, R., & Parsons, N. P. (1997). *Practicing the application of health education skills and competencies.* Boston, MA: Jones and Bartlett.

Kim, S., McLeod, J. H., & Shantzis, C. (1992). Cultural competence for evaluators working with Asian American communities: Some practical considerations. In M. A. Orlandi, R. Weston, & L. G. Epstein (Eds.), *Cultural competence for evaluators.* Rockville, MD: Office of Substance Abuse Prevention.

Kittleson, M. J. (1995). Comparison of the response rate between e-mail and postcards. *Health Values, 19*(2), 27–29.

Kittleson, M. J. (1997). Determining effective follow-up of e-mail surveys. *American Journal of Health Behavior, 21*(3), 193–196.

Kittleson, M. J. (2003). Suggestions for using the web to collect data. *American Journal of Health Behavior, 27*(2), 170–172.

Kline, M. V., & Huff, R. M. (1999). Tips for the practitioner. In R. M. Huff & M. V. Kline (Eds.), *Promoting health in multicultural populations* (pp. 103–111). Thousand Oaks, CA: Sage.

Koffman, D. M., Lee, J. W., Hopp, J. W., & Emont, S. L. (1998). The impact of including incentives and competition in a workplace smoking cessation program on quit rates. *American Journal of Health Promotion, 13*(2), 105–111.

Kotecki, J. E., & Chamness, B. E. (1999). A valid tool for evaluating health-related WWW sites. *Journal of Health Education, 30*(1), 56–59.

Kotecki, J. E., & Siegel, D. (1997). Finding health information via the world wide web: An essential resource for the community health practitioner. *Journal of Health Education, 28*(2), 117–120.

Kotler, P., & Clarke, R. N. (1987). *Marketing for health care organizations.* Englewood Cliffs, NJ: Prentice-Hall.

Kretzmann, J. P., & McKnight, J. L. (1993a). *Building communities from the inside out: A path toward finding and mobilizing a community's assets.* Evanston, IL: Institute for Policy Research.

Kretzmann, J. P., & McKnight, J. L. (1993b). Introduction from *Building communities from the inside out: A path toward finding and mobilizing a community's assets.* Retrieved October 31, 2003, from http://northwestern. edu/ipr/publications/community/introd-building.html

Kreuter, M. W. (1992). PATCH: Its origin, basic concepts, and links to contemporary public health policy. *Journal of Health Education, 23*(3), 135–139.

Kreuter, M. W., Bull, F. C., Clark, E. M., & Oswald, D. L. (1999). Understanding how people process health information: A comparison of tailored and nontailored weight-loss materials. *Health Psychology, 18,* 487–494.

Kreuter, M. W., Farrell, D., Olevitch, L., & Brennan, L. (2000). *Tailoring health messages: Customizing communication with computer technology.* Hillsdale, NJ: Erlbaum.

Kreuter, M. W., Nelson, C. F., Stoddard, R. P., & Watkins, N. B. (1985). *Planned approach to community health.* Atlanta, GA: Centers for Disease Control.

Kreuter, M. W., Vehige, E., & McGuire, A. G. (1996). Using computer-tailored calendars to promote childhood immunization. *Public Health Reports, III* (March/April), 176–178.

Krosnick, J. A., & Petty, R. E. (1995). Attitude strength: An overview. In R. E. Petty & J. A. Krosnick (Eds.), *Attitude strength: Antecedents and consequences* (pp.1–24). Hillsdale, NJ: Erlbaum.

Kumpfer, K., Turner, C., & Alvarado, R. (1991). A community change model for school health promotion. *Journal of Health Education, 22*(2), 94–96, 109–110.

Kviz, F. J., Crittenden, K. S., Madura, K. J., & Warnecke, R. B. (1994). Use and effectiveness of buddy support in a self-help smoking cessation program. *American Journal of Health Promotion, 8*(3), 191–201.

Lalonde, M. (1974). *A new perspective on the health of Canadians: A working document.* Ottawa, Canada: Minister of Health.

Langton, S. (Ed.). (1978). *Citizen participation in america.* Lexington, MA: Lexington Books.

Lefebvre, C. (1992). Social marketing and health promotion. In R. Burton & G. MacDonald (Eds.), *Health promotion: Disciplines and diversity* (pp. 153–181). London: Routledge.

Lefebvre, R. C., & Flora, J. A. (1988). Social marketing and public health intervention. *Health Education Quarterly, 15*(3), 299–315.

LeMaster, P. L., & Connell, C. M. (1994). Health education interventions among native Americans: A review and analysis. *Health Education Quarterly, 21*(4), 521–538.

Leventhal, H., & Cleary, P. D. (1980). The smoking problem: A review of the research and theory in behavioral risk modification. *Psychological Bulletin, 88*(2), 370–405.

Levin, H. M., & McEwan, P. J. (2001). *Cost-effectiveness analysis: Methods and applications.* Thousand Oaks, CA: Sage.

Levine, R. J. (1988). *Ethics and regulations of clinical research* New Haven, CT: Yale University Press.

Lewin, K. (1935). *A dynamic theory of personality.* New York: McGraw-Hill.

Lewin, K. (1936). *Principles of topological psychology.* New York: McGraw-Hill.

Lewin, K., Dembo, T., Festinger, L., & Sears, P. S. (1944). Level of aspiration. In J. Hunt (Ed.), *Personality and the behavior disorders* (pp. 333–378). New York: Ronald Press.

Linkins, R. W., Dini, E. F., Watson, G., & Patriarca, P. A. (1994). A randomized trail of the effectiveness of computer-generated telephone messages in increasing immunization visits among preschool children. *Archives of Pediatric and Adolescent Medicine, 148*(9), 908–914.

Ludman, E. J., Curry, S. J., Meyer, D., & Taplin, S. H. (1999). Implementation of outreach telephone counseling to promote mammography participation. *Health Education & Behavior, 26*(5), 689–702.

Luquis, R. R., & Pe'rez, M. A. (2003). Achieving cultural competence: The challenges for health educators. *American Journal of Health Education, 34*(3), 131–138.

Maccoby, N., & Solomon, D. S. (1981). Heart disease prevention: Community studies. In R. E. Rice, et al. (Eds.), *Public communication campaigns* (pp. 105–125). Beverly Hills, CA: Sage.

Maibach, E., Shenker, A., & Singer, S. (1997). Results of the Delphi survey. *Journal of Health Communication, 2,* 304–307.

Marcarin, S. (Ed.). (1995). *Cumulative index to nursing & allied health literature: CINAHL.* Volume 40, Part A. Glendale, CA.

Marcus, B. H., Emmons, K. M., Simkin-Silverman, L., Linnan, L. A., Taylor, E. R., Bock, B. C., Roberts, M. B., Rossi, J. S., & Abrams, D. B. (1998). Evaluation of motivationally-tailored versus standard self-help physical activity interventions at the workplace. *American Journal of Health Promotion, 12*(4), 246–253.

Marlatt, G. A. (1982). Relapse prevention: A self-control program for treatment of addictive behaviors. In R. B. Sturat (Ed.), *Adherence, compliance, and generalization in behavioral medicine* (pp. 329–377). New York: Brunner/Mazel.

Marlatt, G. A. (1985). Relapse prevention: Theoretical rationale and overview of the model. In G. A. Marlatt & J. R. Gordon (Eds.), *Relapse prevention* (pp. 3–70). New York: Guilford Press.

Marlatt, G. A., & George, W. H. (1998). Relapse prevention and the maintenance of optimal health. In S. A. Shumaker, E. B. Schron, J. K. Ockene, & W. L. McBee (Eds.), *The handbook of health behavior change* (2nd ed., pp. 33–58). New York: Springer.

Marlatt, G. A., & Gordon, J. R. (1980). Determinants of relapse: Implications for maintenance of behavior change. In P. O. Davidson & S. M. Davidson (Eds.), *Behavioral medicine: Changing health lifestyles* (pp. 410–452). New York: Brunner/Mazel.

Mason, J. O., & McGinnis, J. M. (1990). "Healthy people 2000": An overview of the national health promotion and disease prevention objectives. *Public Health Reports, 105*(5), 441–446.

Matson, D. M., Lee, J. W., & Hopp, J. W. (1993). The impact of incentives and competitions on participation and quit rates in worksite smoking cessation programs. *American Journal of Health Promotion, 7*(4), 270–280, 295.

Mausner, J. S., & Kramer, S. (1985). *Epidemiology—An introductory text* (2nd ed.). Philadelphia, PA: W. B. Saunders Company.

McAlister, A. L., Puska, P., Salonen, J. T., Tuomilehot, J., & Koskelia, A. (1982). Theory and action for health promotion: Illustrations from the North Karelia project. *American Journal of Public Health, 72*(1), 43–50.

McCaul, K. D., Bakdash, M. B., Geoboy, M. J., Gerbert, B., et al. (1990). Promoting self-protective health behaviors in dentistry. *Annuals of Behavioral Medicine, 12,* 156–160.

McDermott, R. J., & Sarvela, P. D. (1999). *Health education evaluation and measurement: A practitioner's perspective* (2nd ed.). New York: WCB/McGraw-Hill.

McDowell, I., Newell, C., & Rosser, W. (1989a). Computerized reminders for blood pressure screening in primary care. *Medical Care, 27*(3), 297–305.

McDowell, I., Newell, C., & Rosser, W. (1989b). Computerized reminders to encourage cervical screening in family practice. *Journal of Family Practice, 28*(4), 420–424.

McGinnis, J. M., & Foege, W. H. (1993). Actual causes of death in the United States. *Journal of the American Medical Association, 270,* 2207–2212.

McGinnis, J. M., Williams-Russo, & Knickman, J.R. (2002). The case for more active policy attention to health promotion. *Health Affairs, 21*(2), 78–93.

McGuire, W. J. (1983). A contextual theory of knowledge: Its implications for innovation and reform in psychological research. *Advances in Experimental Social Psychology, 16,* 1–47.

McKenzie, J. F. (1986). Cost-benefit and cost-effectiveness as a part of the evaluation of health promotion programs. *The Eta Sigma Gamman, 18*(2), 10–16.

McKenzie, J. F. (1988). Twelve steps in developing a schoolsite health education/promotion program for faculty and staff. *The Journal of School Health, 58*(4), 149–153.

McKenzie, J. F., Luebke, J., & Romas, J. A. (1992). Incentives: A means of getting and keeping workers involved in health promotion programs. *Journal of Health Education, 23*(2), 70–73.

McKenzie, J. F., Wood, M. L., Kotecki, J. E., Clark, J. K., & Brey, R. A. (1999). Establishing content validity: Using qualitative and quantitative steps. *American Journal of Health Behavior, 23*(4), 311–318.

McKnight, J. L., & Kretzmann, J. P. (1997). Mapping community capacity. In M. Minkler (Ed.), *Community organizing and community building for health.* (pp. 157–172). New Brunswick, NJ: Rutgers University Press.

McLeroy, K. R. (1993). Theory and practice in health education: Which practice, which theory? *American Public Health Association,* *Public Health Education and Health Promotion Section Newsletter,* Summer, 7–8.

McLeroy, K. R., Bibeau, D., Steckler, A., & Glanz, K. (1988). An ecological perspective on health promotion programs. *Health Education Quarterly, 15,* 351–377.

McLeroy, K. R., Steckler, A., Goodman, R. & Burdine, J. N. (1992). Health education research, theory, and practice: Future directions. *Health Education Research, Theory, and Practice, 7*(1), 1–8.

Meyer, J., & Rainey, J. (1994). Writing health education material for low-literacy populations. *Journal of Health Education, 25*(6), 372–374.

Mikanowicz, C. K., & Altman, N. H. (1995). Developing policies on smoking in the workplace. *Journal of Health Education, 26*(3), 183–185.

Miller, R. E., & Golaszewski, T. J. (1992). Analysis of commercial health newsletters by worksite decision makers. *American Journal of Health Promotion, 7*(1), 11–12, 75.

Minino, A. M., & Smith, B. L. (2001). Deaths: *Preliminary data for 2000. National Vital Statistics Report, Vol. 49, No. 12.* Hyattsville, MD: National Center for Health Statistics.

Minkler, M. (Ed.). (1997a). *Community organizing and community building for health.* New Brunswick, NJ: Rutgers University Press.

Minkler, M. (1997b). Introduction and overview. In M. Minkler (Ed.), *Community organizing and community building for health* (pp. 3–19). New Brunswick, NJ: Rutgers University Press.

Minkler, M. (1997c). Community organizing among the elderly poor in San Francisco's Tenderloin district. In M. Minkler (Eds.), *Community organizing and community building for Health.* New Brunswick, NJ: Rutgers University Press.

Minkler, M., & Wallerstein, N. (1997). Improving health through community organization and community building: A health education perspective. In M. Minkler (Ed.), *Community organizing and community building for health* (pp. 30–52). New Brunswick, NJ: Rutgers University Press.

Minkler, M., & Wallerstein, N. B. (2002). Improving health through community organization and community building. In K. Glanz, B. K. Rimer, & F. M. Lewis (Eds.),

Health behavior and health education: Theory, research, and practice (3rd ed., pp. 279–311). San Francisco, CA: Jossey-Bass.

Modell, M. E. (1996). *A professional's guide to system analysis* (2nd ed.). Boston, MA: McGraw-Hill.

Mokdad, A. H., Marks, J. S. Stroup, D. F., & Gerberding, J. L. (2004). Actual causes of death, in the United States, 2000. *Journal of the American Medical Association, 291*(10), 1238–1245.

Mondros, J. B., & Wilson, S. M. (1994). *Organizing for power and empowerment.* New York: Columbia Press.

Montano, D. E., & Kasprzyk, D. (2002). The theory of reasoned action and the theory of planned behavior. In K. Glanz, B. K. Rimer, & F. M. Lewis (Eds.), *Health behavior and health education: Theory, research, and practice* (3rd. ed, pp. 67–98). San Francisco, CA: Jossey-Bass.

Montano, D., Kasprzyk, D., von Haeften, I., & Fishbein, M. (2001). Toward an understanding of condom use behaviors: A theoretical and methodological overview of the project SAFER. *Psychology, Health, & Medicine, 6*(2), 139–150.

Montano, D., Phillips, W,. & Kasprzyk, D. (2000). Explaining physician rates of providing flexible sigmoidoscopy. *Cancer Epidemiology, Biomarkers, & Prevention, 9,* 665–669.

Montano, D., Thompson, B., Taylor, V. M., & Mahloch, J. (1997). Understanding mammography intention and utilization among women in an inner city public hospital clinic. *Prevention Medicine, 26,* 817–824.

Morreale, M. (no date). Understanding public health research: A primer for youth workers. *Issue Brief.* Washington, DC: National Network for Youth.

Morris, L. L., Fitz-Gibbon, C. T., & Freeman, M. E. (1987). *How to communicate evaluation findings.* Newbury Park, CA: Sage.

Moskowitz, J. M. (1989). Preliminary guidelines for reporting outcome evaluation studies of health promotion and disease prevention programs. In M. Braverman (Ed.), *New directions for program evaluation* (pp. 59–74). San Francisco: Jossey-Bass.

National Association of County and City Health Officials (NACCHO). (2001). *Mobilizing for action through planning and partnerships (MAPP).* Washington, DC: Author.

National Association of County Health Officials (NACHO). (1991). *APEX/PH, Assessment protocol for excellence in public health.* Washington, DC: Author.

National Cancer Institute (NCI). (2002). *Making health communication programs work* (NIH Publication No. 02-5145). Washington, DC: U.S. Department of Health and Human Services.

National Commission for Health Education Credentialing, Inc. (NCHEC). (1996). *A competency-based framework for professional development of certified health education specialists.* New York: Author.

National Commission for Health Education Credentialing, Inc. (2003a). *About NCHEC Competencies Update Project.* Retrieved August 29, 2003, from http://www.nchec. org/aboutnchec/cup/press.htm

National Commission for Health Education Credentialing, Inc. (2003b) *Become a CHES: Eligibility for the CHES exam.* Retrieved August 31, 2003, from http://www.nchec. org/becomeches/eligibility.htm

National Dairy Council. (1992). *2000 and counting.* Rosemont, IL: Author.

National Institutes for Health (NIH). (n.d.). *Informed consent and assent.* Retrieved May 25, 2003, from http://www.cc.nih. gov/ccc/protomechanics/chap_3.html# whatareinformca

National Task Force on the Preparation and Practice of Health Educators, Inc. (1985). *A framework for the development of competency-based curricula for entry-level health educators.* New York: Author.

Neiger, B. L. (1998). *Social marketing: Making public health sense.* Paper presented at the annual meeting of the Utah Public Health Association, Provo, UT.

Neiger, B. L., & Thackeray, R. (2002). Application of the SMART Model in two successful social marketing campaigns. *American Journal of Health Education, 33,* 291–293.

Neiger, B. L., Thackeray, R., Merrill, R. M., Miner, K. M., Larsen, L., & Chalkley, C. M. (2001). The impact of social marketing on fruit and vegetable consumption and physical activity among public health employees at the Utah department of health. *Social Marketing Quarterly, 7,* 9–28.

Nelson, D. E., Brownson, R. C., Remington, P. L., & Parvanta, C. (Eds.). (2002). *Communicating public health information effectively: A guide for practitioners.* Washington, DC: American Public Health Association.

Net.MBA. (2003). *CPM-critical path method.* Retrieved November 14, 2003, from http://www.netmba.com/operations/project/cpm/

Newcomer, K. E. (1994). Using statistics appropriately. In J. S. Wholey, H. P. Hatry, & K. E. Newcomer (Eds.), *Handbook of practical program evaluation* (pp. 389–416). San Francisco: Jossey-Bass.

Norwood, S. L. (2000). *Research strategies for advanced practice nurses.* Upper Saddle River, NJ: Prentice-Hall, Inc.

Novelli, W. D. (1988). Marketing health and social issues: What works? In R. Dunmire (Ed.), *Social marketing: Accepting the challenge in public health.* Atlanta, GA: Centers for Disease Control.

Novelli, W. D., & Ziska, D. (1982). Health promotion in the workplace: An overview. *Health Education Quarterly, 9* (suppl.), 20–26.

Nutbeam, D., & Harris, E. (1999). *Theory in a nutshell: A guide to health promotion theory.* Sydney, Australia: The McGraw-Hill Companies, Inc.

Nye, R. D. (1979). *What is B. F. Skinner really saying?* Englewood Cliffs, NJ: Prentice-Hall.

Nye, R. D. (1992). *The legacy of B. F. Skinner: Concepts and perspectives, controversies, and misunderstandings.* Pacific Grove, CA: Brooks/Cole.

O'Donnell, M. (1992). Design of workplace health promotion programs (2nd ed.). Rochester Hills, MI: *American Journal of Health Promotion.*

O'Donnell, M. P. (1996). Editor's notes. *American Journal of Health Promotion, 10*(4), 244.

O'Donnell, M., & Ainsworth, T. (Eds.). (1984). *Health promotion in the workplace.* New York: John Wiley and Sons.

Office of Minority Health (OMH) (2001). *National Standards on Culturally and Linguistically Appropriate Services (CLAS) in Health Care Final Report.* Retrieved November 5, 2003, from http://www.omhrc.gov/clas/ds.htm

Ogbu, J. (1987). Cultural influences on plasticity in human development. In J. L. Gallagher & C. T. Ramey (Eds.), *The malleability of children* (pp. 155–169). Baltimore, MD: Paul H. Brookes.

Olpin, M., & Gotthoffer, D. (2000). *Quick guide to the Internet for health.* Boston: Allyn and Bacon.

Pahnos, M. L. (1992). The continuing challenge of multicultural health education. *Journal of School Health, 62*(1), 24–26.

Parcel, G. S. (1983). Theoretical models for application in school health education research. *Health Education, 15*(4), 39–49.

Parcel, G. S. (1995). Diffusion research: The smart choices project. *Health Education Research: Theory and Practice, 10*(3), 279–281.

Parcel, G. S., & Baranowski, T. (1981). Social learning theory and health education. *Health Education, 12*(3), 14–18.

Parkinson, R. S., & Associates. (1982). *Managing health promotion in the workplace: Guidelines for implementation and evaluation.* Palo Alto, CA: Mayfield.

Pasick, R. J., D'Onofrio, C. N., & Otero-Sabogal, R. (1996). Similarities and differences across cultures: Questions to inform a third generation for health promotion research. *Health Education, 23* (Suppl.), S142–S161.

Pastor, P. N., Makuc, D. M., Reuben, C., & Xia, H. (2002). *Chartbook on trends in health of Americans. Health, United States, 2002.* Hyattsville, MD: National Center for Health Statistics.

Patton, M. Q. (1986). *Utilization-focused evaluation.* Beverly Hills, CA: Sage.

Patton, M. Q. (1988). *How to use qualitative methods in evaluation.* Newbury Park, CA: Sage.

Patton, R. P., Corry, J. M., Gettman, L. R., & Graff, J. S. (1986). *Implementing health/fitness programs.* Champaign, IL: Human Kinetics.

Pavlov, I. (1927). *Conditional reflexes.* Oxford: Oxford University Press.

Pealer, L. N., & Dorman, S. M. (1997). Evaluating health-related web sites. *Journal of School Health, 67*(1), 232–235.

Pellmar, T. C., Brandt, Jr., E. N., & Baird, M. (2002). Health and behavior: The interplay of biological, behavioral, and social influences: Summary of an Institute of Medicine Report. *American Journal of Health Promotion, 16*(4), 206–219.

Penner, M. (1989). Economic incentives to reduce employee smoking: A health insurance surcharge for tobacco using state of Kansas employees. *American Journal of Health Promotion, 4*(1), 5–11.

Pentz, M. A., Johnson, C. A., Dwyer, J. H., MacKinnon, D. M., Hansen, W. B., & Flay, B. R. (1989). A comprehensive community approach to adolescent drug abuse prevention: Effects on cardiovascular disease risk behaviors. *Annals of Medicine, 21*(3), 382–388.

Perlman, J. (1978). Grassroots participation from neighborhood to nation. In S. Langton (Ed.), *Citizen participation in America* (pp. 65–79). Lexington, MA: Lexington Books.

Pescatello, L. S., Murphy, D., Vollono, J., Lynch, E., Bernene, J., & Costanzo, D. (2001). The cardiovascular health impact of an incentive worksite health promotion program. *American Journal of Health Promotion, 16*(1), 16–20.

Petersen, D. J., & Alexander, G. R. (2001). *Needs assessment in public health: A practical guide for students and professionals.* New York, NY: Kluwer Academic/Plenum Publishers.

Petty, R. E., Barden, J., & Wheeler, S. C. (2002). The elaboration likelihood model of persuasion. In R. J. DiClemente, R. A. Crosby, & M. C. Kegler (Eds.), *Emerging theories in health promotion practice and research: Strategies for improving public health.* (pp. 71–99). San Francisco, CA: Jossey-Bass.

Petty, R. E., Wheeler, S. C., & Bizer, G. Y. (1999). Is there one persuasion process or more? Lumping versus splitting in attitude change theories. *Psychology Inquiry, 10,* 156–163.

Pickett, G. E., & Hanlon, J. J. (1990). *Public health: Administration and practice.* St. Louis: Mosby-Year Book, Inc.

Piniat, A. J. (1984). How to put spirit in an incentive program. *National Safety News,* (January), 46–49.

Pollock, M. L., Foster, C., Salisburg, R., & Smith, R. (1982). Effects of a YMCA starter fitness program. *The Physician and Sportsmedicine, 10*(1), 89–91, 95–99, 120.

Poole, K., Kumpfer, K., & Pett, M. (2001). The impact of an incentive-based worksite health promotion program on modifiable health risk factors. *American Journal of Health Promotion, 16*(1), 21–26.

Popham, W. J. (1988). *Educational evaluation.* Englewood Cliffs, NJ: Prentice-Hall.

Price, J. H., Telljohann, S. K., Roberts, S. M., & Smit, D. (1992). Effects of incentives in an inner city junior high school smoking prevention program. *Journal of Health Education, 23* (7), 388–396.

Prochaska, J. O. (1979). *Systems of psychotherapy: A transtheoretical analysis.* Homewood, IL: Dorsey Press.

Prochaska, J. O., & DiClemente, C. C. (1983). Stages and processes of self-change of smoking: Toward an integrative model of change. *Journal of Consulting and Clinical Psychology, 51*(3), 390–395.

Prochaska, J. O., DiClemente, C. C., & Norcross, J. C. (1992). In search of how people change: Applications to addictive behaviors. *American Psychologist, 47*(9), 1102–1114.

Prochaska, J. O., Johnson, S., & Lee, P. (1998). The transtheoretical model of behavior change. In S. A. Shumaker, E. B. Schron, J. K. Ockene, & W. L. McBee (Eds.), *The handbook of health behavior change* (2nd ed., pp. 59–84). New York: Springer.

Prochaska, J. O., Norcross, J. C., Fowler, & J. L., Follick, M. J., & Abrams, D. B. (1992). Attendance and outcome in a worksite weight control program: Processes and stages of change as process and predictor variables. *Addictive Behaviors, 17,* 35–45.

Prochaska, J. O., Redding, C. A., Harlow, L. L., Rossi, J. S., & Velicer, W. F. (1994). The transtheoretical model of change and HIV prevention: A review. *Health Education Quarterly, 21*(4), 471–486.

Prochaska, J. O., Reeding, C. A., & Evers, K. E. (2002). The transtheoretical model and stages of change. In K. Glanz, B. K. Rimer, & R. M. Lewis (Eds.), *Health behavior and health education: Theory, research, and practice* (3rd. ed, pp. 99–120). San Francisco, CA: Jossey-Bass.

Rakich, J. S., Longest, B. B., & O'Donovan, T. R. (1977). *Managing health care organizations.* Philadelphia: W. B. Saunders.

Redding, C. A., Rossi, J. S., Rossi, S. R., Velicer, W. F., & Prochaska, J. O. (1999). Health behavior models. In G. C. Hyner, K. W. Peterson, J. W. Travis, J. E. Dewey, J. J. Foerster, & E. M. Framer (Eds.), *SPM handbook of health assessment tools* (pp. 83–93). Pittsburgh, PA: The Society of Prospective Medicine.

Rice, R. E., & Atkin, C. K. (1989). Trends in communication campaign research. In

R. E. Rice & C. K. Atkin (Eds.), *Public communication campaigns* (2nd ed.). Newbury Park, CA: Sage.

Rich, R. F., & Sugrue, N. M. (1989). Health promotion, disease prevention, and public policy. *Wellness Perspectives: Research, Theory and Practice, 6*(1), 27–35.

Riedel, J. E. (1999). The cost-effectiveness of health promotion. In G. C. Hyner, K. W. Peterson, J. W. Travis, J. E. Dewey, J. J. Foerster, & E. M. Framer (Eds.), *SPM handbook of health assessment tools* (pp. 111–118). Pittsburgh, PA: The Society of Prospective Medicine.

Rifkin, S. B. (1986). Lessons from community participation in health programmes. *Health Policy and Planning, 1*(3), 240–249.

Robbins, L. C., & Hall, J. H. (1970). *How to practice prospective medicine.* Indianapolis, IN: Methodist Hospital of Indiana.

Rogers, E. M. (1962). *Diffusion of innovations.* New York: Free Press of Glencoe.

Rogers, E. M. (1983). *Diffusion of innovations* (3rd ed.). New York: Free Press.

Rogers, E. M. (2002). Diffusion of prevention innovations. *Addictive Behaviors, 6*, 989–993.

Rogers, E. M. (2003). *Diffusion of innovations* (5th ed.). New York, NY: Free Press.

Romer, D., & Kim, S. (1995). Health interventions for African American and Latino youth: The potential role of mass media. *Health Education Quarterly, 22*(2), 172–189.

Rosenstock, I. M. (1966). Why people use health services. *Milbank Memorial Fund Quarterly, 44*, 94–124.

Rosenstock, I. M., Strecher, V. J., & Becker, M. H. (1988). Social learning theory and the health belief model. *Health Education Quarterly, 15*(2), 175–183.

Ross, H. S., & Mico, P. R. (1980). *Theory and practice in health education.* Palo Alto, CA: Mayfield.

Ross, M. G. (1967). *Community organization: Theory, principles, and practice.* New York: Harper & Row.

Rothman, J., & Tropman, J. E. (1987). Models of community organization and macro practice perspectives: Their mixing and phasing. In F. M. Cox, J. L. Erlich, J. Rothman, & J. E. Tropman (Eds.), *Strategies of community organization: Macro practice* (pp. 3–26). Itasca, IL: F. E. Peacock.

Rotter, J. B. (1954). *Social learning and clinical psychology.* New York: Prentice-Hall.

Rubin, H. J., & Rubin, I. S. (1992). *Community organizing and development* (2nd ed.). New York: Macmillan.

Ruof, J., Mittendorf, T., Pirk, O., & von der Schulenberg, J. M. (2002). Diffusion of innovations: Treatment of Alzheimer's disease in Germany. *Health Policy, 1*, 59–66.

Schechter, C., Vanchieri, C., & Crofton, C. (1990). Evaluating women's attitudes and perceptions in developing mammography promotion messages. *Public Health Reports, 105*(3), 253–257.

Schmid, T. L., Pratt, M., & Howze, E. (1995). Policy as intervention: Environmental and policy approaches to the prevention of cardiovascular disease. *American Journal of Public Health, 85*, 1207–1211.

Sciacca, J., Seehafer, R., Reed, R., & Mulvaney, D. (1993). The impact of participation in health promotion on medical costs: A reconsideration of the Blue Cross and Blue Shield of Indiana study. *American Journal of Health Promotion, 7*(5), 374–383, 395.

Scriven, M. (1973). Goal-free evaluation. In E. House (Ed.), *School evaluation: The politics and procedures* (pp. 319–328). Berkeley, CA: McCutchan.

Scriven, M. (2000). *The logic and methodology of checklists.* Retrieved November 20, 2003, from http://www.wmich.edu.evalctr/checklists/papers/logic_methodology.htm

Seffrin, J. R. (1994). America's interest in comprehensive school health education. *Journal of School Health, 64*, 397–399.

Shea, S., & Basch, C. E. (1990). A review of five major community-based cardiovascular disease prevention programs: Part I, rationale, design and theoretical framework. *American Journal of Health Promotion, 4*(3), 203–213.

Shepard, M. (1985). Motivation: The key to fitness compliance. *The Physician and Sportsmedicine, 13*(7), 88–101.

Shim, J. K., & Siegel, J. G. (1994). *Complete budgeting workbook and guide.* New York: New York Institute of Finance.

Silberg, W. M., Lundberg, G. D., & Musacchio, R. A. (1997). Assessing, controlling, and assuring the quality of medical information on the internet. *Journal of the American Medical Association, 277*, 1244–1245.

SilverPlatter. (1992, April). PsycLIT on Silver-Platter.

Simkin, L. R., & Gross, A. M. (1994). Assessment of coping with high-risk situations for exercise relapse among healthy women. *Health Psychology, 13,* 274–277.

Simmons, R. (1998). Quitting by phone. *Health Education & Behavior, 25*(6), 686–687.

Simons-Morton, B. G., Greene, W. H., & Gottlieb, N. H. (1995). *Introduction to health education and health promotion* (2nd ed.). Prospect Heights, IL: Waveland Press.

Simons-Morton, D. G., Simons-Morton, B. G., Parcel, G. S., & Bunker, J. F. (1988). Influencing personal and environmental conditions for community health: A multilevel intervention model. *Family and Community Health, 11*(2), 25–35.

Skinner, B. F. (1953). *Science and human behavior.* New York: Free Press.

Skinner, C. S., Strecher, V. J., & Hospers, H. (1994). Physicians' recommendations for mammography; Do tailored messages make a difference? *American Journal of Public Health, 84*(1), 43–49.

Sloan, R., Gruman, J., & Allegrante, J. (1987). *Investing in employee health.* San Francisco: Jossey-Bass.

Society for Public Health Education (SOPHE). (2003). New advocacy website launched. *News & Views, 30*(1), 6.

Soet, J. E., & Basch, C. E. (1997). The telephone as a communication medium for health education. *Health Education & Behavior, 24*(6), 759–772.

Solomon, D. D. (1987). Evaluating community programs. In F. M. Cox, J. L. Erlich, J. Rolhman, & J. E. Tropman (Eds.), *Strategies of community organization: Macro practices* (pp. 366–368). Itasca, IL: F. E. Peacock.

Sorensen, G., Rigotti, N., Rosen, A., Pinney, J., & Prible, R. (1991). Effects of a worksite nonsmoking policy: Evidence for increased cessation. *American Journal of Public Health, 81*(2), 202–204.

Speers, M. (1992). Preface. *Journal of Health Education, 23*(3), 132–133.

SPM Board of Directors (SPMBoD). (1999). Ethics guidelines for the development and use of health assessments. In G. C. Hyner, K. W. Peterson, J. W. Travis, J. E. Dewey, J. J. Foerster, & E. M. Framer (Eds.), *SPM handbook of health assessment tools* (p. xxiii). Pittsburgh, PA: The Society of Prospective Medicine.

Springett, J. (2003). Issues in participatory evaluation. In M. Minkler & N. Wallerstein (Eds.), Community-Based participatory research for health (pp. 263–288). San Francisco, CA: Jossey-Bass.

Stacy, R. D. (1987). Instrument evaluation guides for survey research in health education and health promotion. *Health Education, 18*(5), 65–67.

Stake, R. E. (1983). Program evaluation, particularly responsive evaluation, In G. F. Madaus, M. Scriven, & D. L. Stufflebeam (Eds.), *Evaluation models* (pp. 287–310). Boston, MA: Kluwer-Nijhoff.

Steckler, A., Goodman, R. M., McLeroy, K. R., Davis, S., & Koch, G. (1992). Measuring the diffusion of innovative health promotion programs. *American Journal of Health Promotion, 6*(3), 214–224.

Steckler, A., McLeroy, K. R., Goodman, R. M., Bird, S. T., & McCormick, L. (1992). Toward integrating qualitative and quantitative methods: An introduction. *Health Education Quarterly, 19*(1), 1–8.

Strecher, V. J., DeVellis, B. M., Becker, M. H., & Rosenstock, I. M. (1986). The role of self-efficacy in achieving health behavior change. *Health Education Quarterly, 13*(1), 73–91.

Strecher, V. J., Kreuter, M. W., Den Boer, D. J., Kobrin, S., Hospers, H. J., & Skinner, C. S. (1994). The effects of computer-tailored smoking cessation messages in family practice. *Journal of Family Practice, 39*(3), 262–270.

Strecher, V. J., & Rosenstock, I. M. (1997). The health belief model. In K. Glanz, F. M. Lewis, & B. K. Rimer (Eds.), *Health behavior and health education: Theory, research, and practice* (pp. 41–59). San Francisco: Jossey-Bass.

Strycker, L. A., Foster, L. S., Pettigrew, L., Donnelly-Perry, J., Jordan, S., & Glasgow, R. E. (1997). Steering committee enhancements on health promotion program delivery. *American Journal of Health Promotion, 11*(6), 437–440.

Stufflebeam, D. L. (1971). The relevance of the CIPP evaluation model for educational accountability. *Journal of Research and Development in Education, 5,* 19–25.

Stufflebeam, D. L. (2000). Lessons in contracting for evaluations. *American Journal of Evaluation, 21,* 293–314.

Stufflebeam, D. L., & Members of the National Study Committee on Evaluation of Phi Delta Kappa. (1971). *Educational evaluation and decision making.* Itasca, IL: F. E. Peacock.

Stunkard, A. J., & Braunwell, K. D. (1980). Worksite treatment for obesity. *American Journal of Psychiatry, 137,* 252–253.

Sullivan, D. (1973). Model for comprehensive, systematic program development in health education. *Health Education Report, 1*(1) (November–December), 4–5.

Svenkerud, P. J., & Singhal, A. (1998). Enhancing the effectiveness of HIV/AIDS prevention programs targeted to unique population groups in Thailand: Lessons learned from applying concepts of diffusion of innovation and social marketing. *Journal of Health Communication, 3,* 193–216.

Syre, T. R., & Wilson, R. W. (1990). Health care marketing: Role evolution of the community health educator. *Health Education, 21*(1), 6–8.

Task Force to Review the National Standards for Diabetes Self-Management Education. (2002). National standards for diabetes self-management education. *Diabetes Care 25,* S140–S147.

Taylor, S. M., Elliott, S., & Riley, B. (1998). Heart health promotion: predisposition, capacity and implementation in Ontario public health units, 1994–1996. *Canadian Journal of Public Health, 6,* 410–414.

Thompson, N. J., & McClintock, H. O. (1998). *Demonstrating your program's worth: A primer on evaluation for programs to prevent unintentional injury.* Atlanta, GA: National Center for Injury Prevention and Control, CDC.

Thorndike, E. L. (1898). Animal intelligence: An experimental study of the associative processes in animals. *Psychological Monographs, 2*(8).

Thorogood, M., & Coombes, Y. (Eds.). (2000). *Evaluating health promotion: Practice and methods.* Oxford, UK: Oxford University Press.

Tillman, H. N. (1997). Evaluating quality on the web [Online]. Available: http://tiac.net/users/hope/findqual.html

Timmreck, T. C. (1997). *Health services cyclopedic dictionary* (3rd. ed.). Boston, MA: Jones & Bartlett.

Timmreck, T. C. (2003). *Planning, program development, and evaluation* (2nd ed.). Boston, MA: Jones & Bartlett.

Torabi, M. R. (1994). Reliability methods and numbers of items in development of health instruments. *Health Values, 18*(6), 56–59.

Toufexis, A. (1985). Giving goodies to the good. *Time* (November 18), 98.

Udinsky, B. F., Osterlind, S. J., & Lynch, S. W. (1981). *Evaluation resource handbook: Gathering, analyzing, reporting data.* San Diego: EdITS.

U.S. Bureau of Census (USBC). (2003). *Statistical abstract of the United States: 2002, The national data book.* Retrieved November 3, 2003, from http://www.census.gov/prod/www/statistical-abstract-02.html

U.S. Department of Health and Human Services (USDHHS), Centers for Disease Control and Prevention (CDC). (no date). *Planned approach to community health: Guide for local coordinator.* Atlanta, GA: Author.

U.S. Department of Health and Human Services (USDHHS), Office of Disease Prevention and Health Promotion. (1997). *Developing objectives for healthy People 2010.* Washington, DC: U.S. Government Printing Office.

U.S. Department of Health and Human Services (USDHHS), Office of Substance Abuse Prevention. (1991). *The fact is . . . you can prepare easy-to-read materials.* Rockville, MD: Author.

U.S. Department of Health and Human Services (USDHHS). (1980). *Promoting health/preventing disease: Objectives for the nation.* Washington, DC: U.S. Government Printing Office.

U.S. Department of Health and Human Services (USDHHS). (1985). *No smoking: A decision maker's guide to reducing smoking at the worksite.* Washington, DC: U.S. Government Printing Office.

U.S. Department of Health and Human Services (USDHHS). (1986a). *Integration of risk factor interventions.* Washington, DC: U.S. Government Printing Office.

U.S. Department of Health and Human Services (USDHHS). (1986b). *The 1990 health objectives for the nation: A midcourse review.* Washington, DC: U.S. Government Printing Office.

U.S. Department of Health and Human Services (USDHHS). (1989). *Making health communication programs work: A planner's guide* (NIH Publication No. 89–1493). Washington, DC: U.S. Government Printing Office.

U.S. Department of Health and Human Services (USDHHS). (1990a). *Healthy People 2000: National health promotion disease prevention objectives* (DHHS Publication No. [PHS] 90–50212). Washington, DC: U.S. Government Printing Office.

U.S. Department of Health and Human Services (USDHHS). (1990b). *Prevention '89/'90.* Washington, DC: U.S. Government Printing Office.

U.S. Department of Health and Human Services (USDHHS). (1994). *Healthy People 2000 Review, 1993* (DHHS Publication No. [PHS] 94–1232-1). Washington, DC: U.S. Government Printing Office.

U.S. Department of Health and Human Services (USDHHS). (1995). *Healthy People 2000: Midourse review and 1995 revisions.* Washington, DC: U.S. Government Printing Office.

U.S. Department of Health and Human Services (USDHHS). (2000). *Healthy People 2010 (CD-ROM Version).* Washington, DC: Author.

U.S. Department of Health and Human Services (USDHHS). (2001). *Healthy people in healthy communities: A community planning guide using healthy people 2010.* Washington, DC: Author.

U.S. Department of Health and Human Services (USDHHS). (2003). *Medical privacy—National standards to protect the privacy of personal health information.* Retrieved May 22, 2003, from http://hhs.gov/hipaa/

United Nations. (1955). *Social progress through community development.* New York, NY: Author.

Valente, T. W. (2002). *Evaluating health promotion programs.* New York, NY: Oxford University Press.

van Ryn, M., & Heaney, C. A. (1992). What's the use of theory? *Health Education Quarterly, 19*(3), 315–330.

Venditto, G. (1997, January). Critic's choice: Six sites that rate the web. *Internet World,* pp. 82–96.

Wagner, E. H., & Guild, P. A. (1989). Choosing an evaluation strategy. *American Journal of Health Promotion, 4*(2), 134–139.

Walker, R. A., & Bibeau, D. (1985/1986). Health education as freeing—Part II. *Health Education, 16*(6), (December/January), 4–8.

Wallerstein, N. (1994). Empowerment education applied to youth. In A. C. Matiella (Ed.), *The multicultural challenge in health education* (pp. 153–176). Santa Cruz, CA: ETR Associates.

Wallerstein, N., & Bernstein, E. (1988). Empowerment education: Freier's ideas adapted to health education. *Health Education Quarterly, 15*(4), 379–394.

Wallerstein, N., Sanchez-Merki, V., & Dow, L. (1997). Freirian praxis in health education and community organizing: A case study of an adult prevention program. In M. Minkler (Ed.), *Community organizing and community building for health* (pp. 195–215). New Brunswick, NJ: Rutgers University Press.

Wallston, K. A. (1992). Hocus-pocus, the focus isn't strictly on locus: Rotter's social learning theory modified for health. *Cognitive Therapy and Research, 16,* 183–199.

Wallston, K. A. (1994). Theoretically based strategies for health behavior change. In M. P. O'Donnell, & J. S. Harris (Eds.), *Health promotion in the workplace* (2nd ed.). (pp. 185–203). Albany, NY: Delmar.

Wallston, K. A., Wallston, B. S., & DeVellis, R. (1978). Development of the multidimensional health locus of control (MHLC) scales. *Health Education Monographs, 6,* 160–170.

Walsh, D. C., Rudd, R. E., Moeykens, B. A., & Moloney, T. W. (1993). Social marketing for public health. *Health Affairs, 12,* 104–119.

Walter, C. L. (1997). Community building practice: A conceptual framework. In M. Minkler (Ed.), *Community organizing and community building for health* (pp. 68–83). New Brunswick, NJ: Rutgers University Press.

Warner, K. E. (1987). Selling health promotion to corporate America: Uses and abuses of the economic argument. *Health Education Quarterly, 14*(1), 39–55.

Warner, K. E., Wickizer, T., Wolfe, R., Schildroth, J., & Samuelson, M. (1988). Economic implications of workplace health promotion programs: Review of literature. *Journal of Occupational Medicine, 30*(2), 106–112.

Washington, R. (1987). Alternative frameworks for program evaluation. In F. M. Cox, J. L. Erlich, J. Rolhman, & J. E. Tropman (Eds.), *Strategies of community organization: Macro practices* (pp. 373–374). Itasca, IL: F. E. Peacock.

Watson, J. B. (1925). *Behaviorism*. New York: W. W. Norton.

Watts, G. F., Donahue, R. E., Eddy J. M. & Wallace, E. V. (2001). Use of an ecological approach to worksite health promotion. *American Journal of Health Studies, 17*(3), 144–147.

Webopedia. (2003). *Critical path method*. Retrieved November 14, 2003, from http://itmanagement.webopdia.com/TERM/C/Critical_Path_Method.html

Weinreich, N. K. (1999). *Hands-on social marketing: A step by step guide*. Thousand Oaks, CA: Sage Publications.

Weinstein, N. D. (1988). The precaution adoption process. *Health Psychology, 7*, 355–386.

Weinstein, N. D., & Rothman, A. J., & Sutton, S. R. (1998). Stage theories of health behavior: Conceptual and methodological issues. *Health Psychology, 17*, 290–299.

Weinstein, N. D., & Sandman, P. M. (1992). A model of the precaution adoption process: Evidence from home radon testing. *Health Psychology, 11*, 170–180.

Weinstein, N. D., & Sandman, P. M. (2002a). The precaution adoption process model. In K. Glanz, B. K. Rimer, & F. M. Lewis (Eds.), *Health behavior and health education: Theory, research, and practice* (3rd. ed., pp. 121–143). San Francisco, CA: Jossey-Bass.

Weinstein, N. D., & Sandman, P. M. (2002b). The precaution adoption process model and its application. In R. J. DiClemente, R. A. Crosby, & M. C. Kegler (Eds.), *Emerging theories in health promotion practice and research: Strategies for improving public health.* (pp. 16–39). San Francisco, CA: Jossey-Bass.

Weiss, C. H. (1984). Increasing the likelihood of influencing decisions. In L. Rutman (Ed.), *Evaluation research methods: A basic guide* (2nd ed.) (pp. 159–190). Beverly Hills, CA: Sage.

Weiss, C. H. (1998). *Evaluation* (2nd ed.). Upper Saddle River, NJ: Prentice-Hall.

Wilbur, C. (1983). Live for life—The Johnson & Johnson program. *Preventive Medicine, 12*(5), 672–681.

Williams, B., & Suen, H. (1998). Formal vs. informal assessment methods. *American Journal of Health Behavior, 22*(4), 308–313.

Williams, J. E., & Flora, J. A. (1995). Health behavior segmentation and campaign planning to reduce cardiovascular disease risk among Hispanics. *Health Education Quarterly, 22*(1), 36–38.

Wilson, M. G. (1990). Factors associated with, issues related to, and suggestions for increasing participation in workplace health promotion programs. *Health Values, 14*(4), 29–36.

Windsor, R. A., Baranowski, T., Clark, N., & Cutter, G. (1984). *Evaluation of health promotion and education programs*. Palo Alto, CA: Mayfield.

Windsor, R., Baranowski, T., Clark, N., & Cutter, G. (1994). *Evaluation of health promotion, health education, and disease prevention programs* (2nd ed.). Mountain View, CA: Mayfield.

Wolfe, R., Slack, T., & Rose-Hearn, T. (1993). Factors influencing the adoption and maintenance of Canadian, facility-based worksite health promotion programs. *American Journal of Health Promotion, 7*(3), 189–198.

Woolf, H. B. (Ed.). (1979). *Webster's new collegiate dictionary*. Springfield, MA: G. & C. Merriam.

Wright, P. A. (Ed.). (1994). *Technical assistance bulletin: A key step in developing prevention materials is to obtain expert and gatekeepers' reviews*. Bethesda, MD: Center for Substance Abuse Prevention (CASP) Communications Team.

Wright, P. A. (Ed.). (1997). *Technical assistance bulletin: Identifying the target audience*. Bethesda, MD: Center for Substance Abuse Prevention (CASP) Communications Team.

Wurzbach, M. E. (Ed.). (2002). *Community health education and promotion: A guide to program design and evaluation* (2nd ed.). Gaithersburg, MD: Aspen Publishers, Inc.

Yamane, T. (1973). *Statistics: An introductory analysis* (3rd ed.). New York, NY: Harper & Row, Publishers.

Name Index

Subject Index